HUMAN CELL CULTURE
Volume VI: Embryonic Stem Cells

Human Cell Culture

Volume 6

The titles published in this series are listed at the end of this volume.

Human Cell Culture

Volume VI

Embryonic Stem Cells

edited by

John R. Masters

University College London, London, UK

Bernhard O. Palsson

University of California, San Diego, CA, USA

and

James A. Thomson

University of Wisconsin, Madison, WI, USA

Springer

A C.I.P. Catalogue record for this book is available from the Library of Congress.

ISBN-13 978-1-4020-5982-7 (HB)
ISBN-13 978-1-4020-5983-4 (e-book)

Published by Springer,
P.O. Box 17, 3300 AA Dordrecht, The Netherlands.

www.springer.com

Printed on acid-free paper

CONTENTS

PREFACE

The aim of this volume is to describe methods for culturing human embryonic stem cells and the culture conditions needed to direct these cells to differentiate into specialized cell types.

Human embryonic stem cells are potentially capable of differentiation into any other cell type, including endoderm, mesoderm, and ectoderm. Consequently there is a great deal of academic and commercial interest in utilizing these cells in the treatment of a wide variety of medical conditions, as well as certain ethical considerations. The maintenance and differentiation of human embryonic stem cells is the focus of many large programs in cell biology and of many groups wishing to translate their research to the clinic. However, human embryonic stem cells are difficult first to establish in culture and second to maintain in an undifferentiated state. The development and optimization of techniques for growing and maintaining stem cells and for directing them to differentiate along specific cell lineages are crucial to the clinical application of these cells and are the focus of this book.

Transplanted organs and tissues are often used to replace those that are diseased or destroyed, but the number of people needing a transplant far exceeds the number of organs available. Pluripotent stem cells offer the possibility of a renewable source of replacement cells and tissues to treat conditions such as Parkinson's and Alzheimer's diseases, spinal cord injury, stroke, burns, heart disease, diabetes, osteoarthritis, and rheumatoid arthritis. This book deals with human embryonic stem cells and the derivation, maintenance, and differentiation of human adult stem cells will be the subject of the next volume.

CHAPTER 1

DEFINED CULTURE MEDIA FOR HUMAN EMBRYONIC STEM CELLS

TENNEILLE LUDWIG[1,2,3] AND JAMES A. THOMSON[1,2,3,4]

[1]*WiCell Research Institute, P.O. Box 7365, Madison, WI 53707*

[2]*National Primate Research Center, University of Wisconsin Graduate School, 1220 Capitol Court, Madison, WI 53705*

[3]*Genome Center of Wisconsin, University of Wisconsin-Madison, 425 Henry Mall, Madison, WI 53706*

[4]*Department of Anatomy, University of Wisconsin Medical School, 470 N. Charter Street, Madison, WI 53706-1509*

Human embryonic stem (ES) cells can differentiate into any tissue type within the body, and thus offer tremendous potential for use in regenerative medicine. However, traditional tissue culture methods employed in their derivation and proliferation jeopardize that potential because of the inclusion of animal-derived products. The improved safety facilitated by the development of defined culture systems that eliminate the need for animal products are key in the transfer of human ES cell technology from the bench to the bedside. Here we describe recent advances in the culture of human ES cells in defined culture medium.

Human ES cells were first isolated using mouse embryonic fibroblast (MEF) feeder layers and bovine serum-containing medium (Thomson et al. 1998). This technique, using serum and feeder layers to support difficult-to-culture cells, was first developed more than half a century ago when Puck used mitotically inactivated feeder cells along with serum to maintain delicate HeLa cells in culture (Puck and Marcus 1955). Years later, the technique was adapted for both murine embryonic carcinoma (EC) (Evans 1972) and ES cell culture (Evans and Kaufman 1981; Martin 1981), and has been used in the derivation of all human ES cell lines that are currently available for federal funding in the USA (see http://stemcells.nih.gov/research/registry). However, use of feeder layers and animal serum products in human ES cell culture carries the risk of cross contamination of xenogenic or allogenic pathogens or cell byproducts. This risk was confirmed when it was found that human ES cells incorporate a nonhuman sialic acid during culture with animal products (Martin et al. 2005). The incorporation of this immunogenic molecule during routine culture raises the specter

J.R. Masters et al (eds.), Embryonic Stem Cells, 1–16.

of immune rejection and renders the resulting cells inappropriate for transplantation therapies unless the antigen is removed.

The inherent risks of culture with animal feeders and serum products were recognized early, and almost as soon as the cell lines were isolated, improved culture systems were being developed. Because serum is highly variable lot to lot, and is known to mask media deficiencies, research to improve the quality of the medium required that it be eliminated from the culture system. Amit and colleagues first discovered that human ES cells could be maintained and clonally propagated on MEFs in the absence of serum using a combination of basic fibroblast growth factor (bFGF) and a commercially available serum replacer (Knockout Serum Replacer, KOSR: Gibco) (Amit et al. 2000). While a substantial improvement over serum products in terms of variability, KOSR contains "Albumax," a poorly defined lipid-rich bovine albumin, making it problematic for culturing cells for clinical use. The same medium supports human ES cells in the absence of direct contact with feeder layers if it is conditioned on MEFs prior to use (Xu et al. 2001). This method became known as "feeder-free" culture, despite the fact that it is not free from potential feeder-layer contaminants, merely free of direct human ES cell contact with MEFs.

In an effort to remove animal products from the culture system, many investigators replaced MEFs with human-sourced feeder cells. Fetal muscle and fetal epithelial (Richards et al. 2002), adult epithelial (Richards et al. 2003), fallopian tube (Richards et al. 2002), marrow (Cheng et al. 2003), foreskin (Amit et al. 2003; Choo et al. 2004; Hovatta et al. 2003), and placental cells (Genbacev et al. 2005) were all used with success. Feeder layers were also derived from differentiated human ES cells (Stojkovic et al. 2004), addressing the limited availability and tremendous variability often seen with primary cell culture material. All but one (Genbacev et al. 2005) of these studies, however, utilized bovine albumin containing KOSR or calf serum, and therefore, did not eliminate all potential sources of human ES cell contamination. Additionally, it is important to note that feeder layers, regardless of the source, are extremely labor-intensive to prepare, and may be the primary factor limiting large-scale culture of human ES cells necessary for therapeutic use. The variability between lots is also a cause of inconsistency in human ES cell culture, and the use of primary human tissues has the potential to introduce human pathogens to the culture. Clearly, a culture system completely independent of feeders of any kind is more desirable.

The role that feeder layers play in maintaining self-renewal in human ES cell culture, however, remains poorly understood. While leukemia inhibitory factor (LIF) activation of the LIF/Stat pathway is sufficient to sustain pluripotency in the absence of feeder layers in murine ES cells, it does not have the same effect in human ES cells (Thomson et al. 1998; Reubinoff et al. 2000; Daheron et al. 2004; Sato et al. 2004), suggesting a role for other pathways in maintaining human ES cells self-renewal. Amit and associates demonstrated a role for transforming growth factor beta (TGFβ), which when combined with bFGF allows feeder-independent growth of human ES cells, but with about a 20% background differentiation rate, leaving open the possibility that the cells in effect make their own feeders (Amit et al. 2004). An increasing body of evidence suggests that bFGF plays a central role in maintaining human ES cell pluripotency, and several investigators have been able to liberate human ES cells from feeders using high concentrations of bFGF in culture (Klimanskaya et al. 2005; Genbacev et al. 2005; Levenstein et al. 2005; Li et al. 2005; Wang et al. 2005; Xu, C. et al. 2005; Xu, R.H. et al. 2005). The precise mechanism of action, however, has not yet been fully elucidated. While feeder-independent culture has been achieved in the presence of high doses of FGF, the majority of these studies included KOSR and mouse matrix products (Amit et al. 2004; Klimanskaya et al. 2005; Levenstein et al. 2005; Wang et al. 2005; Xu, R.H. et al. 2005).

TeSR1 (Ludwig et al. 2006) is a serum-free, feeder-independent, animal-product free, fully disclosed medium specifically formulated for the undifferentiated proliferation of human ES cells *in vitro*. The formulation of TeSR1 medium was based on a program of optimization that included optimization of the physiochemical environment and the medium formulation itself. In developing TeSR1, we tested a variety of media supplements to evaluate their effect on human ES cell proliferation and self-renewal. cDNA microarray expression profiles that identified genes in human ES cell lines that are highly expressed relative to differentiated cell types (Sperger et al. 2003) initially formed our selection of factors for testing. In preliminary screenings, we evaluated 85 individual media supplements, including proteins, vitamins, lipids, nucleic acids, and growth factors. Relying on visual assessment of initial attachment, cell and colony morphology, and cell proliferation, we determined that when added individually, many factors had positive effects on human ES cell culture, including activin A, cholera toxin, dexamethosone, αFGF, bFGF, Flt3 ligand, γ-aminobutyric acid (GABA), heparin, IGF II, lithium chloride (LiCl), noggin, PDGF (α, β, and αβ), pipecolic acid (PA), SDGF (α), somatomammotropin (placental lactogen), TGFβ, and Wnt. When tested in combination, however, positive effects seen individually with many components were reduced or eliminated.

Five of these factors were ultimately included in TeSR1: bFGF, TGFβ, LiCl, GABA, and PA. When any of these individual factors are removed from TeSR1, there is a consistent, statistically significant decrease in culture performance. However, in general, the removal of any of these individual components has only a relatively minor effect during three passages (Ludwig et al. 2006). The exception is bFGF, which had the strongest effect on the undifferentiated proliferation of human ES cells, supporting previous literature that demonstrates high doses of bFGF play a pivotal role in the maintenance of human ES cell pluripotency (Amit et al. 2000; Levenstein et al. 2005; Li et al. 2005; Wang et al. 2005; Xu, C. et al. 2005; Xu, R.H. et al. 2005). TGFβ and LiCl stimulate signaling pathways that have been highlighted in the previous publications on human ES cell culture (Schuldiner 2000; Amit et al. 2003; Sato et al. 2003, 2004; Beattie et al. 2005; James 2005; Vallier et al. 2004, 2005). At lower concentrations of FGFs, both activin and TGFβ have clear strong effects on human ES cells (Schuldiner 2000;

Amit et al. 2004; Beattie et al. 2005; James 2005;), and based on inhibitor studies, it has been suggested that TGFβ/activin signaling is essential for human ES cell self-renewal (Sato et al. 2003; Vallier et al. 2004). At the higher concentrations of bFGF present in TeSR1, the effects of exogenous TGFβ were modest, but statistically significant (Ludwig et al. 2006). LiCl was initially tested because of its ability to inhibit GSK-3 (Klein and Melton 1996) and promote Wnt signaling, as Frizzled receptors are present on human ES cells (Sperger et al. 2003). The specific role of Wnt signaling in human ES cells remains controversial (Sato et al. 2004; Dravid et al. 2005). In our hands, neither purified Wnt3a, nor LiCl were sufficient to sustain human ES cells (unpublished data), but removal of LiCl from TeSR1 did modestly reduce culture performance (Ludwig et al. 2006).

We initially tested GABA because our previous microarray results indicated a high level of expression of the beta-3 subunit of the GABA-A receptor by human ES cells (Ludwig et al. 2006). Recent SAGE results indicate the expression of message for the α, β3, and δ subunits of the GABA-A receptor, and the GABA-B receptor (http://www.transcriptomES.org/). GABA is an inhibitory neurotransmitter of the central nervous system, and there is some evidence it can stimulate proliferation of both neural and nonneural tissues (Owens and Kriegstein 2002; Watanabe et al. 2002). Additionally, both GABA and LiCl affect calcium release, and may impact ES cell proliferation through modulation of intracellular calcium levels. Calcium concentration, and more importantly Ca^{2+}/Mg^{2+} ratio in culture medium, have been shown to affect both *in vitro* embryo development (Lane and Bavister 1998; Lane et al. 1998) and keratinocyte proliferation (Daniels et al. 1995). We tested PA as it has been reported to enhance GABA-A-receptor responses (Charles 1986; Takahama et al. 1986). Removal of either GABA or pipecolic acid from TeSR1 media consistently resulted in a decline in cell number after three passages (Ludwig et al. 2006).

1. PREPARATION OF TeSR1 MEDIUM FOR DEFINED CULTURE OF HUMAN ES CELLS

TeSR1 medium is a defined, feeder-independent, animal-product free medium consisting of a DMEM/F12 base, supplemented with human serum albumin (hSA), vitamins, antioxidants, trace minerals, specific lipids, and cloned growth factors (Table 2). Assembly of TeSR1 medium involves combining commercially available products with additional individual components. Addition of individual components to the TeSR1 formulation involves the preparation of primary stock solutions that are either added directly, or used to create in-house stocks for use. Purchasing information for all ingredients can be found in Table 1.

In most cases, the primary stocks can be stored frozen for a period of 3 months to 1 year (be sure to follow the manufacturers' recommendations for all primary stocks). Secondary stocks (i.e., TeSR serum replacer stock) can be stored only as long as the most labile component. Likewise, TeSR1 medium, once complete, can be stored only as long as the most labile component. Sodium

Table 1. Defined culture media components and matrix proteins listed by manufacturer and catalog number

Component	Supplier	Catalog #
2-Mercaptoethanol	Sigma (St. Louis, MO)	M7522
L-Ascorbic acid 2-phosphate Mg salt	Sigma	A8960
bFGF	PeproTech (Rocky Hill, NJ)	100-18B
Chemically defined lipid concentrate	Invitrogen/GIBCO (Carlsbad, CA)	11905-031
DMEM/F12	Invitrogen/GIBCO	11330-032
GABA	Sigma	A5835
Glutathione (reduced)	Sigma	G6013
Human collagen	Sigma	C-5533
Human fibronectin	Sigma	F-2518
Human holo-transferrin	Sigma	T0665
Human insulin solution	Sigma	I9278
Human laminin	Sigma	L-6274
Human serum albumin	Irvine Scientific (Santa Ana, CA)	9988
Human vitronectin	Sigma	V-8379
L-Glutamine	Sigma	G6392
Lithium chloride (LiCl)	Sigma	L4408
Nonessential amino acids	Invitrogen/GIBCO	11140076
Phosphate buffered saline (Ca/Mg free)	Invitrogen/GIBCO	14190-144
Pipecolic acid	MP Biomedicals (Irvine, CA)	151898
Sodium bicarbonate	Sigma	S3817
Sodium selenite	Sigma	S-5261
TGF beta 1	R&D Systems (Minneapolis, MN)	240-B/CF
Thiamine hydrochloride	Sigma	T1270
Trace elements B	Mediatech/Cellgro (Herndon, VA)	99-175-CI
Trace elements C	Mediatech/Cellgro	99-176-CI

bicarbonate and glutamine are relatively unstable in solution, and breakdown occurs within 2–3 weeks, depending on a variety of factors (temperature, exposure to air and light etc.). They are also known to break down in solution following freezing and thawing. For these reasons, these components should always be prepared and added fresh into the TeSR1 formulation. While many stocks can be frozen and thawed successfully, for best results, completed TeSR1-containing glutamine and bicarbonate should not be frozen, and should be used or discarded within 2 weeks of preparation. Preparation of all noncommercial primary and secondary stocks used in TeSR1 is described below:

1.1 Diluent Stock

Mix together:
99.9 mL Ca-free, Mg-free phosphate buffered saline (–/– PBS)
100 μL human serum albumin
Filter sterilize
Store at 4°C

Table 2. Complete formulation of TeSR1 medium

Component (listed within stock)	Embodiment in stock (mg/L)	Embodiment in medium (mg/L)	mL stock in 1L medium
DMEM/F12			784.314
Biotin	0.0035	2.75 E-03	
Calcium chloride (anhydrous)	116.6	9.15 E + 01	
Choline chloride	8.98	7.04 E-00	
Cupric sulfate ($CuSO_4$ $5H_2O$)	0.0013	1.02 E-03	
D-Calcium pantothenate	2.24	1.76 E-00	
D-glucose	3151	2.47 E + 03	
Ferric nitrate ($Fe(NO_3)_3$ $9H_2O$)	0.05	3.92 E-02	
Ferric sulfate ($FeSO_4$ $7H_2O$)	0.417	3.27 E-01	
Folic acid	2.65	2.08 E-00	
Glycine	18.75	1.47 E + 01	
HEPES	3574.5	2.80 E + 03	
i-Inositol	12.6	9.88 E-00	
L-Alanine	4.45	3.49 E-00	
L-Arginine HCl	147.5	1.16 E + 02	
L-Asparagine H_2O	7.5	5.88 E-00	
L-Aspartic acid	6.65	5.22 E-00	
L-Cysteine HCl H_2O	17.56	1.38 E + 01	
L-Cystine 2HCl	31.29	2.45 E + 01	
L-Glutamic acid	7.35	5.76 E-00	
L-Glutamine	365	2.86 E + 02	
L-Histidine HCl H_2O	31.48	2.47 E + 01	
Linoleic acid	0.042	3.29 E-02	
Lipoic acid	0.105	8.24 E-02	
L-Isoleucine	54.47	4.27 E + 01	
L-Leucine	59.05	4.63 E + 01	
L-Lysine HCl	91.25	7.16 E + 01	
L-Methionine	17.24	1.35 E + 01	
L-Phenylalanine	35.48	2.78 E + 01	
L-Proline	17.25	1.35 E + 01	
L-Serine	26.25	2.06 E + 01	
L-Threonine	53.45	4.19 E + 01	
L-Tryptophan	9.02	7.07 E-00	
L-Tyrosine 2Na $2H_2O$	55.79	4.38 E + 01	
L-Valine	52.85	4.15 E + 01	
Magnesium chloride (anhydrous)	28.64	2.25 E + 01	
Magnesium sulfate ($MgSO_4$)	48.84	3.83 E + 01	
Na Hypoxanthine	2.39	1.87 E-00	
Niacinamide	2.02	1.58 E-00	
Phenol red	8.1	6.35 E-00	
Potassium chloride (KCl)	311.8	2.45 E + 02	
Pyridoxine HCl	2.031	1.59 E-00	
Riboflavin	0.219	1.72 E-01	
Sodium bicarbonate ($NaHCO_3$)	1200	9.41 E + 02	
Sodium chloride (NaCl)	6995.5	5.49 E + 03	
Sodium phosphate, dibasic (anhydrous)	71.02	5.57 E + 01	
Sodium phosphate, monobasic	62.5	4.90 E + 01	

Table 2. Complete formulation of TeSR1 medium—Cont'd.

Component (listed within stock)	Embodiment in stock (mg/L)	Embodiment in medium (mg/L)	mL stock in 1L medium
Sodium putrescine 2HCl	0.081	6.35 E-02	
Sodium pyruvate	55	4.31 E + 01	
Thiamine HCl	2.17	1.70 E-00	
Thymidine	0.365	2.86 E-01	
Vitamin B12	0.68	5.33 E-01	
Zinc sulfate ($ZnSO_4$ $7H_2O$)	0.432	3.39 E-01	
Chemically defined lipid concentrate			1.961
Arachidonic acid	2	3.92 E-03	
Cholesterol	220	4.31 E-01	
DL-Alpha tocopherol-acetate	70	1.37 E-01	
Linoleic acid	10	1.96 E-02	
Linolenic acid	10	1.96 E-02	
Myristic acid	10	1.96 E-02	
Oleic acid	10	1.96 E-02	
Palmitic acid	10	1.96 E-02	
Palmitoleic acid	10	1.96 E-02	
Pluronic F-68	100000	1.96 E + 02	
Stearic acid	10	1.96 E-02	
Tween 80	2200	4.31 E-00	
TeSR Serum Replacer Stock			156.863
Glutathione (reduced)	12.5	1.96 E-00	
L-Ascorbic acid 2-phosphate Mg salt	412.5	6.47 E + 01	
Selenium	0.0875	1.37 E-02	
Thiamine HCl	41.25	6.47 E-00	
Human insulin	125	1.96 E + 01	
Human holo-transferrin	68.75	1.08 E + 01	
Human serum albumin	83750	1.31 E + 04	
$AgNO_3$	0.0010625	1.67 E-04	
$AlCl_3$ $6H_2O$	0.0075	1.18 E-03	
Ammonium metavanadate NH_4VO_3	0.008125	1.27 E-03	
Ba $(C_2H_3O_2)_2$	0.0159375	2.50 E-03	
$CdCl_2$	0.01425	2.24 E-03	
$CoCl_2$ $6H_2O$	0.014875	2.33 E-03	
$CrCl_3$	0.002	3.14 E-04	
GeO_2	0.0033125	5.20 E-04	
KBr	0.00075	1.18 E-04	
KI	0.0010625	1.67 E-04	
Manganous sulfate Mn SO_4 H_2O	0.002125	3.33 E-04	
Molybdic acid, ammonium salt	0.0155	2.43 E-03	
NaF	0.02625	4.12 E-03	
$NiSO_4$ $6H_2O$	0.001625	2.55 E-04	
RbCl	0.0075625	1.19 E-03	
$SnCl_2$	0.0015	2.35 E-04	
Sodium meta silicate Na_2SiO_3 $9H_2O$	1.75	2.75 E-01	
$ZrOCl_2$ $8H_2O$	0.020125	3.16 E-03	

(*Continued*)

Table 2. Complete formulation of TeSR1 medium—Cont'd.

Component (listed within stock)	Embodiment in stock (mg/L)	Embodiment in medium (mg/L)	mL stock in 1L medium
L-Glutamine stock			9.804
L-Glutamine	14600	1.43 E + 02	
2-Mercaptoethanol	779.8	7.65 E-00	
MEM nonessential amino acids			9.804
L-Alanine	890	8.73 E-00	
L-Asparagine H_2O	1320	1.29 E + 01	
L-Aspartic acid	1330	1.30 E + 01	
L-Glutamic acid	1470	1.44 E + 01	
Glycine	750	7.35 E-00	
L-Proline	1150	1.13 E + 01	
L-Serine	1050	1.03 E + 01	
Additional factors			
GABA	51550	1.01 E + 02	1.961
Pipecolic acid	1000	1.27 E-01	0.127
bFGF	50	9.80 E-02	1.961
LiCl	21180	4.15 E + 01	1.961
TGF beta 1	0.3	5.88 E-04	1.961
Sterile water	n/a	n/a	29.284
Other			
Additional sodium bicarbonate	n/a	5.49 E + 02	
Additional NaCl (for osmolarity adjustment)	n/a	variable	
10 N NaOH (For pH adjustment)	n/a	variable	

1.2 Vitamin Stock (100x)

Dissolve:
165 mg thiamine
50 mg reduced glutathione
1,650 mg L-ascorbic acid 2-phosphate Mg salt into
500 mL MilliQ (or sterile) water
Aliquot into tubes (10–50 mL)
Wrap tubes in foil to protect from light
Store stocks at –20°C

1.3 bFGF Stock (50 μg/mL)

Dissolve:
500 μg bFGF into
10 mL "diluent stock" (previously described)
Aliquot into sterile microfuge tubes
Store stocks at –80°C

1.4 TGFβ1 Stock (0.3 μg/mL)

Reconstitute:
30 μg TGFβ1 in
600 μL 4mM HCl
Add:
99.4 mL "diluent stock" (previously described)
Aliquot into sterile microfuge tubes.
Store stocks at –80°C

1.5 Pipecolic Acid Stock

To prepare concentrated stock (100 mg/mL):
Reconstitute:
100 mg pipecolic acid in
1 mL MilliQ water
Aliquot 20 μL/tube (2 mg/tube)
Store concentrated stocks at –80°C
To prepare working stock (1 mg/mL):
Combine:
20 μL concentrated stock with
1980 μL "diluent stock" (previously described)
Aliquot into sterile microfuge tubes
Store working stocks at –80°C

1.6 GABA (γ-aminobutyric acid) Stock (51.55 mg/mL)

Dissolve:
2062 mg GABA into
40 mL sterile water
Aliquot into sterile microfuge tubes
Store at –80°C

1.7 LiCl (lithium chloride) Stock (21.18 mg/mL)

Dissolve:
847.2 mg of LiCl into
40 mL sterile water
Store at 4°C

1.8 Glutamine Stock (14.6 mg/mL)

Dissolve:
146 mg L-glutamine into
10 mL –/– PBS plus
7 μL 2-mercaptoethanol

Use immediately.
Do not freeze stock
Prepare fresh every time

1.9 Selenium Stock (0.07 mg/mL)

Dissolve:
7 mg sodium selenite into
100 mL sterile water
Store at 4°C

1.10 TeSR Serum Replacer Stock (1,000 mL Final Volume)

Mix together:
125 mL vitamin stock (previously described)
1.25 mL selenium stock
12.5 mL trace mineral stock B (commercial)
6.25 mL trace mineral stock C (commercial)
837.5 mL human serum albumin solution (commercial)
12.5 mL human insulin solution (commercial)
68.75 mg human holo-transferrin
5 mL sterile water
Filter sterilize
Store at 4°C

1.11 Assembly of TeSR1 Medium From Stock Solutions (1,020 mL Final Volume)

Mix together:
800 mL DMEM/F12 (commercial)
160 mL TeSR Serum Replacer Stock (previously described)
10 mL L-glutamine stock (previously described)
10 mL MEM NEAA solution (commercial)
2 mL bFGF stock (previously described)
2 mL GABA stock (previously described)
2 mL TGFβ stock (previously described)
2 mL LiCl Stock (previously described)
2 mL Chemically defined lipid concentrate (commercial)
129.7 μL pipecolic acid stock (previously described)
560 mg sodium bicarbonate
29.870 mL research grade water
To achieve a total of 1020 mL TeSR1 medium
Once well mixed, adjust pH to 7.4 using 10N NaOH
Adjust osmolarity to 345 +/– 5mOsMol using NaCl
Filter sterilize medium, store at 4°C for up to 2 weeks

2. TRANSFERRING HUMAN ES CELLS TO DEFINED CULTURE MEDIUM

We recommend that the transition from DMEM/F12-based culture media to TeSR1 medium be done mid-passage. Cells in culture on either MEF-feeder layers or Matrigel-coated 6-well plates can be fed 2 mL/well of TeSR1 medium beginning 3 days prior to passaging the cells. No "adaptation" time is necessary, and medium can be completely switched from any DMEM/F12-based medium to TeSR at normal feeding time. Cells growing in 6-well plates should be fed 2mL TeSR1/well/day, and must be fed daily for best results. At passage, cells can be transferred onto defined human matrix-coated plates or to Matrigel-coated plates (subsequently described). TeSR1 medium should be warmed to 37°C prior to feeding cells, and spent medium should be completely removed at each feeding.

2.1 Preparation of Matrigel-Coated Plate for Culture

When completely defined culture conditions are not required, feeder-independent culture can be obtained using Matrigel-coated plates. We have achieved good success using 0.5 mg Matrigel per 6-well plate.

2.1.1 Plating Matrigel

Dilute Matrigel according to manufacturer's recommendations and aliquot 0.5 mg into 1.5 mL tubes. Store tubes at –80°C. To plate Matrigel, quickly dilute 0.5 mg Matrigel (one vial) into 6 mL DMEM/F12. Plate 1 mL into each well of a 6-well culture plate. Allow plate to incubate at room temperature for at least 1 h prior to use. Plates may be wrapped with parafilm or foil and refrigerated for up to 1 week prior to use without compromising performance. Plates should not be allowed to dry, however, as attachment is compromised. Aspirate excess Matrigel from plate immediately prior to plating cells.

3. PREPARATION OF HUMAN MATRIX-COATED CULTURE PLATES FOR DEFINED CULTURE

TeSR1 medium can be used to successfully culture human ES cells on the commercially available Matrigel matrix (Ludwig et al. 2006). However, because Matrigel is derived from murine tumor cells, therapeutically relevant culture in fully defined conditions requires an alternate matrix. While other investigators report success using human fibronectin or human laminin alone (Xu et al. 2001; Amit et al. 2004; Klimanskaya et al. 2005), we have had difficulty reliably maintaining human ES cells for extended periods using single-protein matrices. Others have found an additive effect of combining individual matrix components (Draper et al. 2004). We obtained the best results using a combination of human-sourced collagen IV, fibronectin, laminin, and vitronectin. These products are readily available commercially, and purchasing information is listed in

Table 1. To assemble the culture plates, first prepare primary stocks of individual matrix components as follows:

3.1 Collagen Stock

Reconstitute:
5 mg human collagen type IV into
1 mL 6M GuHCl
Aliquot 120 µL into 1.5 mL tubes. This will be enough to coat one 6-well plate (20 µL stock/well)
Store at –80°C

3.2 Fibronectin Stock

Reconstitute:
5 mg human fibronectin into
5 mL reagent quality water
Aliquot 300 µL into 1.5 mL tubes. This will be enough to coat one 6-well plate (50 µL stock/well)
Store at –80°C

3.3 Vitronectin Stock

Dissolve:
50 µg human vitronectin into
2.5 mL reagent grade water
Aliquot 600 µL into 1.5 mL tubes. This will be enough to coat one 6-well plate (100 µL stock/well)
Store at –80°C

3.4 Laminin Stock

Thaw prepared solution according to manufacturer's recommendation.
Aliquot 600 µL into 1.5 mL tubes. This will be enough to coat one 6-well plate (100 µL stock/well)
Store at –80°C

3.5 Plating Human Matrices

For each 6-well plate, dilute 120 µL of 5 mg/mL collagen stock (1 vial) into 6 mL calcium and magnesium-free PBS. Filter sterilize the resulting solution using a 0.2 µ PES filter. Plate 1 mL/well into a 6-well plate and incubate plate at room temperature for at least 1 h. Dilute 300 µL of 1 mg/mL fibronectin stock (1 vial), 600 µL of 0.5 mg/mL laminin stock (1 vial) and 600 µL of 20 µg mg/mL vitronectin stock (1 vial) into 4.5 mL –/– PBS solution. Filter sterilize the resulting solution using a 0.2 μ PES filter. Remove excess collagen solution from the 6-well plate. Plate 1 mL/well fibronectin-laminin-vitronectin solution into the collagen-coated 6-well plate and allow mixture to incubate on plate at least 1 h at room temperature prior to plating cells. Remove excess matrix solution from plate immediately prior to plating cells.

4. METHODS FOR SPLITTING CELLS

Passaging techniques used with human ES cells may have a tremendous effect on the stability of the culture. Recent studies demonstrated that techniques that result in the individualization of cells (i.e., use of trypsin or CDB) may accumulate karyotypic abnormalities more readily than cultures passaged manually (Mitalipova et al. 2005). While the cause of these changes are unclear, it may be due to a selective cloning advantage in abnormal cells, allowing them to overtake the culture. Therefore, techniques that allow the passage of human ES cells in clumps, rather than as single cells, may result in greater stability over time. Manual passaging has been recommended to maintain stability (Buzzard et al. 2004; Mitalipova et al. 2005). While it does result in a more consistent colony size at passage, it is labor intensive and incompatible with large-scale culture required for human ES cells to be used clinically. Alternatives to this method include enzyme treatments that allow cells to be primarily passaged in clumps, such as dispase, collagenase, and EDTA. Our best results to date are achieved using dispase, and care must be taken to ensure that colonies are not excessively disrupted.

4.1 Passaging Cells in TeSR1 Medium

Aspirate medium, and incubate cells with 1 mL/well of 0.5 mg/mL dispase (in DMEM/F12) for 5 min at 37°C (2 mg/mL dispase if using Matrigel-coated plates). Following incubation, cells are rinsed on the plate a minimum of three times using warmed DMEM/F12 medium. Cells are then bathed in TeSR1 medium and carefully lifted from the plate by gentle scraping. Cells are then plated directly into a freshly prepared human matrix coated plate. Cells should be passaged at a density of roughly 5×10^6 cells/well for the best results if using a human matrix (3×10^6 if using Matrigel matrix). Cultures will need to be split roughly every 3–5 days if maintained on human matrix plates; every 4–7 days if maintained on Matrigel-coated plates. On-time passaging is critical—more so than in any other medium we have tested—and cells are unforgiving if passaged either too early or allowed to overgrow. Cells should be passaged when the colony centers are roughly 3–4 times denser than the colony edge (Figure 1A). Light reflection will show these dense centers to be bright when viewed using a phase contrast microscope at the appropriate splitting time (Figure 1B, C). There is generally a 24-h window in which to split the cells for maximum attachment and survival. If the culture is passaged prematurely, the cells will not properly

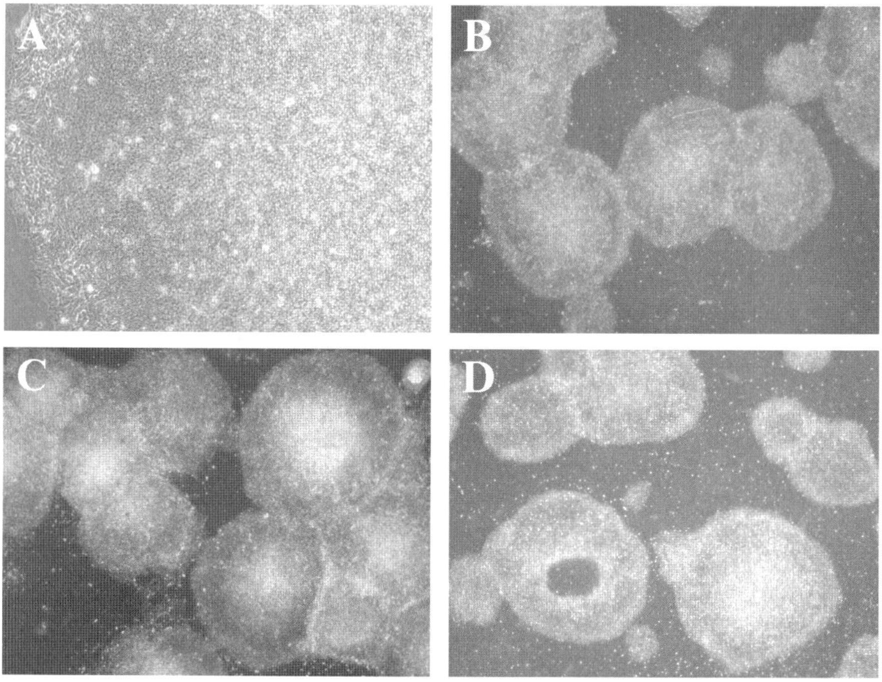

Figure 1. Morphology of TeSR1 cultured cells ready to passage. (A) Colony center is noticeably denser than edge. (B) and (C) Center of colonies are bright compared to colony edge when viewed at ×2 using phase contrast microscopy. (D) Differentiation in the center of a single colony allowed to grow past the optimum passaging timepoint. If not extensive, this differentiation may be aspirated and the remaining culture passaged as usual.

attach when replated. If allowed to overgrow, the dense centers of the colonies will begin to differentiate (Figure 1D). If only a few colonies have differentiated centers, they may be aspirated off from the plate, and the remaining colonies passaged as usual.

5. CONCLUSION

Tremendous potential exists for human ES cells to have a dramatic and lasting impact on human health. That potential is directly linked to the ability to reliably sustain ES cells in culture. TeSR1 medium is serum-free, feeder-independent, animal-product free, fully defined, and disclosed. This allows it to serve as a starting point for further optimization to improve human ES cell culture systems. More importantly, the use of TeSR1 medium in combination with the defined human matrix results in the production of the first therapeutically relevant human ES cell cultures, and enables the widespread application of human ES cell technology in regenerative medicine.

REFERENCES

Amit, M. et al. (2000) Clonally derived human embryonic stem cell lines maintain pluripotency and proliferative potential for prolonged periods of culture. Dev. Biol., 227: 271–278.

Amit, M. et al. (2003) Human feeder layers for human embryonic stem cells. Biol. Reprod., 68: 2150–2156.

Amit, M., Shariki, C., Margulets, V., and Itskovitz-Eldor, J. (2004) Feeder layer- and serum-free culture of human embryonic stem cells. Biol. Reprod., 70: 837–845.

Beattie, G.M. et al. (2005) Activin A maintains pluripotency of human embryonic stem cells in the absence of feeder layers. Stem. Cells, 23: 489–495.

Buzzard, J.J., Gough, N.M., Crook, J.M. and Colman, A. (2004) Karyotype of human ES cells during extended culture. Nat. Biotechnol., 22: 381–382; author reply 382.

Charles, A.K. (1986) Pipecolic acid receptors in rat cerebral cortex. Neurochem. Res., 11: 521–525 (1986).

Cheng, L., Hammond, H., Ye, Z., Zhan, X., and Dravid, G. (2003) Human adult marrow cells support prolonged expansion of human embryonic stem cells in culture. Stem. Cells, 21: 131–142.

Choo, A.B., Padmanabhan, J., Chin, A.C., and Oh, S.K. (2004) Expansion of pluripotent human embryonic stem cells on human feeders. Biotechnol. Bioeng., 88: 321–331.

Daheron, L. et al. (2004) LIF/STAT3 signaling fails to maintain self-renewal of human embryonic stem cells. Stem. Cells, 22: 770–778.

Daniels, J.T., Harris, I.R., Kearney, J.N., and Ingham, E. (1995) Calcium: a crucial consideration in serum-free keratinocyte culture. Exp. Dermatol., 4: 183–191.

Draper, J.S., Moore, H.D., Ruban, L.N., Gokhale, P.J., and Andrews, P.W. (2004) Culture and characterization of human embryonic stem cells. Stem. Cells Dev., 13: 325–336.

Dravid, G. et al. (2005) Defining the role of Wnt/b-catenin signaling in the survival, proliferation and self-renewal of human embryonic stem cells. Stem. Cells Express, 23: 150–165.

Evans, M.J. (1972) The isolation and properties of a clonal tissue culture strain of pluripotent mouse teratoma cells. J. Embryol. Exp. Morphol., 28: 163–176.

Evans, M.J., and Kaufman, M.H. (1981) Establishment in culture of pluripotential cells from mouse embryos. Nature, 292: 154–156.

Genbacev, O. et al. (2005) Serum-free derivation of human embryonic stem cell lines on human placental fibroblast feeders. Fertil. Steril., 83: 1517–1529.

Hovatta, O. et al. (2003) A culture system using human foreskin fibroblasts as feeder cells allows production of human embryonic stem cells. Hum. Reprod., 18: 1404–1409.

James, D., Levine, A., Besser, D., and Hemmati-Brivanlou (2005) TGFβ/activin/nodal signaling is necessary for the maintenance of pluripotency in human embryonic stem cells. Development, 132: 1273–1282.

Klein, P.S. and Melton, D.A. (1996) A molecular mechanism for the effect of lithium on development. Proc. Natl. Acad. Sci. USA, 93: 8455–8459.

Klimanskaya, I. et al. (2005) Human embryonic stem cells derived without feeder cells. Lancet, 365: 1636–1641.

Lane, M. and Bavister, B.D. (1998) Calcium homeostasis in early hamster preimplantation embryos. Biol. Reprod., 59: 1000–1007.

Lane, M., Boatman, D.E., Albrecht, R.M., and Bavister, B.D. (1998) Intracellular divalent cation homeostasis and developmental competence in the hamster preimplantation embryo. Mol. Reprod. Dev., 50: 443–450.

Levenstein, M.E. et al. (2005) Basic FGF support of human embryonic stem cell self-renewal. Stem. Cells.

Li, Y., Powell, S., Brunette, E., Lebkowski, J., and Mandalam, R. (2005) Expansion of human embryonic stem cells in defined serum-free medium devoid of animal-derived products. Biotechnol. Bioeng., 91: 688–698.

Ludwig, T.E. et al. (2006) Derivation of human embryonic stem cells in defined conditions. Nat. Biotechnol., 24: 185–187.

Martin, G.R. (1981) Isolation of a pluripotent cell line from early mouse embryos cultured in medium conditioned by teratocarcinoma stem cells. Proc. Natl. Acad. Sci. USA., 78.

Martin, M.J., Muotri, A., Gage, F., and Varki, A. (2005) Human embryonic stem cells express an immunogenic nonhuman sialic acid. Nat. Med., 11: 228–232.

Mitalipova, M.M. et al. (2005) Preserving the genetic integrity of human embryonic stem cells. Nat. Biotechnol., 23: 19–20.

Owens, D.F. and Kriegstein, A.R. (2002) Is there more to GABA than synaptic inhibition? Nat. Rev. Neurosci. 3: 715–727.

Puck, T.T. and Marcus, P.I. (1955) Rapid method for viable cell titration and clone production with HeLa cells on tissue culture: the use of X-irradiated cells to supply conditioning factors. Proc. Natl. Acad. Sci. USA, 4: 432–437.

Reubinoff, B.E., Pera, M.F., Fong, C.Y., Trounson, A., and Bongso, A. (2000) Embryonic stem cell lines from human blastocysts: somatic differentiation in vitro. Nat. Biotechnol., 18: 399–404.

Richards, M. et al. (2003) Comparative evaluation of various human feeders for prolonged undifferentiated growth of human embryonic stem cells. Stem. Cells, 21: 546–556.

Richards, M., Fong, C.Y., Chan, W.K., Wong, P.C., and Bongso, A. (2002) Human feeders support prolonged undifferentiated growth of human inner cell masses and embryonic stem cells. Nat. Biotechnol., 20: 933–936.

Sato, N. et al. (2003) Molecular signature of human embryonic stem cells and its comparison with the mouse. Dev. Biol., 260: 404–413.

Sato, N., Meijer, L., Skaltsounis, L., Greengard, P., and Brivanlou, A.H. (2004) Maintenance of pluripotency in human and mouse embryonic stem cells through activation of Wnt signaling by a pharmacological GSK-3-specific inhibitor. Nat. Med., 10: 55–63.

Schuldiner, M., Yanuka, O., Itskovitz-Eldor, J., Melton, D.A., and Benvenisty, N. (2000) Effects of eight growth factors on the differentiation of cells derived from human embryonic stem cells. Proc. Natl. Acad. Sci. USA, 97: 11307–11312.

Sperger, J.M. et al. (2003) Gene expression patterns in human embryonic stem cells and human pluripotent germ cell tumors. Proc. Natl. Acad. Sci. USA, 100: 13350–13355.

Stojkovic, P. et al. (2005) An autogeneic feeder cell system that efficiently supports growth of undifferentiated human embryonic stem cells. Stem. Cells, 23: 306–314.

Takahama, K. et al. (1986) Pipecolic acid enhancement of GABA response in single neurons of rat brain. Neuropharmacology, 25: 339–342.

Thomson, J.A. et al. (1998) Embryonic stem cell lines derived from human blastocysts. Science, 282: 1145–1147.

Vallier, L., Alexander, M., and Pedersen, R.A. (2005) Activin/Nodal and FGF pathways cooperate to maintain pluripotency of human embryonic stem cells. J. Cell Sci., 118: 4495–4509.

Vallier, L., Reynolds, D., and Pedersen, R.A. (2004) Nodal inhibits differentiation of human embryonic stem cells along the neuroectodermal default pathway. Dev. Biol., 275: 403–421.

Wang, L., Li, L., Menendez, P., Cerdan, C., and Bhatia, M. (2005) Human embryonic stem cells maintained in the absence of mouse embryonic fibroblasts or conditioned media are capable of hematopoietic development. Blood, 105: 4598–4603.

Watanabe, M., Maemura, K., Kanbara, K., Tamayama, T., and Hayasaki, H. (2002) GABA and GABA receptors in the central nervous system and other organs. Int. Rev. Cytol., 213: 1–47.

Xu, C. et al. (2001) Feeder-free growth of undifferentiated human embryonic stem cells. Nat. Biotechnol., 19: 971–974.

Xu, C. et al. (2005) Basic fibroblast growth factor supports undifferentiated human embryonic stem cell growth without conditioned medium. Stem. Cells, 23: 315–323.

Xu, R.H. et al. (2005) Basic FGF and suppression of BMP signaling sustain undifferentiated proliferation of human ES cells. Nat. Methods, 2: 185–190.

CHAPTER 2

GENERATION OF DISEASE-SPECIFIC HUMAN EMBRYONIC STEM CELL LINES

STEPHEN MINGER

Director of Stem Cell Biology Laboratory, Wolfson Centre for Age-Related Diseases, Kings College London, UK

In addition to the derivation of human embryonic stem (hES) cell lines for potential therapeutic use, drug discovery, and toxicology screening, hES cells can also be used as model systems for understanding human genetic disease, elucidating the pathophysiology of specific genetic disorders as well as providing human cells with endogenous genetic lesions that might be useful for testing novel therapies and identifying new pharmacological strategies.

To date several hES cell lines with specific genetic disorders have been derived, usually from embryos at high risk for genetic disease and screened after *in vitro* fertilisation using preimplantation genetic diagnosis (PGD), although other methods for deriving disease-specific cell lines have also been reported. This chapter will provide an overview of the approaches used to derive such "mutant" cell lines and the special characterisation processes involved in confirming the genetic identity of each cell line.

PGD is a procedure whereby couples at risk of passing on a known genetic disorder to their child can utilise *in vitro* fertilisation as a means of creating embryos which can then be screened using molecular or cytogenetic tools to ascertain the genetic status of each IVF-derived embryo relevant to the genetic disorder in question (for a review see Braude et al. 2002). Diagnosis can be achieved using blastomere biopsy of cleavage-stage embryos (i.e., removal of a single cell from an 8-cell embryo) and subsequent polymerase chain reaction (PCR) using disease-specific primers for simple monogenic disorders, for example Huntington's disease, spinal muscular atrophy (SMA), cystic fibrosis (CF) amongst others. For many X-linked disorders that only result in disease in males, this type of genetic analysis is not generally possible. In many cases, embryos are merely sexed using X- and Y-chromosome-specific probes and only female embryos will be subsequently implanted. Recently, whole genome amplification has been proposed as a means of specifically

J.R. Masters et al (eds.), Embryonic Stem Cells, 17–25.

diagnosing each male embryo (see, e.g., Handyside et al. 2004) though this technology is still under development and is not yet widely used for pre-implantation diagnosis.

Diagnosis of the genetic status or sex of each embryo is obtained 2–3 days post-fertilisation and healthy unaffected embryos are then usually implanted between 4 and 6 days after fertilisation or cryopreserved for subsequent use. Affected embryos from couples that have consented for embryo donation for research are usually then cultured to the blastocyst stage equivalent to 6–7 days post-fertilisation and then processed for hES cell derivation using conventional methods.

1. GENERATION OF DISEASE-SPECIFIC CELL LINES FROM PGD

The use of PGD embryos as a potential source population of embryos for the generation of disease-specific cell lines was first reported in 2003 (Pickering et al. 2003). A total of 44 embryos from eight sets of embryos subjected to PGD and subsequently donated for stem cell derivation were used to attempt to derive mutant hES cell lines. This population of embryos included five sets of embryos screened for X-linked disorders (36 embryos), one set for SMA Type I (2 embryos), and two sets of embryos which were found to have chromosomal translocations (6 embryos). Donated embryos were cultured to the blastocyst stage and the inner cell mass (ICM) was isolated using immunosurgery by selectively lysing the surrounding trophoectoderm. Of the original 44 PGD embryos, 25 successfully progressed to the blastocyst stage (55%) and from these 16 individual ICMs were recovered (36%). The ICMs were placed onto mitomycin-C-treated mouse embryonic fibroblasts in conventional hES cell medium (Reubinoff et al. 2000) containing 20% fetal calf serum and 1,000 units/ml leukaemia-inhibitory factor and the medium was completely replaced every other day. Seven of the 16 ICMs expanded in culture and two of these generated cells with hES cell appearance. Both sets of cells were successfully passaged for approximately 2 months, but one putative cell line was lost due to bacterial contamination prior to characterisation whilst all the colonies from the other line spontaneously arrested after about 50 days and were discarded after 2 months in culture. Nevertheless, and in parallel, a hES cell line from a genetically normal cryopreserved embryo was successfully established by this group (designated WT-3), demonstrating that the procedures and culture conditions used in this study were competent for the derivation of hES cells (Pickering et al. 2003).

The first reports of well-characterised disease-specific hES cell lines successfully derived from PGD embryos were published in 2005 (Pickering et al. 2005; Verlinsky et al. 2005). As part of an ongoing and continuous process of using PGD embryos to attempt to derive disease-specific hES cell lines, two embryos diagnosed by PGD and shown to be homozygous for the delta508 mutation in the cystic fibrosis transmembrane conductance regulator (CFTR) gene, the most common mutation resulting in CF, were donated under informed consent for stem cell derivation (Pickering et al. 2005). The embryos were cultured to blastocyst stage as previously described (Pickering et al. 2003) and although one embryo degenerated at this stage, one of the embryos formed a hatched and expanded blastocyst approximately 6–7 days post-fertilisation. Immunosurgery was performed and the isolated ICM was placed onto inactivated mouse fibroblasts using previously described culture conditions (Pickering et al. 2003). The ICM expanded and after approximately 11 days generated a colony containing cells with prominent hES cell morphology. This colony was dissected into two pieces and transferred to new fibroblast cultures where both pieces expanded and were further subcultured, generating additional colonies, which were subsequently expanded and characterised for hES cell characteristics. The resulting hES cell line, CF-1, displayed all the common characteristics of other published hES cell lines (Thomson et al. 1998; Reubinoff et al. 2000). Undifferentiated CF-1 colonies at passages 7, 15, and 30 expressed high levels of characteristic hES cell surface proteins including stage-specific embryonic antigens SSEA-3 and SSEA-4, the Trafalgar antigens Tra1-60 and Tra-1-81, and the ES cell transcription factor Oct-4, but were negative for the mouse ES (mES) cell surface antigen SSEA-1 (Pickering et al. 2005). Real-time PCR analysis revealed that undifferentiated CF-1 cells also expressed genes characteristic of ES cells, including Oct-4, Nanog, FGF-4, Rex1 and Sox2, and were capable of generating cells of all three germ layers by both spontaneous differentiation and directed differentiation using embryoid body (EB) formation (Pickering et al. 2005). CF-1 cells were also subjected to chromosomal analysis at passages 15, 30, and 45 and shown at each time point to have a normal and stable 46XY karyotype (data not shown) and the presence and maintenance of the delta508 mutation in the CF-1 cell line was also confirmed at passage 28 (Pickering et al. 2005). Also, the CFTR gene was shown to be only expressed in differentiated cells and was absent in undifferentiated CF-1 cells (data not published). Recently, the directed differentiation of CF-1 cells into lung epithelial cells has been obtained by co-culture of CF-1 cells with mature human bronchial epithelial cells (data not published), demonstrating that CF-1 cells are capable of generating lung tissue, an important requirement if this cell line is to be used in future research related to CF. CF-1 thus represents one of the first disease-specific hES cell lines to be generated and may have use in elucidating the role that the CFTR mutation plays in the pathogenesis of CF, as well as use as a target cell line for gene transfer strategies to replace the mutant and misfolded protein with a functional substitute.

Verlinsky and colleagues have also reported the derivation of a large group of putative disease-specific hES cell lines from PGD embryos (Verlinsky et al. 2005) using either conventional immunosurgery to remove the trophectoderm, by plating intact blastocysts onto inactivated fibroblast feeder cells, or by culturing pre-blastocyst morula-stage embryos under the feeder layer (Strelchenko et al. 2004). A total of 15 individual disease-specific hES cell lines were derived from 44 donated PGD embryos and include cell lines homozygous recessive for β-thalassaemia and Fanconi's anaemia (FA), two hES cell lines with expanded CAG repeats that result in Huntington's disease, as well as cell lines harbouring autosomal dominant mutations resulting in Marfan's syndrome, myotonic dystrophy Type I (DM1), and Type I neurofibromatosis (NF), and a series of hES cell lines with X-linked disorders including fragile-X syndrome, adrenoleukodystrophy (ALD), and Becker's muscular dystrophy (BMD). Although this is by far the largest number of disease-specific cell lines published to date, the level of characterisation has been generally poor. The majority of the cell lines have only been characterised at passages 3–8 and not at higher passage number and only cell-surface marker analysis and Oct-4 protein expression was used to validate these cell lines (Verlinsky et al. 2005), which is not sufficient to demonstrate that these are pluripotent hES cell lines. There was no published evidence presented that the cells were capable of multilineage differentiation either *in vitro* using spontaneous or embryoid body-induced differentiation or *in vivo* by injection into SCID mice and subsequent teratoma formation and no karyotype analysis to confirm the chromosomal stability of the cell lines was reported. In addition, important data related to the phenotype of some of the most interesting lines were lacking including the number of the CAG and CTG repeats in the Huntington's disease and myotonic dystrophy (DM) cell lines, respectively. Without such exhaustive characterisation, it is difficult to determine the extent to which these potentially interesting cell lines are truly hES cell lines and at the same time have characteristics that may make them suitable lines for disease-specific investigation.

In contrast, a more complete and standard characterisation of disease-specific hES cell lines from PGD embryos is outlined in a recent manuscript by Mateizel and colleagues (Mateizel et al. 2006). This group isolated three new disease-specific hES cell lines from a total of 14 PGD embryos using conventional embryo handling and culturing methods. All of the hES cell lines were derived from blastocysts that had been subjected to immunosurgery to isolate the ICM and all were derived on inactivated mouse fibroblasts in "knockout" medium including synthetic serum replacement and FGF-2. Each of the cell lines was fully characterised and included positive cell-surface antigen expression for SSEA-3, SSEA-4, Tra-1-60, and Tra-1-81, positive alkaline phosphatase activity, and expression by RT-PCR for known ES cell-specific genes including Oct-4, Nanog, Rex-1, Sox-2, and GDF3. In addition all three cell lines generated cells of all three germ layers when differentiated using EB formation and two of the three cell lines formed teratomas with cells of all three germ layers following injection into SCID mice (Mateizel et al. 2006). The third cell line was being assessed for *in vivo* teratoma formation at the time of publication.

The molecular and genetic phenotype of each of the individual cell lines is unusual and informative of the biology underlying each of the disease states. One cell line was derived from an embryo at risk for DM1. The oocyte donor was affected with the adult form of the disease and shown to have 120 CTG repeats in the dystrophia myotonica-protein kinase (DMPK) gene but the embryo itself was not diagnosed at day 3 following fertilisation due to slow progression through culture. Subsequent genetic examination of the resulting hES cell line at passage 1 identified a very significant expansion of the number of CTG repeats to 470 demonstrating the genetic instability at this locus (Mateizel et al. 2006). Similarly, a hES cell line derived from a gamete donor with 42 CAG repeats (above 38 repeats is considered pathogenic) was found to have 44 CAG repeats at early passage, a small increase compared to that observed in the dystonia cell line (Mateizel et al. 2006). The third cell line was derived from an embryo at risk for CF, and displayed a more complex genetic phenotype than the cell line derived by Pickering et al. (2005). The CF cell line contained one CFTR allele that harboured the delta508 mutation, whilst the other allele was shown to have the intron 8 splice variant 5T of the CFTR which results in congenital bilateral absence of the vas deferens (CBAVD).

1.1 Homologous Recombination

To date, these are the only published reports of disease-specific cell lines obtained from PGD embryos. However, an alternative means of generating mutant hES cell lines is to use gene transfer methodologies to insert disease-specific genes into genetically normal cell lines. The most important technology in this regard is the use of homologous recombination to site-specifically replace the endogenous normal gene with a disease-causal gene. This has the advantage of generating cell lines with mutant genes in their normal physiological and genetic context rather than ectopic gene expression that results from plasmid or viral vector genetic transduction. This also has the advantage that the mutant and normal hES cell lines will have identical genetic backgrounds differing only at the mutant gene locus.

The introduction of exogenous DNA using electroporation has routinely been used in mES cells for gene transfer and to generate transgenic and knockout mice strains. However, similar transduction protocols using hES cells results in poor survival and stable transduction efficiencies of approximately 1 in 10 million cells (Zwaka and Thomson 2003), whereas chemical transfection reagents have proved slightly more successful (Eiges et al. 2001). Initial attempts to use chemical transfection agents to site-specifically knockout the gene encoding the hypoxanthine phosphoribosyltransferase-1 gene (HPRT-1) by homologous recombination proved unsuccessful and no successful targeting events as determined by antibiotic resistance and 6-TG selection for HPRT-1 mutant phenotype were observed (Zwaka and Thomson 2003). A re-evaluation of electroporation technology and several technical modifications in the method of delivering the DNA construct into hES cells ultimately proved more efficient. These modifications included the use of electroporation parameters more suitable for the larger size of individual hES cells compared to mES cells, the replacement of PBS with standard tissue culture medium for the electroporation procedure, and the electroporation of cell clumps rather than completely dissociated cells. These alterations resulted in successful gene-targeting efficiencies that were approximately 100-fold greater than that seen with mES cells (Zwaka and Thomson 2003). Transfection of about 15 million hES cells with the HPRT-1 targeting vector resulted in seven successful targeting events, thus demonstrating that replacement of normal human genes by mutant genes using homologous recombination can be achieved, albeit at relatively low efficiency (Zwaka and Thomson 2003).

Successful homologous recombination of the HPRT-1 gene locus using isogenic DNA to create a human disease model for Lesch-Nyhan disease has also been more recently achieved using a commercially available chemical transfection reagent (Urbach et al. 2004). Successful targeting occurred at a frequency of approximately 10^{-8} transfected cells, and was confirmed not only by antibiotic selection and growth in 6-TG, but also by confirmation that one of the major hallmarks of Lesch-Nyhan disease, the accumulation of uric acid, was significantly increased in the mutant cells compared to parental hES cell lines (Urbach et al. 2004). To date, these are the only published reports of the successful use of homologous recombination in hES cells to create disease-specific cell lines, although attempts are underway to introduce very long Huntington's disease CAG repeats into human ES cell lines to create additional Huntington's disease hES cell lines (Minger and Bates, unpublished data).

1.2 Somatic Cell Nuclear Transfer

Somatic cell nuclear transfer (SCNT) is the process of creating a genetically identical cloned cell line ("therapeutic cloning") or an organism ("reproductive cloning") from a pre-existing cell, animal or individual (for a review see Hochedlinger and Jaenisch 2003). The process involves the removal of the maternal DNA from a donated oocyte, introduction of an adult cell or nucleus into the enucleated oocyte, reprogramming of the adult cell genome by the maternal reprogramming machinery back to an embryonic state, which when successful can then allow for the generation of a cloned embryo which can either be used for ES cell derivation, or when implanted into a recipient uterus may give rise to a clone of the adult cell donor. In most countries reproductive cloning using human somatic cells is not legal and therefore will not be considered in the context of this review. However, SCNT for the purposes of creating cloned hES cells for therapeutic purposes is legal in many countries, including the UK. A license from the Human Fertilisation and Embryology Authority (HFEA) for SCNT is required before this procedure can be employed. An alternative application of SCNT could be the generation of disease-specific hES cell lines from individuals with pre-exiting genetic or acquired disorders, where the DNA content of the affected individual would be expressed in each hES cell. There is considerable interest in generating such cell lines from individuals with rare forms of acquired cancer or from individuals with complex idiopathic disorders, for example motor neurone disease (MND), where the primary cause of the disease is unclear (see, e.g., Wilmut 2004). Once derived, hES cells would be preferentially differentiated into cell types most relevant to the disease in question and subsequently used for basic pathophysiological studies, the development of novel therapies, or new drug development using "diseased" human somatic cells.

The process of human SCNT involves several discrete steps each of which are critical for successful derivation of hES cell lines. The retraction of the published work from the Korean SCNT team means that there has yet to be a successfully cloned hES cell line using SCNT. A number of important details can be gleaned from the Korean work as well as successful generation of cloned primate embryos (Simerly et al. 2004). The first and perhaps most important requirement is a source of high quality fresh human oocytes, preferably from younger women who ideally have not been through a fertility cycle (Stojkovic et al. 2005). The use of young women as oocyte donors for SCNT, which would involve a potentially risky procedure for which no personal medical benefit would be obtained, is an ethically contentious area, particularly as it is uncertain what the actual frequency of successful nuclear transfer using human oocytes and somatic cells is. Partially for this reason, the HFEA has not allowed oocyte donation solely for research purposes, although oocyte sharing for fertility and research has recently been licensed to a group in Newcastle, UK (HFEA website).

One alternative source of oocytes for nuclear transfer which would be ideally suited to the generation of disease-specific cell lines (which would only be used for research) would be to utilise non-human oocytes as recipients for SCNT. Chen et al. (2003) successfully derived cloned hES cell lines using rabbit surrogate oocytes and somatic fibroblasts from human donors ranging from 5–60 years of age. A total of 2,418 rabbit oocytes gave rise to 1,086 successful nuclear transfers which resulted in 158 embryos that progressed to blastocyst stage (14.5%). From these, more than 14 cloned hES cell lines were obtained, four of which were passaged for extended periods (> 28 passages) and rigorously characterised for hES cell characteristics. All four cell lines displayed cell surface marker expression characteristic of hES cells including high levels of alkaline phosphatase and positive immunoreactivity for SSEA-3, SSEA-4, Tra1-10, and Tra-1-85, but were negative for SSEA-1 (Chen et al. 2003). Pluripotency of the cell lines was demonstrated by *in vitro* differentiation through EB formation, with cells from all three primary germ layers present in the differentiated cell populations, although no *in vivo* teratoma formation was reported (Chen et al. 2003). In principle, a wide range of non-human oocytes should support successful SCNT of human cells, including rabbit, sheep, pig, and cow oocytes, which have already been shown to support intra-species SCNT. The latter three species are particularly useful as there are large numbers of ovaries available from these species from abattoirs that could be used for human SCNT.

The enucleation process appears to be crucial for propagation of the embryo following nuclear transfer. Previously, the standard method for removing the meiotic metaphase II spindle apparatus and chromosomes of the oocyte was through extraction by aspiration (see, e.g., Simerly et al. 2003). The aspiration process seems to disrupt the mitotic spindle apparatus, important in chromosomal segregation during cytokinesis, and was thought to be one of the primary reasons for the failure to initially generate primate blastocysts by SCNT (Simerly et al. 2003). An alternative "squish" or extrusion method of enucleation prior to metaphase II arrest appears at least in primate oocytes to be much less deleterious, and successfully cloned blastocysts were obtained using this method, although no viable pregnancies were obtained from 135 implanted blastocysts (Simerly et al. 2004). Although no cloned primate cell lines have been reported to date, progression of nuclear-transferred oocytes to blastocyst stage embryos should allow for the successful derivation of primate ES cell lines with a frequency approaching that of hES cell derivation from *in vitro* fertilization (IVF) embryos.

Following enucleation of the oocyte, the somatic cell or nucleus must then be successfully transferred either through microinjection of the somatic cell or nucleus into the oocyte or by fusion of the oocyte and somatic cell membranes through electrofusion. The now diploid oocyte is then activated using either chemical or electrical means and the resultant embryo is then cultured *in vitro* to the blastocyst stage when isolation of the ICM, propagation on fibroblast feeder cells and generation of a cloned hES cell line would be performed. Between the process of nuclear replacement and activation and subsequent progression of the oocyte to a cleavage stage embryo, one final key process that must occur for successful SCNT is the genetic reprogramming of the adult DNA by maternal reprogramming factors, which essentially resets the adult genome to a developmentally earlier state comparable to that found in the early embryo (for a review see Armstrong et al. 2006). This process, when completed with high fidelity, enables the adult genome to regress to a more primitive and embryonic state, thus allowing the full developmental sequence of embryonic development to occur, which can be utilised in the derivation of hES cells. To date, no disease-specific or normal hES cell lines have been derived by SCNT. However, several groups are proposing to utilise this technique as a means of deriving hES cell lines from individuals with genetic forms of Alzheimer's disease, Parkinson's disease, MND, as well as individuals with major susceptibility genes such as Apolipoprotein E4.

REFERENCES

Armstrong, L., Lako, M., Dean, W., and Stojkovic, M. (2006) Epigenetic modification is central to genome reprogramming in somatic cell nuclear transfer. Stem Cells, 24: 805–814.

Braude, P., Pickering, S., Flinter, F., and Ogilvie, C.M. (2002) Preimplantation genetic diagnosis. Nat. Rev. Genet., 3: 941–953.

Chen, Y., He, Z.X., Liu, A., Wang, K., Mao, W.W., Chu, J.X., Lu, Y., Fang, Z.F., Shi, Y.T., Yang, Q.Z., Chen, D.Y., Wang, M.K., Li, J.S., Huang, S.L., Kong, X.Y., Shi, Y.Z., Wang, Z.Q., Xia, J.H., Long, Z.G., Xue, Z.G., Ding, W.X., and Sheng, H.Z. (2003) Embryonic stem cells generated by nuclear transfer of human somatic nuclei into rabbit oocytes. Cell Res., 13: 251–263.

Eiges, R., Schuldiner, M., Drukker, M., Yanuka, O., Itskovitz-Eldor, J., and Benvenisty, N. (2001) Establishment of human embryonic stem cell-transfected clones carrying a marker for undifferentiated cells. Curr. Biol., 11: 514–518.

Handyside, A.H., Robinson, M.D., Simpson, R.J., Omar, M.B., Shaw, M.A., Grudzinskas, J.G., and Rutherford, A. (2004) Isothermal whole genome amplification from single and small numbers of cells: a new era for preimplantation genetic diagnosis of inherited disease. Mol. Hum. Reprod., 10: 767–772.

Hochedlinger, K. and Jaenisch, R. (2003) Nuclear transplantation, embryonic stem cells, and the potential for cell therapy. N. Engl. J. Med., 349: 275–286.

Mateizel, I., De, T.N., Ullmann, U., Cauffman, G., Sermon, K., Van, d., V, De, R.M., Degreef, E., Devroey, P., Liebaers, I., and Van, S.A. (2006) Derivation of human embryonic stem cell lines from embryos obtained after IVF and after PGD for monogenic disorders. Hum. Reprod., 21: 503–511.

Pickering, S.J., Braude, P.R., Patel, M., Burns, C.J., Trussler, J., Bolton,V., and Minger, S. (2003) Preimplantation genetic diagnosis as a novel source of embryos for stem cell research. Reprod. Biomed. Online, 7: 353–364.

Pickering, S.J., Minger, S.L., Patel, M., Taylor, H., Black, C., Burns, C.J., Ekonomou, A., and Braude, P.R. (2005) Generation of a human embryonic stem cell line encoding the cystic fibrosis mutation deltaF508, using preimplantation genetic diagnosis. Reprod. Biomed. Online, 10: 390–397.

Reubinoff, B.E., Pera, M.F., Fong, C.Y., Trounson, A., and Bongso, A. (2000) Embryonic stem cell lines from human blastocysts: somatic differentiation in vitro [In Process Citation]. Nat. Biotechnol., 18: 399–404.

Simerly, C., Dominko, T., Navara, C., Payne, C., Capuano, S., Gosman, G., Chong, K.Y., Takahashi, D., Chace, C., Compton, D., Hewitson, L., and Schatten, G. (2003) Molecular correlates of primate nuclear transfer failures. Science, 300: 297.

Simerly, C., Navara, C., Hyun, S.H., Lee, B.C., Kang, S.K., Capuano, S., Gosman, G., Dominko, T., Chong, K.Y., Compton, D., Hwang, W.S., and Schatten, G. (2004) Embryogenesis and blastocyst development after somatic cell nuclear transfer in nonhuman primates: overcoming defects caused by meiotic spindle extraction. Dev. Biol., 276: 237–252.

Stojkovic, M., Stojkovic, P., Leary, C., Hall, V.J., Armstrong, L., Herbert, M., Nesbitt, M., Lako, M., and Murdoch, A. (2005) Derivation of a human blastocyst after heterologous nuclear transfer to donated oocytes. Reprod. Biomed. Online, 11: 226–231.

Strelchenko, N., Verlinsky, O., Kukharenko, V., and Verlinsky, Y. (2004) Morula-derived human embryonic stem cells. Reprod. Biomed. Online, 9: 623–629.

Thomson, J.A., Itskovitz-Eldor, J., Shapiro, S.S., Waknitz, M.A., Swiergiel, J.J., Marshall, V.S., and Jones, J.M. (1998) Embryonic stem cell lines derived from human blastocysts [see comments] [published erratum appears in Science 1998 Dec 4;282(5395):1827]. Science, 282: 1145–1147.

Urbach, A., Schuldiner, M., and Benvenisty, N. (2004) Modeling for Lesch-Nyhan disease by gene targeting in human embryonic stem cells. Stem Cells, 22: 635–641.

Verlinsky, Y., Strelchenko, N., Kukharenko, V., Rechitsky, S., Verlinsky, O., Galat, V., and Kuliev, A. (2005) Human embryonic stem cell lines with genetic disorders. Reprod. Biomed. Online, 10: 105–110.

Wilmut, I. (2004) Human cells from cloned embryos in research and therapy. BMJ, 328: 415–416.

Zwaka, T.P. and Thomson, J.A. (2003) Homologous recombination in human embryonic stem cells. Nat. Biotechnol., 21: 319–321.

CHAPTER 3

CHARACTERIZATION AND DIFFERENTIATION OF HUMAN EMBRYONIC STEM CELLS

ANDREW L. LASLETT[1,2], ADELIA LIN[3], AND MARTIN F. PERA[1,3,4]
[1] *The Australian Stem Cell Centre*
[2] *Department of Anatomy and Cell Biology, Monash University, Clayton, Australia*
[3] *Monash Institute of Medical Research, Monash University, Clayton, Australia*
[4] *Center for Stem Cell and Regenerative Medicine, Keck School of Medicine, University of Southern California*

1. INTRODUCTION

This chapter will discuss the characterization and differentiation of human embryonic stem cell (hESC) lines. The first derivation of hESC lines was reported in 1998 (Thomson et al. 1998). Subsequently hundreds of hESC lines have been derived in many countries necessitating the development of standard methodologies for characterization and comparison of cell lines cultured under different conditions and in different laboratories. This chapter will describe selected methods for the characterization and differentiation of hESC from ours and other laboratories.

2. KARYOTYPE AND MICROBIOLOGICAL ASSAYS FOR CONTAMINATION

Karyotype: hESC cultures should be examined regularly for normal G-banded karyotype. This is best performed by a qualified cytogenetics laboratory; simple estimation of chromosome numbers from metaphase spreads is not adequate for assessment of genetic status of hESC cultures. It should be remembered that gross karyotypic analysis only provides a low-resolution read-out of the genetic stability of a cell line and that small mutations will escape detection unless a high-resolution approach such as array comparative genomic hybridization is used (Pinkel and Albertson 2005). A number of recent publications have noted the development of grossly karyotypically abnormal hESC lines detected by G-banded karyotype (Cowan et al. 2004; Draper et al. 2004; Enver et al. 2005; Herszfeld et al. 2006). The CD30 antigen is present on karyotypically abnormal hESC and Herszfeld et al. (Herszfeld et al. 2006) have reported that CD30

J.R. Masters et al (eds.), Embryonic Stem Cells, 27–40.

antigen expression provides a simple means for detecting abnormal hESC even at low frequencies in mixed cultures by flow cytometry.

The true frequency of development of karyotypic or other genetic abnormalities in hESC culture is not known, but it is almost certainly a function of culture methodology and passage level. Karyotypic abnormalities that persist in culture are often accompanied by changes in cellular growth, differentiation, and survival, rendering interpretation of any data on affected cell lines problematic. It is important to recognize that even grossly aneuploid human embryonal carcinoma cell lines show very similar patterns of antigen and gene expression to hESC and may even retain a feeder cell requirement and extensive differentiation capability (Pera et al. 1989), similar to many lines of mouse embryonal carcinoma.

Microbiological contamination: Standard good practice in mammalian cell culture should be followed to prevent and detect contamination with bacteria, fungi, and mycoplasms. Many commonly used hESC lines have been tested for contamination with a range of viral pathogens. Such assays, alongside of transmission electron microscopy, are not routinely carried out in most laboratories. The supplier of the line may provide documentation of absence of viral contaminants, but it is advisable to perform these tests on newly derived stem cell lines. Although human embryonal carcinoma cell lines have been reported to contain retroviral-like particles (Lower et al. 1996), the biological significance of these structures, which are also observed in normal human placental tissues, is unknown, and to date they have not been detected in hESC (International Stem Cell Initiative, unpublished results).

3. IMMUNOCHARACTERIZATION OF hESC

The identification, isolation, and characterization of specific cell types derived from hESC whether differentiated or undifferentiated can be effectively carried out using antibodies to hESC. Antibodies which detect antigenic epitopes expressed on hESC are listed in Table 1. These antibodies allow the characterization and comparison of different hESC lines and the cell surface markers

Table 1A. Cell surface hESC markers*

Antibody	Type	Antigen	Reference
GCTM-2	IgM	KSPG – protein core	(Laslett et al. 2003; Pera et al. 2003)
Tra 1-60	IgM	KSPG – carbohydrate side chain	(Andrews et al. 1984; Cooper et al. 2002)
Tra 1-81	IgM	KSPG – carbohydrate side chain	(Andrews et al. 1984; Cooper et al. 2002)
PHM-5	IgG1	podocalyxin	(Kerjaschki et al. 1986)
P1/33/2	IgG1	CD9	(Laslett et al. 2003; Pera et al. 2003)
SSEA3	IgM	Globoseries glycolipid	(Kannagi et al. 1983)
SSEA4	IgG3	Globoseries glycolipid	(Kannagi et al. 1983)
TG343	IgM	KSPG – protein core	(Cooper et al. 2002)
20-202S	IgG2a	HSPA8	(Son et al. 2005)

Table 1B. Transcription factor hESC markers*

Antibody	Type	Antigen	Reference
Oct4 (C-10)	IgG2b	Oct4	(Laslett et al. 2003; Pera et al. 2003)
nanog	Goat polyclonal	Nanog	(Hyslop et al. 2005)

*That have readily available antibodies.

listed (Table 1A) enable isolation of defined populations of live cells. It is important to realize that all of the markers listed in Table 1 are not entirely specific for undifferentiated hESC (reactivity is also seen in differentiated mature cell types) hence these markers are only useful within a limited context of hESC differentiation. In heterogeneous cell cultures (most likely all cultures involving hESC or differentiated cell types) it is critical to use combinations of markers to definitively identify discrete cell types. This is especially true for the identification of cells differentiated from hESC.

3.1 hESC Markers

Epitopes recognized by antibodies directed against the cell surface of hESC are not all fully characterized in molecular terms and in a number of instances the proteins that carry the epitopes and the gene that encodes them have not been identified.

Many of the antibodies used in the characterization of hESC lines are directed either against cell surface epitopes expressed at discrete stages of mouse embryonic development or against epitopes displayed on human embryonal carcinoma cells. The stage-specific embryonic antigens 1, 3, and 4 are globoseries glycolipids recognized by monoclonal antibodies originally raised by immunization of mice with embryos. While mouse ES (mES) cells are characterized by expression of SSEA-1, hESC express SSEA-3 and SSEA-4, and express SSEA-1 only upon differentiation. A second group of antibodies reactive with hESC, generated by immunization of mice with human embryonal carcinoma cells or cell extracts, all react with a set of epitopes associated with a highly immunogenic pericellular matrix keratan sulphate/chondroitin sulphate proteoglycan. These antibodies (TRA-1-60, TRA-1-81, GCTM-2, and TG-343) do not bind to mouse cells (Andrews et al. 1984; Pera et al. 1988; Cooper et al. 2002; Oka et al. 2002). Undifferentiated hESC also express the tetraspanin molecule CD9, similar to mES cells (Oka et al. 2002; Pera et al. 2003), podocalyxin (Kerjaschki, 1986), and heat shock 70-kD protein 8 isoform 1 (HSPA8) (Son 2005). Expression of the above markers characterizes the hESC culture population, however within that population there are subsets of cells that express these markers to different degrees (Laslett et al. 2007). It is important to reiterate that none of these markers are absolutely specific for hESC, but within the narrow context of hESC differentiation in vitro, they are useful for detection, quantiation, and isolation of stem cells by immunofluorescence, flow cytometry, or immunomagnetic techniques. Use of multiple markers in labelling techniques enhances specificity of stem cell detection.

4. IMMUNOCHEMICAL CHARACTERIZATION OF hESC

Indirect immunofluorescence: hESC are transferred to glass microscope slides after dissociation using enzymatic or non-enzymatic methods. We routinely use dispase (Dispase II, Roche Diagnostics), non-enzymatic dissociation buffer (Sigma) or TrypLE Express (Invitrogen) to harvest hESC prior to plating onto gelatin pretreated, mouse embryonic fibroblast (mEF) coated glass or plastic slides. hESC are then cultivated until fixation is required. For cell surface glycolipid antigens we use 90% acetone:10% water v/v for 5 min as the fixation method of choice. Alternatively, for intracellular transcription factors such as Oct4 we use either methanol:acetone 1:1 v/v or 4% paraformaldehyde in phosphate buffer solution (PBS), both at room temperature for 5 min. Methanol acetone slides need to be air-dried directly after fixation, and paraformaldehyde-fixed slides should be rinsed with water before air drying. The most common fixative employed in our laboratory is ice-cold absolute ethanol which works well with most cell-surface and intracellular antigens, and should be applied for 5 min after which slides should be air-dried. Slides can be stored for at least 6 months at –20°C.

Antibodies are added to the hESC on slides in a humidified chamber for 30 min then rinsed with PBS followed by secondary detection reagents, which may be conjugated to fluorochromes or enzymes. We routinely use indirect immunofluorescence as we think it provides more detailed information about localization of antigens and a better signal-to-noise ratio above background staining. The Alexa Fluor range of conjugated isotype-specific secondary antibodies (Molecular Probes) provide a simple means for multicolour fluorescence detection of more than one antigenic epitope as long as the antibodies used are of distinct isotypes (e.g., IgG2a and IgM). An alternative method is to directly conjugate primary antibodies (or purchase directly conjugated antibodies) to the desired fluorchromes using commercially available kits. After the secondary antibody incubation, the slides are rinsed again in PBS and then mounted. To enable rapid localization of cells we recommend that nuclei be counterstained with a DNA-binding dye such as DAPI or Hoechst 33258; this also allows easy discrimination between human and mouse feeder cells (the latter show a speckled appearance of chromatin after staining with these dyes, whilst the former show a more uniform nuclear staining).

5. CONFOCAL MICROSCOPY

Confocal microscopy is an alternative method to conventional optical microscopy that may be useful for the characterization of hESC. It offers several advantages over the traditional optical microscope including the ability to obtain serial optical sections from thick specimens, reduction of background noise from specimens, as well as the capability to image both live and fixed tissue. As ES cell colonies often vary in thickness, confocal microscopy is especially informative when seeking information on the spatial expression of particular antigens within a colony or an embryoid body.

hESC are cultured either on multiwell slides, chamber well slides or coverslips in a 12-well plate. Thereafter, cells are fixed and stained with the antibodies of interest using the methodology described above and visualized using a confocal microscope.

6. FLOW CYTOMETRY

Flow cytometry is a technique used to quantify populations of cells expressing antigenic and molecular markers of interest in a hESC population and as such, is a useful technique for characterization of these cells. In order for flow cytometry to be performed, cells must be in a single-cell suspension. However, the process of dissociating cells results in a significant degree of cell death and thus it is useful to employ gentler methods of cell dissociation during harvesting. It is also advisable to monitor cell viability during the procedure.

Cells are first washed twice with PBS to remove Mg^{2+} and Ca^{2+} ions. For hESC cultured as pieces in a 12-well tissue culture plate, this is then followed by the addition of 10 mg/mL Dispase (Gibco) dissolved in complete culture media and incubation at 37°C for 5 min at 5% CO_2. Dispase is a neutral protease that does not damage cell membranes and acts by allowing hES cells to be lifted off as an intact colony. Whole colonies are then gently lifted off by nudging with a 1,000μL pipette and transferred into a microcentrifuge tube with PBS to dilute dispase activity. The PBS is aspirated and colonies are washed once more with PBS. Non-enzymatic cell dissociation buffer is then added and the cells are dispersed into small clumps by trituration with a 1,000μL pipette tip. In the case of hESC cultured in bulk in tissue culture flasks, it is not practical to use mechanical methods to dislodge cells. In this case, it is possible to use 1 mg/mL collagenase IA made up in basal medium, in place of Dispase. After washing with PBS, cells are incubated with just enough collagenase to cover the surface area of the culture vessel and incubated at 37°C for 5 min at 5% CO_2. The collagenase is then aspirated and the cells are gently rinsed with culture medium. At this stage, tapping the flask aids in the dislodgement and dispersal of cells into single-cells. A third alternative method of cell dissociation that can be used for cells cultured either as pieces or in bulk is the use of TrypLE Express (Invitrogen). TrypLE Express can be substituted for 0.25% trypsin and is gentler on cells thereby increasing viability. In addition, inactivation by trypsin inhibitors is not necessary. Single cell suspensions are produced by trituration of cell clumps resuspended in dissociation buffer or TrypLE Express.

Before commencement of the staining procedure, single-cell suspensions are washed once in blocking solution, usually 1% goat serum in PBS, and pelleted by centrifugation at 2,000 for 2 min. The wash buffer is removed and cells are then resuspended in 300μL of the antibody of interest at the appropriate dilutions along with the class matched negative controls for 30 min on ice. At the end of the incubation, cells are pelleted by centrifugation again and washed twice with blocking solution followed by incubation for 30 min with 300μL of the secondary antibody with the appropriate isotype for the primary antibody, conjugated to a fluorophore such as Alexafluor 488 (Molecular Probes). Incubations are carried out in the dark to prevent photobleaching of the fluorophore.

Cells are then washed free of the secondary antibodies as mentioned above and resuspended in 300μL of blocking buffer. The cell suspension is then transferred to a tube for flow cytometric analysis. It is beneficial to add propidium iodide at a final concentration of 0.1mg/mL just before analysis to allow live and dead cells to be distinguished. The cell membrane integrity of dead cells is compromised and results in the uptake of propidium iodide. Cells are now ready to be analysed by flow cytometry.

7. FLUORESCENCE ACTIVATED CELL SORTING (FACS)

Live populations of hESC and their derivatives expressing particular antigenic markers of interest can be isolated from the global cell population via fluorescence activated cell sorting (FACS). These isolated populations can then be propagated for differentiation studies either in vitro or in vivo or further characterized for gene expression.

hESC are harvested and stained with the antibodies of interest as described above. However, in order for live cells to be isolated, antibodies used in the staining procedure must recognise antigens located on the cell surface and should not contain sodium azide. The use of antibodies that recognize cytoplasmic or nuclear antigens requires fixation of the cells and permeabilization of the cell membrane, which results in cell death.

8. CHARACTERIZATION OF hES CELLS USING GENE EXPRESSION ANALYSES

Genes characteristically found in hESC which have limited expression elsewhere in the developing embryo such as OCT4, GDF3, Nanog, and Cripto are known. Gene expression analysis is a valuable technique in the characterization of hESC and their differentiated derivatives.

However, when designing gene expression experiments, there are a few caveats to take note of. Firstly, the presence of a mRNA transcript may not always indicate that the translated protein product is functional or even that the transcript is translated. Often, proteins require post-translational modifications in order to function. Likewise, the lack of a gene transcript does not necessarily signify the absence of the protein product as well, since proteins tend to degrade at a slower rate than transcripts. Secondly, the assumption that gene expression patterns in differentiating hESC will always parallel those observed in the developing embryo is not proven. Therefore, experiments using patterns of expression of specific genes associated with particular stages of mouse embryonic development to characterize cell populations in hESC cultures should be subject to cautious interpretation. Nonetheless, careful design of gene expression experiments coupled with consideration for these caveats will yield useful results.

9. RNA ISOLATION

There are various methods that can be employed for the isolation of total or messenger RNA from cells. Many of these are commercially available and are presented in the form of kits. RNA isolation kits work by initially lysing cell membranes and inactivating endogenous ribonucleases with guanidinium thiocyanate solution. Cell lysates are then applied to a RNA-binding column containing a glass fibre filter. Proteins, DNA, and other contaminants are removed through a series of wash steps and the RNA is finally eluted. Depending on the number of cells from which RNA is to be extracted from, kits with RNA-binding columns of various binding capacities are available. It is advisable to select an appropriate column for the amount of starting material as overloading or underloading a column is likely to greatly decrease the RNA yield. Alternatively, RNA can be extracted using TRIzol Reagent (Invitrogen), a solution of guanidinium isothiocyanate and phenol. Cells are first lysed with TRIzol Reagent and chloroform is then added to the lysate resulting in the separation of the solution into an aqueous and an organic phase. RNA exists solely in the aqueous phase. Removal of the aqueous phase is then followed by the subsequent precipitation of the RNA with isopropanol. The disadvantage of using TRIzol Reagent compared to using the commercially available kits is the need for the addition of chloroform, which is potentially hazardous. In addition, TRIzol Reagent is not especially effective when working with less than 5×10^6 cells. After RNA isolation, it is recommended that RNA samples be treated with DNase 1 to remove any possible contamination with genomic DNA.

Regardless of what method is employed to isolate RNA from cells, it is desirable to measure RNA concentration using a spectrophotometer and to assess the purity of the RNA by A 260/280 ratio. Good quality RNA has an A 260/280 ratio of 1.6–1.8.

10. REVERSE TRANSCRIPTION

Total RNA is incubated with 1μL of random primers and 1μL of dNTPs (10mM) at 65°C for 5 min followed by quenching on ice for 1 min. The amount of total RNA used in the reverse transcription is variable and depends on RNA concentration. After this incubation, 6 μL of 5× FS buffer, 2 μL of 0.1M dithiothreitol, 0.5 μL (20U) of RNaseOUT (Invitrogen) and 1 μL (×U) of SuperScriptIII Reverse Transcriptase (Invitrogen) are added. The reaction volume is then made up to 30 μL with water and incubated at 50°C for 1 h for the reverse transcription to occur. This is followed by inactivation of the reverse transcriptase at 70°C for 15 min.

Reverse transcription can also be performed using the Applied Biosystems High-Capacity cDNA Archive Kit. This methodology employs a 96-well plate format and the Applied Biosystems 7500 real-time PCR machine and is carried out according to the manufacturer's instructions.

10.1 Polymerase Chain Reaction (PCR)

The polymerase chain reaction (PCR) is carried out with 1 μL of the reverse transcription reaction in a total reaction volume of 12.5 μL. The PCR reaction contains 1.25 μL of 10× PCR buffer, 0.5 μL of 50 mM $MgCl_2$, 0.25 μL of 10 mM dNTPs, 0.5 μL (1 μM) of each PCR primer, and 0.625U of Taq polymerase (Invitrogen). The reaction volume is made up to 12.5 μL with water. Samples are amplified by incubation at 94°C for 2 min followed by cycles of denaturation at 94°C for 45 s, annealing at an appropriate temperature (usually between 50 and 60°C) for 45 s and an extension temperature of 72°C for 1 min. This is then followed by a final extension at 72°C for 5 min. Amplified products of the PCR are then separated and visualized by running on a 1–2% (w/v) agarose gel stained with ethdium bromide and product sizes are elucidated by comparison with molecular weight standards.

Although PCR can yield results of the expression status of genes, it is limited by its inability to provide quantification of gene expression levels. When characterizing hESC and its differentiated derivatives, the population of cells to be analysed is often heterogeneous. As such, investigating the presence and/or absence of gene transcripts alone is not sufficient and quantitative PCR (QPCR) needs to be employed. QPCR allows either relative or absolute levels of gene expression to be quantified. It is based on the detection of a fluorescent reporter molecule that accumulates with each amplification cycle. There are two chemistries that can be utilized for detection of amplified QPCR products, SYBR Green I dye and TaqMan probes. SYBR Green I is a dye that binds double stranded DNA. As the number of double-stranded DNA molecules increases during each amplification step, there is also an increase in fluorescence levels due to the binding of SYBR Green I to more double-stranded DNA products. The fluorescence is detected by the instrument and quantified. Conversely, TaqMan probes function using a fluorescent reporter and a quencher that is attached to the 5′ and 3′ end of the probe respectively. The probe binds specifically to the DNA strand to be amplified and when the probe is intact, the proximity of the quencher to the fluorescent reporter prevents any emission of fluorescence. However, during the process of amplification, DNA polymerase cleaves the reporter from the probe. This releases the reporter from the quencher and results in fluorescence which is detected by the instrument and quantified.

There are several advantages to using the TaqMan probe-based chemistry over SYBR Green I to detect amplified QPCR products. SYBR Green I dye binds non-specifically to all double-stranded DNA. Therefore, a dissociation curve analysis needs to be performed in order to identify non-specific products. Conversely, TaqMan probes bind specifically to the DNA to be amplified and reduce the likelihood of false positives. In addition, optimized assays are often available for commercial purchase which reduces the amount of time required for optimization.

The QPCR reaction mix using the SYBR Green I dye involves the addition of 10 μL of Low Rox Mix (containing the SYBR Green I dye), 0.5 μL of each primer (1 μM) and 1 μL of cDNA template. The reaction volume is then made up to 20 μL with water. QPCR performed using the TaqMan probe chemistry requires 5 μL of 10× Universal Master Mix (Applied Biosystems), 0.5 μL of 20× OnDemand Mix (Applied Biosystems) and 0.5 μL of cDNA template to be added per reaction. Water is then added to each reaction to make up the final volume to 10 μL. Both methods of QPCR amplification and detection are performed on the Applied Biosystems 7500 real-time PCR machine using the default-cycling parameters. When analysing relative gene expression, gene expression is normalized against a housekeeping gene and plotted on a logarithmic scale with a control population of cells as the calibrator. When absolute levels of gene expression are sought, gene expression is normalized against a housekeeping gene and compared to a standard curve.

11. MICROFLUIDIC CARD AND MICROARRAY ANALYSES

Microfluidic card and microarray analyses are becoming increasingly useful in the field of hESC research. As noted above, studies involving hESC and cells derived from them often entail working with a heterogeneous population of cells. In order to gain a better understanding of the identity of these cells and their differentiation status, large-scale examination of the pattern of gene expression is often required. Both microfluidic cards and microarrays allow high-throughput gene expression studies to be carried out on hESC. Microfluidic cards such as those available from Applied Biosystems function as a low-density custom array. It allows up to 384 genes selected by the operator to be analysed and runs on the Applied Biosystems 7900HT Sequence Detection System using the TaqMan probe chemistry. There are many different commercially available microarray chips that can be purchased. Microarrays provide a larger scale, genome-wide view of gene expression in a given cell type or population and commonly used platforms are those of Affymetrix and recently Illumina. The Illumina Gene Expression system encompasses the human genome using 48,000 transcripts and provides the highest built-in feature redundancy of any array platform to date.

12. DIFFERENTIATION OF hESC

Since the initial report of the derivation of the first hESC lines (Thomson et al. 1998), there has been some progress made with regards to our ability to direct differentiation of hESC towards the ectoderm, mesoderm, and endoderm lineages. A number of protocols are now in place with which to direct the in vitro differentiation of hESC towards each of these lineages. The most rigorous technique available at present for the assessment of the ability of hESC to differentiate into each of the three germ layers is that of teratoma formation, because the capability of hESC to undergo differentiation into multiple types of mature tissue is most clearly revealed in this assay. We discuss this assay first, then some exemplary protocols for in vitro differentiation of hESC into mesodermal, endodermal, and ectodermal derivatives.

12.1 Differentiation in vivo: Teratoma Formation

The ability of hESC to form teratomas when injected into the testis of SCID mice is at present the best means of ascertaining pluripotency. The protocol below describes the inoculation of hESC beneath the testis capsules of SCID mice to allow tumours to form (approximately 6–8 weeks later). The tumours are then investigated for the presence of tissues representative of all three germ layers. Others have used implantation under the kidney capsule or into the hindlimb muscle. Advantages of the testicular assay include ease of the procedure and the ability to obtain tumours even with relatively low numbers of cells.

The operation is performed in a laminar flow cabinet using aseptic technique. Immunodeprived (e.g., NOD.CB17-*Prkdc*^{scid}/J) mice 6–8 weeks of age are anesthetized with avertin. The abdomen is opened with a short (1.2 cm) longitudinal incision around the level of the thigh. The remainder of the procedure is carried out under a dissecting microscope with overhead illumination. The testis is squeezed up into the abdominal cavity, the fat pad that surrounds the testis is located through the incision, and with traction, the testis is exteriorized. A small hole in the testis capsule, well away from blood vessels, is created using a 27 gauge syringe. Clumps of cells, or a cell suspension in a slurry, are introduced beneath the capsule of the testis through this opening using a drawn out capillary. Up to 100 μL may be introduced without causing the tubules to spill out, but should this happen, no attempt to repair the damage is necessary. The testis is returned into the abdomen and the procedure repeated on the contralateral gonad. The abdominal wall is closed with several sutures (4/0 silk) and the skin closed with a wound clip. Tumours will appear around 5 weeks after injection, and they are recognizable by palpating the testis. Sometimes large cystic lesions may form, and the testis may remain in the abdomen. The animal should be humanely killed when the tumour reaches a size that would cause pain or suffering; investigators should always follow local animal experimentation ethics committee guidelines concerning acceptable practice.

At autopsy, remove the testis carefully and include it and any unidentifiable surrounding tissue for fixation and processing. It may prove necessary to section extensively through the testis to ensure that the teratoma is located and representative sections are obtained. Hematoxylin and eosin staining will generally reveal what tissues are present, but inexperienced workers should consult with a histopathologist to assist in interpretation. No embryonal carcinoma, or other malignant elements should be present, but immature tissues are often seen. Immunohistochemical staining for ubiquitously expressed human structural proteins, such as mitochondrial or nuclear constituents, will aid in confirming the human origin of specific tissues, and staining for lineage specific or differentiation markers may aid in the identification of immature tissues.

12.2 Differentiation *in vitro* to Mesoderm: Hematopoietic Cells

Protocols to direct hESC differentiation towards mesoderm, namely blood and cardiomyocytes, have been established. Recently, Ng and colleagues (Ng et al. 2005) reported that hESC can be directed towards hematopoietic differentiation by using a method of forced aggregation of hESC . In this protocol, hESC were trypsinized into single cells and seeded into low attachment, round-bottomed 96 well plates (Nunc) containing chemically defined serum-free medium as described by Johansson and Wiles (Johansson and Wiles 1995). The chemically defined medium was also supplemented with the growth factors hMNP4, hVEGF, hSCF, HFlt3 ligand, hIL-6, and hIGF-II. Optimal blood formation was observed when 1,000 cells were seeded per well. The plates were then centrifuged at 1,500 rpm for 4 min at 4°C to allow the cells to aggregate and form embryoid bodies (EB) before incubation at 37°C, 5% CO_2 for 10–12 days. After this, the EB were transferred onto 96-well flat bottomed tissue culture plates (NUNC) that had been pre-coated with gelatin, containing the same chemically defined media supplemented with hVEGF, hSCF, hFli3 ligand, hIL-3, and Darbepoeitin, a derivative of erythropoietin. This is an improved method compared to previous reported protocols employing the use of EB as it utilizes known numbers of cells thereby resulting in the consistent yield of both EB formation and hematopoietic differentiation.

12.3 Differentiation *in vitro* to Endoderm: Hepatic and Other Cell Types

The derivation of definitive endodermal cell types from hESC has proven to be a somewhat elusive goal and is hampered by the absence of a specific single marker to distinguish definitive endoderm from extra-embryonic endoderm. Extraembryonic endoderm represents the second differentiation lineage in mammalian embryogenesis and is often an early end point of mESC and hESC differentiation in vitro. A recent publication outlines a differentiation protocol and identification strategy that appears to have overcome this issue. D'Amour et al. (D'Amour et al. 2005) used a combination of low serum and activin A to produce cells enriched for definitive endoderm. Undifferentiated hESC were maintained on mEF in DMEM/F12 supplemented with 20% knockout serum replacement (Gibco), non-essential amino acids, Glutamax, penicillin/streptomycin, 2-mercaptoethanol and 4ng/ml recombinant human FGF-2. Differentiation was carried out in RPMI supplemented with Glutamax, penicillin/streptomycin and different concentrations of fetal bovine serum. D'Amour et al. (2005) showed that by adding Activin A (100ng/ml) to hESC for 5 days in the presence of 0.5% FBS followed by FACS selection for CXCR4 resulted in the upregulation of SOX17, MIXL1, GSC, and FOXA2 gene expression by QPCR but not Oct4, SOX7, MEOX1, or ZIC1. These results were confirmed by immunostaining, flow cytometric analysis, and western blotting for a number of these markers. The conclusion that they had produced definitive endoderm is based on the presence of SOX17/FOXA2 double positive cells and the finding that the SOX17 positive population arose from a brachyury positive cell population.

12.4 Differentiation *in vitro* to Ectoderm: Neural Progenitors

There are many protocols for the induction of neural differentiation of hESC. Our laboratory reported that inhibition of endogenous BMP signalling with the antagonist noggin could induce efficient conversion of hESC into neural progenitors (Pera et al. 2004). hESC were cultured in 20% serum-containing medium on mitomycin-C-treated mEF (mEFs, seeded at $6\times10^4/cm^2$) and passaged weekly by mechanical dissociation. For neural induction, 500ng/ml recombinant noggin (R&D Systems) was added to hESC medium at the time of colony transfer onto mEFs (day 0) and cells were cultured for 14 days without passage; noggin-medium was replaced every other day (adapted from methods previously described, (Pera et al. 2004)). After noggin treatment, colonies were cut into small pieces using a 27 gauge needle and pieces transferred to individual wells in a non-adherent 96-well plate to allow neurosphere formation. Neurospheres were cultured in suspension in neural basal medium (NBM) with supplements, as described by Reubinoff and colleagues (Reubinoff et al. 2001), for 1–2 weeks. Subsequent differentiation was carried out by plating the spheres onto laminin or fibronectin for adherent culture under conditions previously described for neural or glial differentiation respectively (Reubinoff et al. 2001).

13. CONCLUSIONS

Research with hESC is still at an early developmental stage, and improvements to culture systems and differentiation protocols are reported on a regular basis in the literature. It is essential to carry out basic characterization protocols on a regular basis during stem cell maintenance, and particularly during adoption of new methodologies for stem cell culture, to ensure that the cells under study represent diploid pluripotent stem cell populations.

REFERENCES

Andrews, P.W., Banting, G., Damjanov, I., Arnaud, D., and Avner, P. (1984) Three monoclonal antibodies defining distinct differentiation antigens associated with different high molecular weight polypeptides on the surface of human embryonal carcinoma cells. Hybridoma, 3: 347–361.

Cooper, S., Bennett, W., Andrade, J., Reubinoff, B.E., Thomson, J., and Pera, M.F. (2002) Biochemical properties of a keratan sulphate/chondroitin sulphate proteoglycan expressed in primate pluripotent stem cells. J. Anat., 200: 259–265.

Cowan, C.A., Klimanskaya, I., McMahon, J., Atienza, J., Witmyer, J., Zucker, J.P., Wang, S., Morton, C.C., McMahon, A.P., Powers, D., and Melton, D.A. (2004) Derivation of embryonic stem-cell lines from human blastocysts. N. Engl. J. Med., 350: 1353–1356.

D'Amour, K.A., Agulnick, A.D., Eliazer, S., Kelly, O.G., Kroon, E., and Baetge, E.E. (2005) Efficient differentiation of human embryonic stem cells to definitive endoderm. Nat. Biotechnol., 23: 1534–1541.

Draper, J.S., Smith, K., Gokhale, P., Moore, H.D., Maltby, E., Johnson, J., Meisner, L., Zwaka, T.P., Thomson, J.A., and Andrews, P.W. (2004) Recurrent gain of chromosomes 17q and 12 in cultured human embryonic stem cells. Nat. Biotechnol., 22: 53–54.

Enver, T., Soneji, S., Joshi, C., Brown, J., Iborra, F., Orntoft, T., Thykjaer, T., Maltby, E., Smith, K., Dawud, R.A., et al. (2005) Cellular differentiation hierarchies in normal and culture-adapted human embryonic stem cells. Hum. Mol. Genet., 14: 3129–3140.

Herszfeld, D., Wolvetang, E., Langton-Bunker, E., Chung, T.L., Filipczyk, A.A., Houssami, S., Jamshidi, P., Koh, K., Laslett, A.L., Michalska, A., et al. (2006) CD30 is a survival factor and a biomarker for transformed human pluripotent stem cells. Nat. Biotechnol., 24: 351–357.

Hyslop, L., Stojkovic, M., Armstrong, L., Walter, T., Stojkovic, P., Przyborski, S., Herbert, M., Murdoch, A., Strachan, T., and Lako, M. (2005) Downregulation of NANOG induces differentiation of human embryonic stem cells to extraembryonic lineages. Stem Cells, 23: 1035–1043.

Johansson, B.M. and Wiles, M.V. (1995) Evidence for involvement of activin A and bone morphogenetic protein 4 in mammalian mesoderm and hematopoietic development. Mol. Cell. Biol., 15: 141–151.

Kannagi, R., Cochran, N.A., Ishigami, F., Hakomori, S., Andrews, P.W., Knowles, B.B., and Solter, D. (1983) Stage-specific embryonic antigens (SSEA-3 and -4) are epitopes of a unique globo-series ganglioside isolated from human teratocarcinoma cells. EMBO J., 2: 2355–2361.

Kannagi, R., Levery, S.B., Ishigami, F., Hakomori, S., Shevinsky, L.H., Knowles, B.B., and Solter, D. (1983) New globoseries glycosphingolipids in human teratocarcinoma reactive with the monoclonal antibody directed to a developmentally regulated antigen, stage-specific embryonic antigen 3. J. Biol. Chem., 258: 8934–8942.

Kerjaschki, D., Poczewski, H., Dekan, G., Horvat, R., Balzar, E., Kraft, N., and Atkins, R.C. (1986) Identification of a major sialoprotein in the glycocalyx of human visceral glomerular epithelial cells. J. Clin. Invest., 78: 1142–1149.

Laslett, A.L., Filipczyk, A.A., and Pera, M.F. (2003) Characterization and culture of human embryonic stem cells. Trends Cardiovasc. Med., 13: 295–301.

Laslett, A.L., Grimmond, S., Gardiner, B., Stamp, L., Lin, A., Hawes, S.M., Wormald, S., Nikolic-Paterson, D., Haylock, D., and Pera, M.F. (2007) Transcriptional analysis of early lineage commitment in human embryonic stem cells. BMC Dev. Biol., 7: 12.

Lower, R., Lower, J., and Kurth, R. (1996) The viruses in all of us: characteristics and biological significance of human endogenous retrovirus sequences. Proc. Natl. Acad. Sci. USA, 93: 5177–5184.

Ng, E.S., Davis, R.P., Azzola, L., Stanley, E.G., and Elefanty, A.G. (2005) Forced aggregation of defined numbers of human embryonic stem cells into embryoid bodies fosters robust, reproducible hematopoietic differentiation. Blood, 106: 1601–1603.

Oka, M., Tagoku, K., Russell, T.L., Nakano, Y., Hamazaki, T., Meyer, E.M., Yokota, T., and Terada, N. (2002) CD9 is associated with leukemia inhibitory factor-mediated maintenance of embryonic stem cells. Mol. Biol. Cell, 13: 1274–1281.

Pera, M.F., Andrade, J., Houssami, S., Reubinoff, B., Trounson, A., Stanley, E.G., Ward-van Oostwaard, D., and Mummery, C. (2004) Regulation of human embryonic stem cell differentiation by BMP-2 and its antagonist noggin. J. Cell Sci., 117: 1269–1280.
Pera, M.F., Blasco-Lafita, M.J., Cooper, S., Mason, M., Mills, J., and Monaghan, P. (1988) Analysis of cell-differentiation lineage in human teratomas using new monoclonal antibodies to cytostructural antigens of embryonal carcinoma cells. Differentiation, 39: 139–149.
Pera, M.F., Cooper, S., Mills, J., and Parrington, J.M. (1989) Isolation and characterization of a multipotent clone of human embryonal carcinoma cells. Differentiation, 42: 10–23.
Pera, M.F., Filipczyk, A.A., Hawes, S.M., and Laslett, A.L. (2003) Isolation, characterization, and differentiation of human embryonic stem cells. Meth. Enzymol., 365: 429–446.
Pinkel, D. and Albertson, D.G. (2005) Comparative genomic hybridization. Annu. Rev. Genomics Hum. Genet., 6: 331–354.
Reubinoff, B.E., Itsykson, P., Turetsky, T., Pera, M.F., Reinhartz, E., Itzik, A., and Ben-Hur, T. (2001) Neural progenitors from human embryonic stem cells. Nat. Biotechnol., 19: 1134–1140.
Son, Y.S., Park, J.H., Kang, Y.K., Park, J.S., Choi, H.S., Lim, J.Y., Lee, J.E., Lee, J.B., Ko, M.S., Kim, Y.S., et al. (2005) Heat shock 70-kDa protein 8 isoform 1 is expressed on the surface of human embryonic stem cells and downregulated upon differentiation. Stem Cells, 23: 1502–1513.
Thomson, J.A., Itskovitz-Eldor, J., Shapiro, S.S., Waknitz, M.A., Swiergiel, J.J., Marshall, V.S., and Jones, J.M. (1998) Embryonic stem cell lines derived from human blastocysts. Science, 282: 1145–1147.

CHAPTER 4

GENETIC MODIFICATION OF HUMAN EMBRYONIC STEM CELLS

THOMAS P. ZWAKA

Baylor College of Medicine, Center for Cell and Gene Therapy and Department of Molecular and Cellular Biology, Houston, Texas, USA

1. INTRODUCTION

Embryonic stem (ES) cells are derived from an early embryonic stage during which the cellular machinery is geared toward rapid expansion and diversification, simultaneously possess both the ability for unlimited self-renewal and the potential to differentiate into derivatives of all three germ layers (Pedersen 1986). Even after months and years of growth in the laboratory, ES cells retain the ability to form varied cell types, including muscle cells, heart cells, neurons, and hematopoietic cells (Thomson et al. 1998; Amit et al. 2000; Odorico et al. 2001).

The initial isolation of murine ES cells over 25 years ago (Evans and Kaufman 1981; Martin 1981) paved the way for subsequent isolation of primate ES cells (Thomson et al. 1995, 1996), and finally that of human ES cells in 1998 (Thomson et al. 1998). Much of the anticipated potential surrounding human ES cells was extrapolated from pioneer experiments in the mouse system. However, recent results in human ES cells have supported the notion that human ES cells will have an important impact on medical science. These advances include (a) the differentiation of human ES cells into various cells types, comprising neurons, cardiac cells, vascular cells, hematopoietic cells, pancreatic cells, hepatic cells, and placental cells (reviewed in Keller 2005); (b) the derivation of new ES cell lines under various conditions (Cowan et al. 2004; Ludwig et al. 2006); and (c) the establishment of protocols that allow genetic modification of these cells (Eiges et al. 2001; Zwaka and Thomson 2003; Urbach et al. 2004).

Genetic manipulation is an essential tool and was a key to the success of mouse ES cell research. Many of the mouse-based techniques have proven amenable to translation to human ES cell systems, with varied levels of success. Here, we provide an overview of the recent strategies and successes in the genetic manipulation of human ES cells.

J.R. Masters et al (eds.), Embryonic Stem Cells, 41–52.

2. EXOGENOUS GENE EXPRESSION IN HUMAN ES CELLS

Genes have been introduced into human ES cells by both transfection and infection techniques. Transient transfection, the simplest method for introducing new genes into various cell types, may be achieved using liposomes and other cationic/lipid-based particles, brief electric shocks (electroporation), or other strategies. However, the expression of transiently transfected DNA tends to be poorly controlled and the DNA tends to disappear within days or weeks, or in rare cases may integrate randomly into the host DNA. Thus, researchers have also used in vitro drug selection strategies to isolate and expand stably transfected ES cells expressing the newly introduced gene. The virus most frequently used in human ES cells is lentivirus.

3. TRANSIENT TRANSFECTION

Biotech companies have developed a huge arsenal of transfection tools that allow the introduction of circular plasmids into virtually any cell type, including human ES cells. The first study describing the introduction of plasmid DNA into human ES cells compared the use of three commercially available transfection reagents, Lipofectamine, Fugene-6, and ExGen 500 (Eiges et al. 2001). Lipofectamine was found to be ineffective for transfecting human ES cells, whereas ExGen 500 was the most effective among the three tested reagents. Subsequently, other companies tested their transfection reagents in mouse and human ES cells and have shown that many of the new transfection reagents, such as Lipofectamine 2000, can be used to successfully transfect human ES cells with efficiencies of 10–50% (Vallier et al. 2004 and unpublished observation).

Typically, when DNA is introduced by transient transfection, it is transferred in the form of a circular plasmid (Weintraub et al. 1986). Under these conditions transcription is initiated within a few hours after transfection and maximal transgenic protein expression is observed within 1–3 days. The number of plasmids taken up by each cell may vary from a single plasmid to hundreds or more. Consequently, expression levels may vary dramatically among individual cells, complicating the interpretation of some transient overexpression experiments. Expression levels may also vary based on the utilized promoter contained within the transgene-encoding plasmid. Most promoter sequences that were previously used in mouse ES cells have proven useful to some degree in human ES cells. The widely used cytomegalovirus (CMV) promoter, which is present in most eukaryotic expression vectors, is relatively silent in human ES cells and generates only minimal expression (Ma et al. 2003). However, although the EF1α promoter has proven sufficient to drive transgene expression in human ES cells, this promoter may exhibit silencing effects due to an intrinsic CpG island.

4. STABLE TRANSFECTION

Stably transfected cells are generally obtained through transient transfection of cells with plasmids harboring an antibiotic resistance gene in addition to the target transgene. The transfected cells are then subjected to antibiotic selection beginning with 1–2 days of transfection and continuing for 2–3 weeks, yielding resistant, stably transfected clones. A standard protocol for chemical transfection of human ES cells is described as follows. Human ES cells can be trypsinized and plated on Matrigel and cultured with fibroblast-conditioned medium. Typically 2 days later the cells are transfected using one of the chemical transfection reagents, according to the provided protocols. Briefly, the vector is co-incubated with the DNA and added to each well. In experiments using ExGen 500, the 6-well plates must be gently centrifuged after addition of the DNA/ExGen mixture (300 g for 5 min). The media must be changed 4 h posttransfection and antibiotic selection (G418; dosage determined based on a previously generated dose-response killing curve) is initiated 2 days posttransfection. Chemical methods such as these yield a stable (drug-selectable) transfection rate of ~5–10% for human ES cells (Eiges et al. 2001), which is higher than that obtained by electroporation (Lakshmipathy et al. 2004).

5. VIRUS-MEDIATED TRANSDUCTION

Exogenous gene expression may also be induced by infection with viral vectors containing the target DNA (Robertson et al. 1986). Engineered viruses can be used to introduce almost any genetic information into cells. Some viruses (e.g., retroviruses) can only effectively infect dividing cells, whereas others (e.g., lentiviruses) do not require active division. In most cases, the genomic information carried by the virus is stably integrated in the host cell genome. If such integration is random, the system may suffer from mutations leading to malignant transformation and/or serious gene dysfunction. However, random integration has the benefit of often integrating multiple copies of the target gene, allowing increased expression and/or avoidance of positional effects (decreased expression due to integration into a transcriptionally inactive area of the genome) and gene silencing (decreased expression due to progressive inactivation of an exogenous gene by the host cell). Gene silencing and positional effects often impact exogenous gene expression in stem cell systems, since the gene activity is subject to multiple changes during differentiation of these cells. Thus, researchers have optimized existing viral vector systems for use in human ES cells by a variety of methods, such as the introduction of additional genomic control and insulator regions, yielding more robust, consistent transgene expression in these cells (Gropp et al. 2003; Ma et al. 2003; Zaehres et al. 2005).

6. EPISOMAL PLASMID STABILIZATION

In some gene transfer systems (chemical transfection or viral) the foreign transgene does not integrate at a high rate, instead remaining outside of the host genomic DNA as an episome (Aubert et al. 2002). Researchers have identified proteins capable of stabilizing these episomal DNA fragments, and some viruses (e.g., adenovirus) have been found to persist in the cell as stable episomes for some time. Recently, episomal systems have been applied to various stem cells (Aubert et al. 2002). The major disadvantage is the necessity of introducing the DNA plasmid stabilization sequence into the plasmids and the viral protein into the cells.

7. TARGETED GENETIC MODIFICATION VIA HOMOLOGOUS RECOMBINATION

Historically, researchers have either analyzed naturally occurring mutants, or applied random mutagenesis strategies and studied the resulting phenotypes. However, although these experiments have yielded many interesting insights over the years, their outcomes vary widely and generally defy prediction. In the modern laboratory setting, it is more desirable to create specific and controlled genetic modifications.

In recent years, homologous recombination has been used to alter genomes in living cells (Smithies et al. 1985; Thomas et al. 1986; Thomas and Capecchi 1987). Briefly, DNA homologous to the target sequence in the host cell is altered in vitro and introduced into the cell by transfection or infection techniques. The altered fragment recombines with the homologous genomic sequence, replacing the normal genomic DNA with recombinant DNA carrying the genetic modification(s). As homologous recombination is a very rare event in cells, a powerful selection strategy is necessary to select properly recombinant cells (Mansour et al. 1988; Stacey et al. 1994). Thus, the introduced gene construct usually encodes an antibiotic resistance gene, along with the thymidine kinase (TK) gene from the herpes simplex virus. Antibiotic resistance is used to identify cells that have incorporated the recombinant DNA. In contrast, the absence of TK expression (detected by gancyclovir sensitivity) is used to identify homologous recombination events, as this gene is spliced out of the expression construct during homologous recombination. This strategy, called gene targeting, has been used extensively in mouse ES cells to investigate gene function and create mouse models of human diseases (Doetschman et al. 1987; Smithies 1993).

There are two main types of gene-targeting vectors, the insertion vector and the replacement vector (Deng et al. 1993; Bronson and Smithies 1994). Insertion gene-targeting vectors mediate a single homologous recombination event with a circular DNA vector, leading to duplication of the homologous region. The replacement strategy, which is more commonly used for gene disruption (knockout) or introduction of new genes (knock-in), involves the use of vectors containing two homologous regions separated by marker genes, leading to a one-for-one exchange of genetic material. Gene-targeting experiments were originally complicated by the issues discussed above, namely the low frequency of homologous recombination events (Vasquez et al. 2001) and the inefficiency of DNA delivery into cells (Nairn et al. 1993; Yanez and Porter 1999). However, homologous recombination was undertaken in mouse ES cells over 20 years ago and has proven useful for investigating gene function and creating mouse models of human diseases (Thomas et al. 1986; Doetschman et al. 1987; Thomas and Capecchi 1987; Smithies 1993). However, differences between mouse and human ES cells initially limited the application of homologous recombination techniques in human ES cells. Specifically, the electroporation protocols widely used for transfection of mouse ES cells were relatively ineffective in human ES cells, and researchers found it difficult to achieve high stable transfection efficiencies in human ES cells (Zwaka and Thomas 2003). In addition, whereas mouse ES cells may be easily cloned from single cells, human ES cells cannot, making it difficult to screen the cells for rare homologous recombination events (Amit et al. 2000). However, researchers have recently reported successful gene targeting in human ES cells, using newly optimized vectors and transfection protocols (Zwaka and Thomas 2003; Urbach et al. 2004).

8. OPTIMIZING ELECTROPORATION FOR HUMAN ES CELLS

Many parameters influence the transfection rate obtained by electroporation (Potter et al. 1984; Baum et al. 1994), and must be optimized for each individual cell line; this is particularly important in the highly sensitive human ES cells (Amit et al. 2000). Human and mouse ES cells differ in terms of multiple parameters (i.e., diameter, protein content, etc.) with the result that typical mouse ES cell transfection protocols yield very low transfection rates in human ES cells ($\sim 10^{-7}$), making recovery of homologous recombinant clones almost impossible (Fehling et al. 1994).

In recent years, however, electroporation protocols have been successfully adapted to the special needs of human ES cells (Zwaka and Thomas 2003). For example, studies have shown that removal of human ES cells as intact small clumps (~100–500 cells) instead of trypsinization, along with high-density plating after electroporation, allow a higher frequency of cell survival. In addition, the use of medium instead of phosphate buffer saline (PBS) as an electroporation buffer has also increased the human ES cell survival rate. These changes, along with alterations in the physical parameters of the electric fields and the use of room temperature electroporation, have combined to yield stable human ES cell transfection rates up to 100-fold higher than those obtained using the standard mouse ES cell electroporation procedures.

9. GENE-TARGETED ABLATION OF HPRT1 IN HUMAN ES CELLS ("KNOCKOUT")

The first gene ablated (or "knockedout") by gene targeting in both mouse and human ES cells was the gene encoding HPRT1, located on the X chromosome. Due to its location, a single homologous recombination event was able to induce a complete loss of function in XY cells, making this gene an ideal target for initial homologous recombination experiments in ES cells (Doetschman et al. 1987; Kuehn et al. 1987; Thomas and Capecchi 1987). In addition, the HPRT1-deficient cells could be selected based on their resistance to 6-Thioguanine, 2-amino-6-Mercaptopurine (6-TG), allowing easy estimation of the frequency of homologous recombination (Albertini 2001). In one instance the optimized gene-targeting vector for the human HPRT1 gene was constructed by substitution of the last three exons (exons 7–9) with a neoresistance cassette under control of the TK promoter (Zwaka and Thomas 2003). Numerous studies have shown that the length of the homologous region is a critical factor for determining the effectiveness of homologous recombination (Thomas and Capecchi 1987; Hasty et al. 1991; Thomas et al. 1992). Targeting was found to require at least 500 bp of sequence, and targeting efficiency increased exponentially as the homologous sequence increased from 2 to 10 kb, although further increases were less dramatic with regions longer than 14 kb (Deng and Capecchi 1992). In one particular report targeting the HPRT locus in human ES cells was accomplished with 10 and 1.9 kb homologous arms in the 5′ and 3′ directions, respectively. At the end of the 3′ homologous arm the TK gene was added for negative selection (Mansour et al. 1988). Previous studies have described problems with nonisogenic genomic DNA in mouse experiments (Deng and Capecchi 1992). The requirement for isogenic DNA in ES cell gene targeting has been disputed, although homologous DNA isogenic to the utilized human ES cell line was used in the initial report. This DNA was obtained by long-distance, high-fidelity genomic protein/creatinine ratio (PCR) and subcloned into a PCR cloning vector.

Gene targeting should be possible with vectors using the stable transfection protocols as discussed above. In our laboratory, for example, human ES cells are treated with collagenase to generate clumps, and then washed with culture media and resuspended. A small amount of PBS containing linearized targeting vector DNA is added, and cells are electroporated at room temperature. Following electroporation, the cells are incubated for 10 min at room temperature, and then plated at high density on Matrigel (Xu et al. 2001). After 2 days, G418 selection is applied. Notably, it is vital to generate an appropriate drug selection killing curve, since even different passage numbers of the same human ES cell line show remarkable differences in their resistances to G418 (ranging from 12.5 to 200 μg/ml). After 1 week of culture in the presence of the initial dose of G418, the concentration can be doubled and 6-TG selection is initiated. After 3 weeks the surviving colonies are picked, transferred to 48-well plates as cell clusters and analyzed individually by PCR using primers specific for the selection cassette and gene sequences just upstream of the 5′ homologous region. PCR-positive clones are then rescreened by Southern blot analysis using appropriate cutter-digested DNA and a probe 3′ of the neo cassette.

10. INTRODUCTION OF NEW DNA BY HOMOLOGOUS RECOMBINATION ("KNOCK-IN")

Homologous recombination may also be used to add, or "knock-in" an exogenous gene. This technique may be used, for example, to monitor gene expression patterns of a cell type-specific gene through expression of a reporter gene (e.g., enhanced green fluorescence protein (EGFP)). In human ES cells, knock-in technology has been used to generate cell lines with a selectable marker introduced into a locus with a tissue-specific expression pattern, allowing purification of ES cell-derived cells from a mixed population (Mountford et al. 1994; Wernig et al. 2002; Xian et al. 2003; Ying et al. 2003). Representative examples of this approach include introducing a reporter gene into the human Oct4 or tyrosine hydroxylase (TH) genes via homologous recombination, as described below.

11. Oct4 EGFP/NEO KNOCK-IN

Oct4 belongs to the POU (Pit, Oct, Unc) transcription factor family. It is expressed exclusively in the pluripotent cells of the embryo, where it acts as a central regulator of pluripotency (Nichols et al. 1998; Niwa et al. 1998). In our laboratory, we introduced two promoterless reporter/selection cassettes into the 3′ untranslated region (UTR) of the human Oct4 gene (Takeda et al. 1992). The first cassette contained the internal ribosomal entry site (IRES) sequence of the encephalomyocarditis virus (Jang and Wimmer 1990) and a gene encoding the EGFP (Zhang et al. 1996). The second cassette included the same IRES sequence and a gene encoding neomycin resistance (neo). These cassettes were flanked by two homologous arms in the 5′ and 3′ directions, respectively (Zwaka and Thomas 2003). Human ES cells were electroporated with the linearized targeting vector to generate G418-resistant clones. PCR and Southern blotting demonstrated homologous recombination. Similar transfection experiments using FuGene-6 with the same Oct4 gene-targeting vector yielded G418-resistant clones, but none of these resulted from homologous recombination. The resulting genetically modified human ES cells showed EGFP expression that could be turned off by various stimuli, allowing assessment of Oct4 downregulation. In addition, these undifferentiated ES cells could be purified from a mixed, partially differentiated cell population using either drug selection or flow cytometry for EGFP expression. These knock-in cells are useful for studying Oct4 gene expression during differentiation in vitro, and for optimizing human ES cell culture conditions. However, other experiments require knock-in of genes not normally expressed in ES cells.

12. TH EGFP KNOCK-IN

TH, the rate-limiting enzyme of dopamine synthesis, is one of the most common markers used for dopaminergic neurons (Haavik and Toska 1998). In order to achieve bicistronic expression of both TH and EGFP in neuronal cells derived from ES cells we designed a targeting vector that introduced an IRES–EGFP reporter gene cassette into the 3′ UTR region in the last exon of the TH gene. The cassette is flanked by a short homologous arm 5′ of this exon and a long homologous arm in the 3′ region of the last exon. The long arm follows the TK gene, allowing for negative selection of randomly integrated, stably transfected clones. Between the long homologous arm and the IRES–EGFP cassette, a phosphoglycerine kinase (PGK)-driven neo resistance cassette was embedded between two loxP sites. Human ES cells were transfected with this vector, yielding five PCR-confirmed homologous recombinant clones after double selection with G418 and gancyclovir. In these clones, the positive selection marker (a neo cassette under the control of the PGK promoter) was still present. As this could alter the expression level of the TH gene itself or the IRES–EGFP reporter gene, two of the TH–EGFP knock-in cell lines were transfected with a plasmid containing the phage Cre recombinase under the control of the EF1α promoter, along with an IRES–EGFP cassette for identification of Cre-expressing cells. EGFP-positive cells were purified by fluorescence activated cell sorting (FACS) and analyzed for successful recombination of the two loxP sites, which led to excision of the neo cassette.

13. GENE SILENCING BY RNAi ("KNOCKDOWN")

In addition to gene targeting, endogenous gene expression may be silenced to a greater or lesser degree through the use of RNA interference, which acts post-transcriptionally. As double-stranded RNA is targeted for specific mRNA degradation, introduction of short complementary RNA-interfering (RNAi) molecules or their encoding vectors via transient or stable transfection can lead to targeted gene silencing (Fire et al. 1998; Billy et al. 2001; Elbashir et al. 2001). The underlying mechanisms that cause gene silencing by RNAi are specific to a particular target gene and may cause unwanted cellular side effects, such as differentiation or cell death. However, RNAi has been successfully used in mouse and human ES cells to knockdown expression of Oct4 (Vallier et al. 2004; Zaehres et al. 2005).

14. CONCLUSIONS AND PERSPECTIVES

Genetic modification of human ES cells is vital to the study of gene function in vitro, and will be particularly important in cases where the human and mouse genes show clinically significant differences and/or diseases in which mouse models have proven inadequate. For example, although mutations in the gene encoding

HPRT have been associated with Lesch–Nyhan syndrome in humans, HPRT-deficient mice fail to demonstrate Lesch–Nyhan like phenotypes (Finger et al. 1988). Thus, in vitro neural differentiation of human HPRT-defective ES cells or transplantation of human HPRT-defective ES cell-derived neural tissue into animal models could provide new insights into the pathogenesis of Lesch–Nyhan syndrome. Another example could be found in human ES cell-derived cardiomyocytes bearing mutations or polymorphisms in specific ion channels. Such genetic changes may confer increased risks for severe arrhythmia and/or sudden death in humans, but mice generated from correspondingly mutated ES cells often have normal hearts (London 2001). Thus, homologous recombination in human ES cells is a vital next step for developing workable models of certain pathologies showing species-specific differences between humans and mice.

Genetic manipulation of human ES cells may also have important therapeutic applications. For example, introduction of reporter genes could be useful for purifying specific ES cell-derived differentiated cell types from a mixed population (Odorico et al. 2001). It is also possible that future work will enable researchers to alter the antigenicity of human ES cells through homologous recombination or other genetic alterations. Studies have shown already that human ES cells may be given new properties, such as viral resistance or directed differentiation into a particular lineage.

Although we appear to be poised on the brink of major advancements in stem cell research, major problems remain to be overcome. For example, the more specific and extensive the required genetic modifications are, the longer the ES cells have to remain in vitro. Although most ES cells remain remarkably stable in culture, they progressively accumulate harmful genetic and epigenetic changes. Sporadic chromosomal abnormalities have been reported in human ES cell culture (Buzzard et al. 2004; Cowan et al. 2004; Draper et al. 2004; Mitalipova et al. 2005), suggesting that it will be necessary to further optimize the culture conditions, explore new human ES cell lines, and monitor existing cell lines for instability (Ludwig et al. 2006). Introduction of a genetically abnormal stem cell into a patient could cause great harm. Similarly, harm could be caused by the introduction of incompletely differentiated ES cells that have the potential to form teratomas. Protocols are currently being developed to ensure the complete depletion of undifferentiated ES cells prior to use. It is clear that further research is essential to determine the full potential of genetic modifications in ES cells and ensure safe use.

REFERENCES

Albertini, R.J. (2001) HPRT mutations in humans: biomarkers for mechanistic studies. Mutat. Res., 489: 1–16.

Amit, M., Carpenter, M.K., Inokuma, M.S., Chiu, C.P., Harris, C.P., Waknitz, M.A., Itskovitz-Eldor, J., and Thomson, J.A. (2000) Clonally derived human embryonic stem cell lines maintain pluripotency and proliferative potential for prolonged periods of culture. Dev. Biol., 227: 271–278.

Aubert, J., Dunstan, H., Chambers, I., and Smith, A. (2002) Functional gene screening in embryonic stem cells implicates Wnt antagonism in neural differentiation. Nat. Biotechnol., 20: 1240–1245.

Baum, C., Forster, P., Hegewisch-Becker, S., and Harbers, K. (1994) An optimized electroporation protocol applicable to a wide range of cell lines. Biotechniques, 17: 1058–1062.

Billy, E., Brondani, V., Zhang, H., Muller, U., and Filipowicz, W. (2001) Specific interference with gene expression induced by long, double-stranded RNA in mouse embryonal teratocarcinoma cell lines. Proc. Natl. Acad. Sci. USA, 98: 14428–14433.

Bronson, S.K. and Smithies, O. (1994) Altering mice by homologous recombination using embryonic stem cells. J. Biol. Chem., 269: 27155–27158.

Buzzard, J.J., Gough, N.M., Crook, J.M., and Colman, A. (2004) Karyotype of human ES cells during extended culture. Nat. Biotechnol., 22: 381–382; author reply 382.

Cowan, C.A., Klimanskaya, I., McMahon, J., Atienza, J., Witmyer, J., Zucker, J.P., Wang, S., Morton, C.C., McMahon, A.P., Powers, D., et al. (2004) Derivation of embryonic stem-cell lines from human blastocysts. N. Engl. J. Med., 350: 1353–1356.

Deng, C. and Capecchi, M.R. (1992) Reexamination of gene targeting frequency as a function of the extent of homology between the targeting vector and the target locus. Mol. Cell Biol., 12: 3365–3371.

Deng, C., Thomas, K.R., and Capecchi, M.R. (1993) Location of crossovers during gene targeting with insertion and replacement vectors. Mol. Cell Biol., 13: 2134–2140.

Doetschman, T., Gregg, R.G., Maeda, N., Hooper, M.L., Melton, D.W., Thompson, S., and Smithies, O. (1987) Targeted correction of a mutant HPRT gene in mouse embryonic stem cells. Nature, 330: 576–578.

Draper, J.S., Smith, K., Gokhale, P., Moore, H.D., Maltby, E., Johnson, J., Meisner, L., Zwaka, T.P., Thomson, J.A., and Andrews, P.W. (2004) Recurrent gain of chromosomes 17q and 12 in cultured human embryonic stem cells. Nat. Biotechnol., 22: 53–54.

Eiges, R., Schuldiner, M., Drukker, M., Yanuka, O., Itskovitz-Eldor, J., and Benvenisty, N. (2001) Establishment of human embryonic stem cell-transfected clones carrying a marker for undifferentiated cells. Curr. Biol., 11: 514–518.

Elbashir, S.M., Harborth, J., Lendeckel, W., Yalcin, A., Weber, K., and Tuschl, T. (2001) Duplexes of 21-nucleotide RNAs mediate RNA interference in cultured mammalian cells. Nature, 411: 494–498.

Evans, M.J. and Kaufman, M.H. (1981) Establishment in culture of pluripotential cells from mouse embryos. Nature, 292: 154–156.

Fehling, H.J., Swat, W., Laplace, C., Kuhn, R., Rajewsky, K., Muller, U., and von Boehmer, H. (1994) MHC class I expression in mice lacking the proteasome subunit LMP-7. Science, 265: 1234–1237.

Finger, S., Heavens, R.P., Sirinathsinghji, D.J., Kuehn, M.R., and Dunnett, S.B. (1988) Behavioral and neurochemical evaluation of a transgenic mouse model of Lesch–Nyhan syndrome. J. Neurol. Sci., 86: 203–213.

Fire, A., Xu, S., Montgomery, M.K., Kostas, S.A., Driver, S.E., and Mello, C.C. (1998) Potent and specific genetic interference by double-stranded RNA in *Caenorhabditis elegans*. Nature, 391: 806–811.

Gropp, M., Itsykson, P., Singer, O., Ben-Hur, T., Reinhartz, E., Galun, E., and Reubinoff, B.E. (2003) Stable genetic modification of human embryonic stem cells by lentiviral vectors. Mol. Ther., 7: 281–287.

Haavik, J. and Toska, K. (1998) Tyrosine hydroxylase and Parkinson's disease. Mol. Neurobiol., 16: 285–309.

Hasty, P., Rivera-Perez, J., and Bradley, A. (1991) The length of homology required for gene targeting in embryonic stem cells. Mol. Cell Biol., 11: 5586–5591.

Jang, S.K. and Wimmer, E. (1990) Cap-independent translation of encephalomyocarditis virus RNA: structural elements of the internal ribosomal entry site and involvement of a cellular 57-kD RNA-binding protein. Genes Dev., 4: 1560–1572.

Keller, G. (2005) Embryonic stem cell differentiation: emergence of a new era in biology and medicine. Genes Dev., 19: 1129–1155.

Kuehn, M.R., Bradley, A., Robertson, E.J., and Evans, M.J. (1987) A potential animal model for Lesch–Nyhan syndrome through introduction of HPRT mutations into mice. Nature, 326: 295–298.

Lakshmipathy, U., Pelacho, B., Sudo, K., Linehan, J.L., Coucouvanis, E., Kaufman, D.S., and Verfaillie, C.M. (2004) Efficient transfection of embryonic and adult stem cells. Stem Cells, 22: 531–543.

London, B. (2001) Cardiac arrhythmias: from (transgenic) mice to men. J. Cardiovasc. Electrophysiol., 12: 1089–1091.

Ludwig, T.E., Levenstein, M.E., Jones, J.M., Berggren, W.T., Mitchen, E.R., Frane, J.L., Crandall, L.J., Daigh, C.A., Conard, K.R., Piekarczyk, M.S., et al. (2006) Derivation of human embryonic stem cells in defined conditions. Nat. Biotechnol., 24: 185–187.

Ma, Y., Ramezani, A., Lewis, R., Hawley, R.G., and Thomson, J.A. (2003) High-level sustained transgene expression in human embryonic stem cells using lentiviral vectors. Stem Cells, 21: 111–117.

Mansour, S.L., Thomas, K.R., and Capecchi, M.R. (1988) Disruption of the proto-oncogene int-2 in mouse embryo-derived stem cells: a general strategy for targeting mutations to non-selectable genes. Nature, 336: 348–352.

Martin, G.R. (1981) Isolation of a pluripotent cell line from early mouse embryos cultured in medium conditioned by teratocarcinoma stem cells. Proc. Natl. Acad. Sci. USA, 78: 7634–7638.

Mitalipova, M.M., Rao, R.R., Hoyer, D.M., Johnson, J.A., Meisner, L.F., Jones, K.L., Dalton, S., and Stice, S.L. (2005) Preserving the genetic integrity of human embryonic stem cells. Nat. Biotechnol., 23: 19–20.

Mountford, P., Zevnik, B., Duwel, A., Nichols, J., Li, M., Dani, C., Robertson, M., Chambers, I., and Smith, A. (1994) Dicistronic targeting constructs: reporters and modifiers of mammalian gene expression. Proc. Natl. Acad. Sci. USA, 91: 4303–4307.

Nairn, R.S., Adair, G.M., Porter, T., Pennington, S.L., Smith, D.G., Wilson, J.H., and Seidman, M.M. (1993) Targeting vector configuration and method of gene transfer influence targeted correction of the APRT gene in Chinese hamster ovary cells. Somat. Cell Mol. Genet., 19: 363–375.

Nichols, J., Zevnik, B., Anastassiadis, K., Niwa, H., Klewe-Nebenius, D., Chambers, I., Scholer, H., and Smith, A. (1998) Formation of pluripotent stem cells in the mammalian embryo depends on the POU transcription factor Oct4. Cell, 95: 379–391.

Niwa, H., Burdon, T., Chambers, I., and Smith, A. (1998) Self-renewal of pluripotent embryonic stem cells is mediated via activation of STAT3. Genes Dev., 12: 2048–2060.

Odorico, J.S., Kaufman, D.S., and Thomson, J.A. (2001) Multilineage differentiation from human embryonic stem cell lines. Stem Cells, 19: 193–204.

Pedersen, R.A. (1986) Potency, lineage and allocation in preimplantation mouse embryos. In: Experimental Approaches to Mammalian Embryonic Development (Ed.: Rossant, J. and Pedersen, R.A.), Cambridge University Press, New York, pp. 3–33.

Potter, H., Weir, L., and Leder, P. (1984) Enhancer-dependent expression of human kappa immunoglobulin genes introduced into mouse pre-B lymphocytes by electroporation. Proc. Natl. Acad. Sci. USA, 81: 7161–7165.

Robertson, E., Bradley, A., Kuehn, M., and Evans, M. (1986) Germ-line transmission of genes introduced into cultured pluripotential cells by retroviral vector. Nature, 323: 445–448.

Smithies, O. (1993) Animal models of human genetic diseases. Trends Genet., 9: 112–116.

Smithies, O., Gregg, R.G., Boggs, S.S., Koralewski, M.A., and Kucherlapati, R.S. (1985) Insertion of DNA sequences into the human chromosomal beta-globin locus by homologous recombination. Nature, 317: 230–234.

Stacey, A., Schnieke, A., McWhir, J., Cooper, J., Colman, A., and Melton, D.W. (1994) Use of double-replacement gene targeting to replace the murine alpha-lactalbumin gene with its human counterpart in embryonic stem cells and mice. Mol. Cell Biol., 14: 1009–1016.

Takeda, J., Seino, S., and Bell, G.I. (1992) Human Oct3 gene family: cDNA sequences, alternative splicing, gene organization, chromosomal location, and expression at low levels in adult tissues. Nucleic Acids Res., 20: 4613–4620.

Thomas, K.R. and Capecchi, M.R. (1987) Site-directed mutagenesis by gene targeting in mouse embryo-derived stem cells. Cell, 51: 503–512.

Thomas, K.R., Deng, C., and Capecchi, M.R. (1992) High-fidelity gene targeting in embryonic stem cells by using sequence replacement vectors. Mol. Cell Biol., 12: 2919–2923.

Thomas, K.R., Folger, K.R. and Capecchi, M.R. (1986) High frequency targeting of genes to specific sites in the mammalian genome. Cell, 44: 419–428.

Thomson, J.A., Itskovitz-Eldor, J., Shapiro, S.S., Waknitz, M.A., Swiergiel, J.J., Marshall, V.S., and Jones, J.M. (1998) Embryonic stem cell lines derived from human blastocysts. Science, 282: 1145–1147.

Thomson, J.A., Kalishman, J., Golos, T.G., Durning, M., Harris, C.P., Becker, R.A., and Hearn, J.P. (1995) Isolation of a primate embryonic stem cell line. Proc. Natl. Acad. Sci. USA, 92: 7844–7848.

Thomson, J.A., Kalishman, J., Golos, T.G., Durning, M., Harris, C.P., and Hearn, J.P. (1996) Pluripotent cell lines derived from common marmoset (*Callithrix jacchus*) blastocysts. Biol. Reprod., 55: 254–259.

Urbach, A., Schuldiner, M., and Benvenisty, N. (2004) Modeling for Lesch–Nyhan disease by gene targeting in human embryonic stem cells. Stem Cells, 22: 635–641.

Vallier, L., Rugg-Gunn, P.J., Bouhon, I.A., Andersson, F.K., Sadler, A.J., and Pedersen, R.A. (2004) Enhancing and diminishing gene function in human embryonic stem cells. Stem Cells, 22: 2–11.

Vasquez, K.M., Marburger, K., Intody, Z., and Wilson, J.H. (2001) Manipulating the mammalian genome by homologous recombination. Proc. Natl. Acad. Sci. USA, 98: 8403–8410.

Weintraub, H., Cheng, P.F., and Conrad, K. (1986) Expression of transfected DNA depends on DNA topology. Cell, 46: 115–122.

Wernig, M., Tucker, K.L., Gornik, V., Schneiders, A., Buschwald, R., Wiestler, O.D., Barde, Y.A., and Brustle, O. (2002) Tau EGFP embryonic stem cells: an efficient tool for neuronal lineage selection and transplantation. J. Neurosci. Res., 69: 918–924.

Xian, H.Q., McNichols, E., St Clair, A., and Gottlieb, D.I. (2003) A subset of ES-cell-derived neural cells marked by gene targeting. Stem Cells, 21: 41–49.

Xu, C., Inokuma, M.S., Denham, J., Golds, K., Kundu, P., Gold, J.D., and Carpenter, M.K. (2001) Feeder-free growth of undifferentiated human embryonic stem cells. Nat. Biotechnol., 19: 971–974.

Yanez, R.J. and Porter, A.C. (1999) Influence of DNA delivery method on gene targeting frequencies in human cells. Somat. Cell Mol. Genet., 25: 27–31.

Ying, Q.L., Stavridis, M., Griffiths, D., Li, M., and Smith, A. (2003) Conversion of embryonic stem cells into neuroectodermal precursors in adherent monoculture. Nat. Biotechnol., 21: 183–186.

Zaehres, H., Lensch, M.W., Daheron, L., Stewart, S.A., Itskovitz-Eldor, J., and Daley, G.Q. (2005) High-efficiency RNA interference in human embryonic stem cells. Stem Cells, 23: 299–305.

Zhang, G., Gurtu, V., and Kain, S.R. (1996) An enhanced green fluorescent protein allows sensitive detection of gene transfer in mammalian cells. Biochem. Biophys. Res. Commun., 227: 707–711.

Zwaka, T.P. and Thomson, J.A. (2003) Homologous recombination in human embryonic stem cells. Nat. Biotechnol., 21: 319–321.

CHAPTER 5

HEMATOPOIETIC DIFFERENTIATION

CHANTAL CERDAN, VERONICA RAMOS-MEJIA, AND MICKIE BHATIA

Stem Cell and Cancer Research Institute (SCC-RI), Michael G. DeGroote School of Medicine, Department of Biochemistry, McMaster University, 1200 Main Street, MDCL 5029 Hamilton, Ontario, L8N 3Z5, Canada

1. INTRODUCTION

Human embryonic stem cells (hESCs) spontaneously and randomly differentiate into multiple ectodermal, endodermal, and mesodermal cell types, in the absence of fibroblast growth factor (FGF) which sustains their undifferentiated state. These human pluripotent cells provide therefore a powerful model system to understand the cellular and molecular basis of human embryonic hematopoietic development. Differentiation methodologies of hESCs are largely adapted from methodologies used for mouse ESC differentiation and include two main approaches: coculture on supportive stromal cell layers (Kaufman et al. 2001; Tian et al. 2004, 2006; Narayan et al. 2005; Qui et al. 2005; Vodyanik et al. 2005; Woll et al. 2005; Slukvin et al. 2006) or formation of embryoid bodies (EB) (Chadwick et al. 2003; Cerdan et al. 2004; Tian et al. 2004; Wang et al. 2004, 2005; Zhan et al. 2004; Ng et al. 2005; Zambidis et al. 2005; Bowles et al. 2006; Cameron et al. 2006). Combination (Kim et al. 2005; Wang J. et al. 2005a) and side-by-side comparison (Tian et al. 2004) of both strategies have also been used.

Despite the different procedures applied in studying hematopoietic development from hESCs, different groups have achieved common outcomes. First, different groups independently found that hematopoietic development from hESCs displays a spatial and temporal pattern (Kaufman et al. 2001; Chadwick et al. 2003; Wang et al. 2004; Zhan et al. 2004; Vodyanik et al. 2005; Zambidis et al. 2005). Second, during early hESC differentiation, hematopoietic cells are derived from CD45 negative (CD45$^-$) precursors that coexpress CD31 and CD34 surface markers (Kaufman et al. 2001; Chadwick et al. 2003; Wang et al. 2004; Vodyanik et al. 2005; Zambidis et al. 2005). Two groups have identified an immature endothelial population giving rise to hematopoiesis from

J.R. Masters et al (eds.), Embryonic Stem Cells, 53–83.

hESCs (Wang et al. 2004; Zambidis et al. 2005). Through clonal experiments our group (Wang et al. 2004) demonstrated that a rare resident population within human embryoid bodies (hEBs) was able to generate both the endothelial and hematopoietic lineages, suggesting that this population contains cells with "hemangioblastic" properties. These combined findings recapitulate observations from human embryos (Tavian et al. 1999, 2001; Oberlin et al. 2002), further illustrating that hESCs can be applied as a model for studies of early human development.

The validity of ESCs as a model for adult hematopoiesis is controversial, because long-term engrafting hematopoietic stem cells (HSCs) have been difficult to demonstrate from mouse ESCs. However, preliminary data from Wang et al. (2005b) and others (Narayan et al. 2005; Tian et al. 2006) suggest that hESC-derived hematopoietic cells have HSC properties. However, the ability to generate fully functional hESC-derived HSCs, capable of long-term multilineage reconstitution of mouse models and ultimately patients, remains a challenge and will depend upon further understanding of intrinsic gene regulation and extrinsic environmental cues.

Here, we review the various methodologies applied to the in vitro derivation of mature, functional hematopoietic cell lineages from hESCs. We compare in the following sections (listed below) and appended tables, the main interests, limitations, and overlap of these methodologies for differentiation of hESCs and their hematopoietic derivatives in a controlled, robust, and reproducible manner.

1. Coculture of hESCs with stromal cells
2. Formation of hEBs and direct growth factor exposure
3. Combination and side-by-side comparison of coculture- and hEB-based systems
4. Derivation of hemogenic endothelium during hEB differentiation
5. Derivation of erythroid lineages
6. Derivation of lymphoid lineages and immune cells
7. Derivation of hESC-derived hematopoietic cells capable of repopulating animal models

2. COCULTURE OF hESCs WITH STROMAL CELLS

It is thought that bone marrow (BM) stromal cells create distinct microenvironments, known as "stem cell niches," that provide support for hematopoiesis. In all cases of stroma support used for hESC-derived hematopoiesis, the first step of differentiation did not require any supplementation with exogenous hematopoietic cytokines/growth factors, but fetal bovine serum (FBS) was used. Of the murine cell lines, OP9 cells have been reported to be the most efficient in inducing hematopoietic differentiation from hESCs.

2.1 Hematopoietic Colony-Forming Cells Derived from Human Embryonic Stem Cells (Kaufman et al. 2001)

Culture methods and media supplements: hESCs were allowed to differentiate for 17 days on irradiated murine BM cell line S17 or yolk sac endothelial cell line C166, using Dulbecco Modified Eagle Medium (DMEM) (Gibco) medium supplemented with 20% FBS (Hyclone or Gencyte), 2 mM L-glutamine, 1% nonessential amino acids, and 0.1 mM β-mercaptoethanol, in the absence of exogenous hematopoietic growth factors (HGF). Medium was changed every 2–3 days. Colony forming unit (CFU) assays were performed by replating single-cell suspensions of hESCs in Methocult GF+ medium (Stem Cell Technologies) consisting of 1% methylcellulose, 30% FBS, 1% BSA, 50 ng/mL SCF, 20 ng/mL GM-CSF, 20 ng/mL IL-3, 20 ng/mL IL-6, 20 ng/mL G-CSF, and 3U/mL EPO. After 14 days, CFUs were scored according to standard criteria. To support the growth of CFU-Mk (megakaryocytes), H1/S17 cells were cultured in MegaCult-C media (Stem Cell Technologies) consisting of 1.1% collagen, 1% BSA, 10 μg/mL bovine pancreatic insulin, 40 μg/mL low-density lipoproteins (Sigma), 200 μg/mL human transferrin, 2 mM L-glutamine, 0.1 mM β-mercaptoethanol, 50 ng/mL TPO, 10 ng/mL IL-6, and 10 ng/mL IL-3. After 10–14 days, cells were fixed, dried, and stained with a CD41 antibody specific for megakaryocytes and platelets. Cellular morphology of individual colonies was examined with Diff-Quick (a modified Wright–Giemsa staining, Dade).

Results: Precursors, comprising 1–2% of cells expressing CD34 but lacking CD45 and CD38 were generated in either coculture conditions. Roughly 50% of $CD34^+$ cells also expressed PECAM-1/CD31. Regardless of the stroma cell line used, these cells generated hematopoietic progenitor cells in CFU assays that displayed the morphology and surface markers characteristic of myeloid (CD15) (CFU-M, CFU-G, and CFU-GM), erythroid (glycophorin A) (BFU-E and CFU-E), megakaryocytic (CD41) (CFU-Mk) colonies, and occasionally mixed colonies (CFU-GEMM). Temporal development of CFUs was observed between 14 and 28 days, with a peak of production at 17–18 days and no production at 28 days. H1/S17 and H1/C166 cocultured cells gave rise to 30.4 (plating efficiency: 1 in 3290) and 4.3 (plating efficiency: 1 in 23255) total CFUs per 10^5 input cells, respectively. In the case of H1/S17 cocultures, CD34 selection enriched for hematopoietic cells, giving rise to 270 CFUs per 10^5 input cells, while the CD34-depleted populations gave rise to only 10 CFUs per 10^5 input cells. The plating efficiency (1 in 370) of the $CD34^+$ hESC population was similar to that of CD34 selection from adult BM or umbilical cord blood (UCB) cells.

By using semiquantitative RT-PCR, H1/S17 cocultures were shown to express mRNAs for the hematopoietic transcription factors SCL/TAL-1 and GATA-2, as early as day 7, before the appearance of CFUs. GATA-2 was no longer detectable after day 21, corresponding to the loss of CFU generation. RNA prepared from H1/S17-derived erythroid colonies showed expression of α, β, and δ globins but not the embryonic ε, ζ, or fetal γ globins, showing that hESC-derived erythroid colonies can express mature, adult-type globins.

Main interests and limitations

- The differentiated precursors generated in this system lacked CD45 expression.
- Although a side-by-side comparison of the supportive role of S17 and C166 was not provided, CFU plating efficiency was superior with S17.
- The erythroid colonies expressed adult but not embryonic/fetal globins.
- The following conditions did not lead to generation of CFUs:
  (i) differentiation in serum-free media without HGFs
  (ii) differentiation on mouse embryonic fibroblasts (MEFs)

2.2 Human Embryonic Stem Cell-Derived CD34+ Cells: Efficient Production in Coculture With OP9 Stromal Cells and Analysis of Lymphohematopoietic Potential (Vodyanik et al. 2005)

Culture methods and media supplements: HESC lines were cocultured on the mouse BM stromal feeder layers OP9, S17, or MS-5, at 3×10^5/4 mL per well of a 6-well plate in α-MEM supplemented with 10% FBS (Hyclone), 100 μM monothioglycerol (MTG, Sigma). Cocultures were maintained for up to 10 days with half-medium changed on day 4, 6, and 8. $CD34^+$ cells were isolated from day 8 to 9 hESC/OP9 cocultures with CD34 paramagnetic monoclonal antibodies using Direct CD34 Progenitor Isolation Kit (Miltenyi Biotech). Generation of simultaneous lymphomyeloid differentiation from $CD34^+$ cells generated in the OP9 coculture system was performed by coculture on MS-5, at a cell density of 5×10^4/well of 6-well plates for 21 days in serum-free expansion medium (SFEM) (Stem Cell Technologies) or α-MEM containing 10% FBS, 100 μM MTG in the presence of 50 ng/mL SCF, 50 ng/mL Flt3L, 10 ng/mL IL-3, and 20 ng/mL IL7. Separate cultures were additionally supplemented with IL15 to allow for NK cell maturation. Half of the medium was changed every fifth day with complete medium without IL-3.

Short-term cultures of isolated $CD34^+$ cells (at a density of 2.5×10^4 cells/mL) on MS-5 were grown for 5 days in SFEM or α-MEM containing 10% FBS, 400 μM MTG, and 100 ng/mL SCF, 100 ng/mL Flt3L, 50 ng/mL TPO, 5 ng/mL VEGF (Peprotech), and 10 ng/mL BMP-4 (R&D systems).

CFU assays were performed in MethoCult GF+H4435 semisolid medium (Stem Cell Technologies) consisting of 1% methycellulose, 30% FBS, 1% BSA, 50 ng/mL SCF, 20 ng/mL GM-CSF, 20 ng/mL IL-3, 20 ng/mL IL-6, 20 ng/mL G-CSF, and 3U/mL EPO (Peprotech). Supplementation with 20 ng/mL IL15 was performed to induce NK cell maturation. Sorted $CD34^+$ cells were plated at 2×10^3/mL while unsorted cells were plated at different densities depending on the day of differentiation: 2×10^5/mL from day 1 to 5, 1×10^5/mL at day 6, 5×10^4/mL from day 7 to 8, and 2×10^4/mL from day 9 to 10.

Results: Coculture on OP-9 is superior to both S17 or MS-5 for the production of CD34$^+$ cells (15–20% vs 2% after 8–9 days coculture) and CFU plating efficiency (1 in 66 vs 1 in 1,000). Up to 10^7 CD34$^+$ cells with >95% purity could be isolated, and 88.5% ± 3.5 of CD34$^+$ cells coexpressed PECAM-1/CD31.

CD34$^+$ cells first appeared on day 3 and gradually peaked at day 7. The temporal kinetics of CD31$^+$ cells closely followed that of CD34$^+$ cells, with emergence starting 1 day earlier than CD34. CD45$^+$ cells emerged at day 7 to 9, occurring a week earlier when compared to the S17 or MS-5 cocultures.

CFU-Es were induced on day 4 of coculture, followed by myeloid (GM, M) and mixed (GEMM) CFUs. The hESC-derived hematopoietic progenitors were restricted mostly to the CD34$^+$ population, as all CFUs except CFU-Es were enriched in the CD34$^+$ population and minimal numbers of CFU-M and CFU-GM were found in the CD34$^-$ population. The level of GATA-1 and GATA-2 transcription factors was also higher in this population, and coincident with the appearance of CD34 (day 2 to 3), while that of SCL/Tal-1 was detected a day later.

After 21 days, isolated CD34$^+$ cells gave rise to 58.5% ± 3.4 CD45$^+$ cells of total cells in coculture. This population contained not only myeloid cells (CD14$^+$HLA$^-$DR$^+$ macrophages and CD10$^+$CD66b$^+$ mature granulocytes) but also lymphoid cells that were identified both morphologically on cytospins and phenotypically (expression of CD19 for B cells and CD56 for NK cells). The addition of IL-15 generated perforin-expressing CD56$^+$ cells. Expression of transcripts for VpreB and Igα, cell receptor complex as well as for CD3ε, δ, and ζ, known to be expressed in embryonic and fetal NK cells, corroborated the characterization of B and NK cells, respectively. Pre-Tα receptor was not detected, suggesting that a different differentiation system is required to direct the differentiation of CD34$^+$ cells into T lymphocytes. Short-term cultures of CD34$^+$ cells on MS-5 in SFEM medium containing HGFs allowed for a similar expansion of total cells (about fivefold) than in the presence of serum (10% FBS), but a twofold less expansion of CFUs. In addition, the cells maintained a more primitive phenotype – no CD38 expression (1.8% ± 0.9), coexpression of CD34 and CD45 – and retained multilineage CFU-GEMM potential (300 ± 220), while in the presence of serum-containing media, cells were mostly CD45$^+$CD34$^-$, acquired a high level of CD38 expression (76% ± 9.4), and were enriched in CFU-Ms with a loss in CFU-GEMMs.

Main interests and limitations

- Coculture of hESCs with OP9 appears superior to that with S17 or MS-5 in terms of production of CD34$^+$ cells, CFU plating efficiency, and temporal emergence of CD45$^+$ cells. Therefore, OP9 may be suitable for studying the earliest stages of hematopoietic differentiation within CD45$^-$ populations.
- CD34$^+$ cells generated in the OP9 coculture system possess the capacity to generate at least phenotypically, both myeloid and lymphoid cells (except T cells).

- OP9 cells are very sensitive to variations in maintenance conditions, including medium source and serum lot, which can affect the ability of OP9 to support hematopoiesis.

2.3 Differentiation of Human Embryonic Stem Cells into Hematopoietic Cells by Coculture with Human Fetal Liver Cells Recapitulates the Globin Switch that Occurs Early in Development (Qiu et al. 2005)

Culture methods and media supplements: Two stromal cell layers, a human fetal liver-derived cell line FH-B-hTERT, and the mouse BM stromal cell line S17 were used to differentiate hESCs into hematopoietic cells. Cocultures were performed for 8–21 days, in DMEM (Invitrogen) medium supplemented with 20% FBS, 2 mM L-glutamine, and 1% MEM-nonessential amino acids. Medium was changed every 2–3 days. Immunomagnetic beads were used (Miltenyi Biotech) for CD34 cell separations. CFU assays were performed in Methocult GF media H4434 (Stem Cell Technologies) and colonies were scored according to their morphologies after 14 days. For analysis of the erythroid differentiation, please refer to section 6.2.

Results: The pattern of differentiation between the two feeders was different: differentiation initiated almost exclusively from the middle of the colonies for FH-B-hTERT/hESC cocultures, while multiple foci of differentiation were observed in S17/hESC cocultures. At day 8 and 11, both feeder systems produce equivalent total number of cells, but subsequently the total number of cells decreased for S17 but continued to increase until at least day 17 for FH-B-hTERT ($1.5–3 \times 10^6$ vs $<5 \times 10^5$ at day 17). The total cell yield at day 17 could be more than tenfold higher with FH-B-hTERT compared with S17. The frequency of about 3% (ranging from 1.9 to 9% on FH-B-hTERT) of $CD34^+$ cells peaked at day 14 and was similar for both feeders. Almost, no CD45 or CD38 could be detected prior to day 17 of coculture. The frequency of $CD34^+CD45^+$ or $CD34^+CD38^+$ cells remained <0.2% up to day 21. At all time points, the frequency of total CFUs (predominantly CFU-E, BFU-E, CFU-M, and CFU-GM), first detected after 8 days coculture, was the highest at day 14 after coculture with FH-B-hTERT compared to S17. At day 14, the total number of CFUs per 250,000 cells plated were about 250 for FH-B-hTERT and 100 for S17.

Main interests and limitations

Coculture of hESCs with immortalized human fetal liver-derived cells (FH-B-hTERT) is superior to mouse BM stromal cells (S17), in terms of total yield of hematopoietic precursors and CFU plating efficiency.

3. FORMATION OF HUMAN EMBRYOID BODIES AND DIRECT GROWTH FACTOR EXPOSURE

Human EBs are formed from aggregation of hESCs and possess the capacity to spontaneously and randomly differentiate into cell types of all three germ layers: ectoderm, mesoderm, and endoderm. This capacity can be promoted to some extent by the addition of exogenous growth factors or overexpression of regulatory genes. Some technical aspects and time course of hEB development vary in several critical ways from mouse ESC models. In contrast to mouse EBs that initiate from single cells, development of hEBs involves clusters of cells that aggregate in suspension, and acquire differentiated properties when treated with media including specialized lots of FBS, with or without a variety of HGFs. Interestingly, hEBs contain hemogenic endothelium or blood islands analogous to those found in the embryonic yolk sac (Wang et al. 2004; Zambidis et al. 2005), therefore recapitulating at least partially several events of early human development.

3.1 Cytokines and BMP-4 Promote Hematopoietic Differentiation of Human Embryonic Stem Cells (Chadwick et al. 2003)

Culture methods and media supplements: HEB were differentiated for 15 days in ultra-low attachment 6-well plates using differentiation medium consisting of knockout DMEM (KO-DMEM), supplemented with 20% FBS (Hyclone), 1% nonessential amino acids, 1 mM L-glutamine, 0.1 mM β-mercaptoethanol, and the following HGFs—300 ng/mL SCF (Amgen), 300 ng/mL Flt3L (R&D systems), 10 ng/mL IL-3 (R&D systems), 10 ng/mL IL-6 (R&D systems), and 50 ng/mL G-CSF (Amgen). In some experiments, 50 ng/mL of the ventral mesoderm inducer BMP-4 (R&D systems) was also added or used alone. Media and supplements were changed every 3 days.

CFU assays were performed by plating unsorted hEBs ($1–2 \times 10^5$) or sorted hEB populations (6×10^3 to 3.4×10^5) into methylcellulose H4230 (Stem Cell Technologies), supplemented with the following HGFs: 50 ng/mL SCF, 3 U/mL EPO (Amgen), 10 ng/mL GM-CSF (Novartis), and 10 ng/mL IL-3. After 10–14 days, colonies were scored based on standard criteria (clusters of greater than 50 cells).

Results: Spontaneous hematopoietic differentiation within hEBs (control: 20% FBS only) was compared to conditions supplemented with the mixture of HGFs (cytokines: SCF, Flt3-L, IL-3, IL-6, and G-CSF); or HGFs in combination with BMP-4 (HGFs + BMP-4); or BMP-4 alone without cytokine addition (BMP-4). No $CD45^+$ cells were detectable at 3, 7, or 10 days of HGFs + BMP-4 treatment. The detection of $CD45^+$ cells at day 15 was influenced by HGFs treatment, with or without BMP-4 addition. Under control conditions or BMP-4 alone, 1.4% ± 0.7 of cells expressed CD45, while the addition of HGFs increased this frequency to 8.0% ± 3.9. Addition of BMP-4 together with HGFs gave a frequency of 9.3% ± 1.2 $CD45^+$ cells. The frequency of $CD34^+$ cells was similarly modulated to patterns of $CD45^+$ cells, with a fivefold increase in the frequency of $CD45^+CD34^+$ cells upon HGFs treatment, while addition of HGFs + BMP-4 increased the frequency by sixfold. Undifferentiated hESCs expressed RUNX-1, but were devoid of detectable levels of GATA-1 or PU.1. Control hEB cultures did not upregulate these factors, whereas HGFs treatment with or without BMP-4 induced GATA-1 expression as early as day 3, and PU.1 expression by day 15. RUNX-1 expression was unaffected by treatment.

Based on CD45 expression, single-cell suspensions of hEBs were sorted by FACS. For both HGFs and HGFs + BMP-4 treated hEBs, only the $CD45^+$ subset contained clonogenic hematopoietic progenitors detected by CFU assay. Using Wright–Giemsa staining and flow cytometry, the CFUs generated included macrophage (CFU-M), granulocyte (CFU-G), and erythroid colonies, as well as multipotent colonies (CFU-GEMM). CFU-M, -G, -GM comprised cells expressing CD45, CD33, and CD13 while lacking glycophorin A expression. Colonies scored as erythroid contained cells characteristic of immature nucleated and mature enucleated erythrocytes and expressed glycophorin A, in the absence of expression of both CD45 and myeloid markers. Control hEBs or hEBs treated with BMP-4 alone produced an average of 68–72 CFU per 10^5 input cells, whereas HGFs-treated hEBs produced an average of 165 colonies. The addition of BMP-4 to HGFs further enhanced progenitor capacity, producing an average of 237 colonies. In the absence of FBS but with HGFs, as described in section 5.1 (hematopoietic culture (Hem-culture)), hEB cultures gave rise to an average of 100 CFU per 10^5 hEBs, suggesting that hematopoietic differentiation is not dependent on serum, and HGFs are sufficient in replacing complex mixture of factors present in the FBS. At day 10 of hEB development, a small number of CFUs was detectable with a clonogenic efficiency <1 in 50,000 cells, whereas at day 15 the clonogenic efficiency was 1 in 262.

Main interests and limitations

- A robust promotion of hematopoietic development (up to 90% at day 22 of hEB development) is achieved with this combination of HGFs and BMP-4.
- Although BMP-4 has little effect on hematopoietic progenitor formation, it supports secondary CFU replating, suggesting a role in self-renewal of hematopoietic progenitors.
- Similar to their somatic counterparts, hematopoietic progenitor function is restricted to the $CD45^+$ population.
- This study suggests that cells remain uncommitted to the hematopoietic cell fate prior to day 10 of hEB development.

3.2 Forced Aggregation of Defined Numbers of Human Embryonic Stem Cells into Embryoid Bodies Fosters Robust, Reproducible Hematopoietic Differentiation (Ng et al. 2005)

Culture methods and media supplements: Known numbers of single hESCs (300–10,000) were deposited in round bottomed, low adherence, 96-well plates and then aggregated into hEBs by centrifugation (spin hEBs), in serum-free medium (SFM) supplemented with 10 ng/mL BMP4, 5 ng/mL VEGF, 20 ng/mL SCF, 5 ng/mL Flt3-L, 5 ng/mL IL-6, and 5 ng/mL IGF-II (all from R&D systems). After 8–12 days, hEBs were allowed to differentiate further in 96-well, flat bottomed tissue culture plates, precoated with gelatin in SFM supplemented with 5 ng/mL VEGF, 20 ng/mL SCF, 5 ng/mL Flt3-L, 5 ng/mL TPO (R&D

systems), and 5U/mL Darboprotein (Amgen). CFU colonies were generated by plating 2.5×10^4–10^5 dissociated hEB cells in Iscove Modified Dulbecco Medium (IMDM) medium containing 1% methylcellulose, supplemented with 10% FBS, 25% D4T endothelial cell conditioned medium, 25 µg/ml ascorbic acid, and 2 mM L-glutamine. May–Grunwald–Giemsa stainings were performed at day 19.

Results: Efficient hematopoietic differentiation required an excess of 500 hESCs per 96-well, and optimal erythropoiesis was observed at 1,000 cells seeded per well. At the molecular level, spin hEBs passed through a transient in vitro "gastrulation" stage based on the expression of MIXL1 and Brachyury mesodermal genes (from day 4 to 8), followed by the emergence of $CD34^+$ cells at day 10, and RUNX-1 at day 20.

Efficiency of differentiation assessed by flow cytometry showed 23% $CD34^+$ cells and 11% $CD38^+$ cells at day 11, while at day 26, 29% $CD45^+$ cells were generated. Using chimeric hEBs generated from mixtures of GFP+ (ENVY) and GFP-hESCs in a clonogenic assay, hematopoietic precursor frequency was estimated to be ~1 in 500 input cells. May–Grunwald–Giemsa-stained cytospins showed that hEBs generated both myeloid cells (neutrophils, macrophages, mast cells) and erythroid cells. Although most erythroid cells were nucleated, occasional cells undergoing enucleation were observed. Total CFU numbers generated from spin hEBs were 92 per 10^4 cells at day 6, and 23 per 10^4 cells at day 10.

Main interests and limitations

- Despite a quite complex methodology, reproducible formation of uniform-size hEBs is achieved, providing a foundation for monitoring directed differentiation of hESCs.
- Determines the minimum number of hESCs (500) required for derivation of hematopoietic lineages in SFM, with an average of 91.8% ± 7.8 wells containing blood cells.
- Suggests that a higher number of hESCs is necessary for inducing optimal erythropoiesis.
- Requires more rigorous characterization of the cell types derived.

3.3 Improved Development of Human Embryonic Stem Cell-Derived Embryoid Bodies by Stirred Vessel Cultivation (Cameron et al. 2006)

Culture methods and media supplements: HESC colonies were cultured in low-adherent dishes in DMEM media containing 15% FBS (Hyclone), 1% MEM-nonessential amino acids (Invitrogen) and 0.1 mM β-mercaptoethanol (Sigma), and allowed to proceed with hEB formation for 24 h in static culture (initial concentration of ~100–200 colonies/mL). After 24 h, equal portions were aliquoted into either spinner flasks or static suspension cultures at equivalent cell and hEB concentrations. CFU assays were performed in Methocult GF+ media (Stem Cell Technologies) consisting of 1% methylcellulose, 30% FBS,

1% BSA, 50 ng/mL SCF, 20 ng/mL GM-CSF, 20 ng/mL IL-3, 20 ng/mL IL-6, 20 ng/mL G-CSF, and 3U/mL EPO.

Results: HEB-derived cells in spinner flask cultures proliferated at a faster rate, reaching concentrations approximately fourfold greater than hEBs in static suspension, at day 21 of the culture period. Cumulatively, this represented a 15-fold expansion in total cell numbers over the initial cell seeding value. In both static and stirred cultures, the $CD34^{+}CD31^{+}$ cell population reached a maximum of 5–6% at day 14, and the $CD34^{+}CD45^{+}$ cell population reached a maximum of 1–2.5% at day 17. Both cultures produced similar numbers of myeloid and erythroid CFUs at day 17, consistent with the development of $CD34^{+}CD45^{+}$ cells.

Main interests and limitations

Stirred suspension cultures of hEBs appear to be a more suitable method to increase total cell expansion from hEBs than static cultures.

Compared to static cultures, morphology and size of hEBs have little impact on hematopoietic differentiation, as hEBs is either (1) large and cystic, (2) small and compact, or (3) agglomerated—possess a hematopoietic phenotype that does not differ >1–2%.

3.4 Generation of Hematopoietic Repopulating Cells from Human Embryonic Stem Cells Independent of Ectopic HOXB4 Expression (Wang et al. 2005b)

Culture methods and media supplements: HEB differentiation was performed as described in section 3.1 and generation of $CD45^{-}$PFV hemogenic precursors as described in section 5.1. Full-length human HOXB4 cloned upstream enhanced GFP reporter gene into MIEV retroviral vector was used. $CD45^{-}$PFV cells were cultured under Hem-culture conditions for 3 days, as described in section 5.1, and then transferred into 96-well plates that had been pre-coated with 10 $\mu g/cm^2$ fibronectin (Sigma) for 4 h before the first retroviral exposure. Three consecutive exposures to virus-containing supernatants harvested from confluent PG13-MIEV retroviral producers were performed. The day after the third viral exposure, viral supernatants were aspirated and cells resuspended in Hem-culture conditions.

Results: Although quantitative RT-PCR confirmed that HOXB4 expression was 60-fold greater in HOXB4-transduced $CD45^{-}$PFV cells than in the vector-transduced cells, ectopic expression of HOXB4 increased the total expansion of hESC-derived hematopoietic cells by about 2.5-fold. HOXB4 did not affect the developmental capacity of these cells, as progenitor frequency and lineage development analyzed by CFU assays and phenotype were similar from HOXB4- and vector-transduced hESCs: 20–25 total CFUs per 15,000 $CD45^{-}$PFV-derived hematopoietic cells plated in both cases, and 2.6% vs 4% of $CD34^{+}CD45^{+}$ cells for HOXB4- and vector-transduced cells, respectively.

Main interests and limitations

First report of the functionality of HOXB4 overexpression on the in vitro expansion of hESC-derived hematopoietic cells. Although the effect is relatively modest, it falls in the same range as that of somatic UCB-derived $Lin^{-}/CD34^{+}$ cells.

3.5 HOXB4 Overexpression Promotes Hematopoietic Development by Human Embryonic Stem Cells (Bowles et al. 2006)

Culture methods and media supplements: Lipofection of HOXB4 cDNA (in the pTP6 vector) into hESCs (HOXB4-hESCs) generated stable expression of HOXB4 transgene for at least 15 passages (the maximum stage studied here). As a control, GFP (GFP-hESCs) was lipofected in place of HOXB4. Three individual HOXB4-hESCs clones were examined—HOXB4.1, HOXB4.2, and HOXB4.3. Hematopoietic differentiation was analyzed during the 20 days after hEB formation in serum containing medium (20% FBS), without additional HGFs or with the same mixture of HGFs and BMP-4 described in section 3.1. CFU assays were performed in Methocult GF+ media (Stem Cell Technologies) consisting of 1% methylcellulose, 30% FBS, 1% BSA, 50 ng/mL SCF, 20 ng/mL GM-CSF, 20 ng/mL IL-3, 20 ng/mL IL-6, 20 ng/mL G-CSF, and 3U/mL EPO.

Results: In the absence of HGFs but with FBS, no difference in total cell numbers was detected in HOXB4 overexpressing cells, at day 10 of hEB differentiation. Glycophorin A was expressed by 1.0% ± 0.1 of HOXB4.1-hESCs, 8.3% ± 1.2 of HOXB4.2-hESCs, and 5.2% ± 1.2 of HOXB4.3-hESCs, compared with 0.1% ± 0.1 of GFP-hESCs. At day 20, CD45 was expressed by 4.2% ± 0.3 of HOXB4.1-hESCs, 21.1% ± 3.3 of HOXB4.2-hESCs, and 9.1% ± 1.9 of HOXB4.3-hESCs, compared with 0.7% ± 0.1 of GFP-hESCs.

In the presence of HGFs and 20% FBS, HOXB4 augmented hematopoietic development additively to the effects of HGFs. At day 15 of hEB development, there was a 15-fold increase in $CD45^+$ cells from HOXB4-hESCs as compared with GFP-hESCs, and a threefold increase compared with HOXB4-hESCs cultured in the absence of HGFs. After 20 days of differentiation there was a 12-fold increase in $CD45^+$ cells from HOXB4-hESCs compared with GFP-hESCs, and a further fivefold increase over HOXB4-hESCs cultured in the absence of HGFs. Analyzed by Q-RT-PCR, the expression of SCL/Tal-1 and GATA-1 mRNAs was increased in HOXB4-hESCs, with a maximum increase of 90-fold for SCL/Tal-1 and 350-fold for GATA-1 at day 20.

On day 10 of differentiation, there were significant increases in the total number of CFUs in HOXB4-hESCs: HOXB4.1-hESCs 83 ± 15, HOXB4.2 233 ± 40, and HOXB4.3 460 ± 89, compared with no colonies from wild-type- or GFP-hESCs. On day 15, the mean numbers of CFUs were: HOXB4.1-hESCs 167 ± 22, HOXB4.2 1083 ± 131, and HOXB4.3 795 ± 84, compared to 24 ± 10 from wild-type-hESCs and 32 ± 10 from GFP-hESCs. On day 20, the mean numbers were: HOXB4.1-hESCs 206 ± 24, HOXB4.2 592 ± 77, and HOXB4.3 498 ± 42, compared to 68 ± 34 from wild-type-hESCs and 83 ± 17 from GFP-hESCs. In all three HOXB4-expressing clones, erythroid development peaked at day 10, whereas myeloid (CFU-GM and CFU-M) development peaked at day 15 to 20.

Main interests and limitations

- Very low baseline levels of in vitro hematopoietic differentiation from hESCs.
- Analysis of three different clones with a consistent supportive role of HOXB4 overexpression.

- Suggests that HOXB4 may act independently of HGFs to enhance in vitro hematopoietic development.
- No in vivo assessment of HOXB4 gain of function.

4. COMBINATION AND SIDE-BY-SIDE COMPARISON OF COCULTURE- AND HEB-BASED SYSTEMS

Two main approaches presented in sections 2 and 3 have been used so far to increase the overall efficiency of hematopoietic differentiation from hESCs: coculture with stromal cells and hEB formation. In this section, we review the efforts of a few groups (Tian et al. 2004; Kim et al. 2005; Wang et al. 2005a) to combine or compare these two methodologies side-by-side.

4.1 Cytokine Requirements Differ from Stroma and Embryoid Body-Mediated Hematopoiesis from Human Embryonic Stem Cells (Tian et al. 2004)

Culture methods and media supplements: HESC cocultures were grown with the S17 cell line, using DMEM medium supplemented with 20% FBS (Hyclone), 2 mM L-glutamine, 0.1 mM β-mercaptoethanol, 1% MEM-nonessential amino acids. Medium was changed every 2–3 days. For SFM, StemLine (Sigma) or QBSF60 (Quality Biologics) medium supplemented with 4 mM L-glutamine and SCF, TPO, Flt3L (each added at 20 ng/mL), VEGF, and BMP-4 (each added at 50 ng/mL). HEB formation was performed either in serum-containing medium: DMEM supplemented with 15% FBS, 1% L-glutamine, 1% MEM-nonessential amino acids, and 0.1 mM β-mercaptoethanol or in StemLine serum-free medium supplemented with 4 mM L-glutamine and HGFs added at the same concentration as cocultures. CFU assays were performed in semisolid medium Methocult GF+ (Stem Cell Technologies) consisting of 1% methycellulose, 30% FBS, 1% BSA, 50 ng/mL SCF, 20 ng/mL GM-CSF, 20 ng/mL IL-3, 20 ng/mL IL-6, 20 ng/mL G-CSF, and 3U/mL EPO. CFUs were scored after 14 days, using Wright–Giemsa (HEMA3 stain set, Fisher) staining.

Results

Coculture with S17 in media containing FBS but no HGFs: $CD34^+$ appeared at day 7 with some $CD31^+$ cells but no CD45. Most $CD34^+$ cells coexpressed CD31 but lacked CD38. $CD34^+CD45^+$ cells emerged at day 14, increased until about 19 days, then diminished. More mature hematopoietic population ($CD34^-CD45^+$) markedly increased between 27 and 32 days. The emergence of CFUs correlated with emergence and maintenance of $CD34^+CD45^+$ cells. Sorting to enrich for either single $CD34^+$, $CD45^+$, $CD31^+$ cells or double $CD34^+CD45^+$ cells increased the frequency of both myeloid and erythroid CFUs.

Direct stroma cell contact (hESCs were cocultured on MEFs and fed with S17-conditioned media) was not absolutely required for derivation of

$CD34^+CD45^+$, $CD31^+$, glycophorin A+ cells and CFUs, but improved by two- to threefold the frequency of these populations. Transwell cultures that prevent the direct contact of hESCs with S17 or MEFs in 20% FBS-containing media gave rise to as many or more CFUs compared to those grown in direct contact with S17 cells.

Coculture on S17 cells in two serum-free media formulations (StemLine and QBSF60) gave rise to little development of $CD34^+CD45^+$ cells (0.32–0.59% vs 0.01%) or CFUs (25 per 10^5 cells vs 0) compared to serum-containing media. Addition of SCF, TPO, and Flt3L to either of the serum-free media led to increased derivation of CFUs (40–50 per 10^5 cells) to a degree essentially the same or superior to when serum (FBS) was used.

Differentiation of hEBs: Timing of hematopoietic differentiation of hEBs cultured in the presence of FBS was similar to development on stromal cocultures. However, when hEBs were allowed to differentiate in serum-free medium, considerably fewer $CD34^+CD45^+$, glycophorin A+ cells, and CFUs were generated. A significant difference between the two systems of hematopoietic differentiation is that soluble SCF, TPO, and Flt3L did not compensate for the absence of serum and did not lead to increased development of $CD34^+CD45^+$ (0.10% vs 0.13 with SFM alone and vs 0.4% with FBS), and CFUs (<5 CFUs per 10^5 cells vs 15–20 with FBS). However, the addition of the mesodermal-inducing factors, VEGF and BMP-4 to the three HGFs in the serum-free hEB system, induced significantly more CFUs (10–15 per 10^5 cells). Serum-induced differentiation of hEBs appeared to give rise to more glycophorin A+ cells compared to the S17-coculture system (1.24% vs 0.5%). In both the stromal- and hEB-based systems, the emergence of CFUs closely correlates to development of $CD34^+$, $CD45^+$, and $CD34^+CD45^+$ cells.

Main interests and limitations

Comparison of hEB formation and coculture methodologies reveals that serum can be substituted by a combination of SCF, Flt3L, and TPO in the coculture but not the hEB system. Although more HGFs are required to support hematopoiesis in the hEB system, it remains more effective in the presence of serum.

4.2 Hematopoietic Differentiation of Embryoid Bodies Derived from Human Embryonic Stem Cell Line SNUhES3 in Coculture with Human Bone Marrow Stromal Cells (Kim et al. 2005)

Culture methods and media supplements: HEB formation was performed in low-adherence dishes in DMEM/F12 supplemented with 20% FBS (Hyclone), 1% nonessential amino acids (Invitrogen), 0.1 mM β-mercaptoethanol (Sigma), and were allowed to differentiate for 10 days. HEBs were either maintained in 20% FBS (EB group) or transferred into EB media containing 40% FBS (EB/high FBS group). Alternatively, after 2 days of culture in EB medium, hEBs were transferred onto irradiated human BM stromal cells and cultured in differentiation medium composed of IMDM (Invitrogen), 12.5% FBS, 12.5% horse serum, and L-glutamine (EB/BM coculture group). CFU assays were performed in Methocult H4444 medium (Stem Cell Technologies), composed of 1% methylcellulose, 30% FBS, 1% BSA, 50 ng/mL SCF, 10 ng/mL GM-CSF, 10 ng/mL IL-3, and 3U/mL EPO.

Results: There were no significant differences in the frequency of $CD34^+CD45^-$ cells between the three groups at day 3 and 5. However, at day 10 of differentiation, the frequency was 3.8% ± 0.58 in the EB/BM coculture group, compared to 0.28% ± 0.23 and 0.35% ± 0.11 for the EB and EB/high FBS groups, respectively. The frequency of $CD34^+CD38^-$ cells also increased from day 5 to 10 of culture in the EB/BM coculture group (5.81% ± 1.19), compared to <0.5% in both the EB and EB/high FBS groups. The frequencies of $CD34^+CD45^+$ or $CD34^+CD38^+$ cells was <0.1% in the three groups regardless of culture duration.

In both the EB and EB/high FBS groups, the total number of CFUs was <5 per 10^5 cells plated at day 7 and 10, while a higher number was observed in the EB/BM coculture group (11 ± 5.14 and 20.6 ± 7.4 at day 7 and 10, respectively).

Main interests and limitations

The hEB/BM coculture leads to more efficient hematopoietic differentiation than the other groups, suggesting that human BM stromal cells might play a role in supporting hematopoietic differentiation from hEBs.

4.3 In vitro Hematopoietic Differentiation of Human Embryonic Stem Cells Induced by Coculture with Human Bone Marrow Stromal Cells and Low-dose Cytokines (Wang et al. 2005a)

Culture methods and media supplements: HESCs were transferred onto low attachment dishes and cultured for 4 days in EB medium consisting of KO-DMEM, supplemented with 15% KO serum replacement, 2 mM L-glutamine, 0.1 mM β-mercaptoethanol, and 1% nonessential amino acids (all from Gibco).

At day 4 of culture, hEBs were transferred to:

- Group 1 = same EB medium
- Group 2 = EB medium +100 ng/mL SCF + 100 ng/mL Flt3L + 10 ng/mLVEGF
- Group 3 = EB medium + 100 ng/mL SCF + 100 ng/mL Flt3L + 10 ng/mL VEGF+ mitomycin C-treated human fetal bone marrow stem cells (hBMSCs)
- Group 4 = EB medium + hBMSCs

Single-cell suspensions of cell clusters were seeded in semisolid medium containing 1% methylcellulose, and 50 ng/mL SCF, 25 ng/mL IL-3, 25 ng/mL IL-6, 50 ng/mL GM-CSF, and 2 U/mL EPO.

Results: In groups 1 and 2, hEBs spread soon after attaching to the culture dish, and underwent differentiation to form large, epithelial-like cells, but not clusters (the authors did not mention the procedure). When the hEBs were cocultured on hBMSCs with or without HGFs (groups 3 and 4), a few clusters of cells had morphological features of hematopoietic blast cells on day 8. Some clusters were surrounded by endothelial-like cells, forming structures similar to embryonic blood islands, while others contained cells that had the morphology of cobblestone-like cells. By semiquantitative RT-PCR, the expression of Flk-1/KDR and SCL/Tal-1 mRNAs was detected and remained high for 2–8 days after cluster formation, whereas the expression of RUNX-1 tended to be down-regulated by day 8. Flow cytometric analysis revealed that the clusters contained 8.81% Flk-1/KDR+ cells, 9.94% $CD34^+$ cells, and 25.7% $CD45^+$ cells.

Colonies with morphology similar to CFU-GEMM were observed. The most potent group is group 3 in terms of numbers of CFU-GEMM with ~30, 8, and 4 times more than groups 1, 2, and 4, respectively.

Main interests and limitations

- First report that provides some evidence for the enhancement of hematopoietic differentiation from hESCs supported by a combination of hEB formation, treatment with HGFs, and coculture with human BM stromal cells.
- A more rigorous characterization of the hESC derivatives produced is still required to demonstrate the efficiency of this system.

5. DERIVATION OF HEMOGENIC ENDOTHELIUM DURING HEB DIFFERENTIATION

The comparisons and observations between mouse and human ESC differentiation illustrate important cellular differences of mouse and human specification toward the hematopoietic lineages (Table 1). Surface markers that have been successfully applied to identify early hematopoietic progeny during mouse ESC development seem unsuitable for hESC differentiation since many of the homologous markers are expressed on cells within the hESC cultures prior to differentiation (Wang et al. 2004; Zambidis et al. 2005). For example, Flk-1/KDR+ cells only emerge after mouse ESC differentiation (Nishikawa et al. 1998), giving rise to either endothelial or hematopoietic lineages (Choi et al. 1998; Nishikawa et al. 1998; Cho et al. 2001; Chung et al. 2002). However, the frequencies of Flk-1/KDR+ cells in undifferentiated hESCs and differentiated hEBs are similar, suggesting that Flk-1/KDR is not an appropriate marker for early hematopoietic progeny of hESCs. A similar distinctive profile of expression of CD105 (endoglin), an accessory receptor for members of the TGF-β family, has been shown between mouse and human ESCs/EBs (Table 1). CD41 antigen has been demonstrated as a reliable marker for early hematopoiesis in mouse ESC (Mitjavila-Garcia et al. 2002; Emambokus and Frampton 2003; Mikkola et al. 2003), but very few cells expressed CD41 during hESC hematopoietic development (Wang et al. 2004) (Table 1).

As those markers cannot be used for identification of hemogenic precursors in the hEB system, CD31/PECAM-1, a marker associated with cells capable of

Table 1. Main differences between mESC and hESC-derived hematopoietic differentiation

Expression/property	mESCs	hESCs
KDR/Flk1	–	+
CD41	+	–
CD105 (endoglin)	–	+
CD135/Flt-3	–	+
Hemangioblast emergence (in vitro)	Between day 2.5 and 4	Between day 7 and 10
HOXB4-induced in vivo hematopoietic reconstitution	+	–

early hematopoietic potential in the human embryo has proven to be useful in two independent studies described in this section.

Increasing evidence from avian and mouse models suggests that HSCs are produced from an endothelial intermediate designated as "hemangioblast" or "hemogenic endothelium." The limited number of studies using human embryos have shown the emergence of hematopoietic cells in close association with vascular endothelial cells. Using the hEB differentiation system, two groups including ours have described primitive endothelial precursors capable of giving rise to both hematopoietic and endothelial cells (Wang et al. 2004; Zambidis et al. 2005).

5.1 Endothelial and Hematopoietic Cell Fate of Human Embryonic Stem Cells Originates from Primitive Endothelium with Hemangioblastic Properties (Wang et al. 2004)

Culture methods and media supplements: HEB formation was performed as described in section 3.1. Preparation of single CD45$^-$PFV and remaining day 10 hEB cells was performed by single-cell dissociation of day 10 hEBs, followed by sequential staining with Flk1/KDR (Research Diagnostics), PECAM-1-FITC (PharMingen), CD45-APC (Becton Dickinson), and 7AAD (Immunotech). Stained subpopulations or single cells were sorted on a FACSVantage. CD45$^-$PFV and remaining cells were seeded in fibronectin-coated plates at a density of 5×10^4 cells/cm^2 and cultured for 7 days in serum-free Hem-culture conditions. Hem-culture consists of IMDM medium supplemented with BSA/Insulin/Transferrin (9500 BIT, Stem Cell Technologies), 2 mM L-glutamine (Invitrogen), 0.1 mM β-mercaptoethanol (Sigma), 300 ng/mL SCF (R&D systems), 50 ng/mL G-CSF (Amgen), 300 ng/mL Flt-3L (R&D systems), 10 ng/mL IL-3 (Novartis), and 10 ng/mL IL-6 (R&D systems). They were then assessed for hematopoietic commitment by CD45 expression and CFU assays, as described in section 3.1. Alternatively, CD45$^-$PFV and remaining hEB cells were plated for 7 days at the same density in endothelial culture conditions (Endo-culture), consisting of Medium-199 (Invitrogen) supplemented with 20% FBS (Hyclone), 50 μg/mL endothelial cell growth supplement (Bovine pituitary extract, Invitrogen), 10

IU/mL heparin (Leo Pharma Inc.), and 5 ng/mL VEGF-A_{165} (R&D systems). In both Hem-culture and Endo-culture, medium was changed at day 2, 4, and 6.

Results: CD31 was first detectable around day 3 of hEB development, significantly increased from day 7 to 15, eventually accounting for ~8% of total hEB cells. Based on coexpression of CD31/PECAM-1, Flk-1/KDR, and VE-Cadherin and the lack of expression of CD45, PECAM-1^+ cells have been termed $CD45^-$PFV. They possess the ability to uptake acetylated low-density lipoprotein (Dil-LDL), and lack hematopoietic CFU capacity. Mature features of functional endothelium such as expression of vWF and eNOS were not detected. Genes associated with both endothelial and hematopoietic potential were highly expressed, including FLT-1, FLK-1, SCL/TAL-1, FLT-4, FOG-1, RUNX-1, and HEX, suggesting that $CD45^-$PFV precursors may possess both hematopoietic and endothelial lineage developmental potential.

After 7 days of Hem-culture, up to 98.5% $CD45^-$PFV cells became $CD45^+$, with 8.3% ± 0.7 of these cells coexpressing CD34. Overall, the number of $CD45^+$ hematopoietic cells generated from $CD45^-$PFV cells was 28.7 ± 8.2-fold higher than that from unsorted cells. The frequency of CFU was 124-fold higher than that from unsorted cells. Similar to human peripheral blood (PB), UCB, and BM, $CD45^+CD34^+$ subpopulation was highly enriched for CFUs with a clonogenic efficiency of 1 in 50, in contrast to 1 in 1,069 for $CD45^+CD34^-$ subpopulation derived from the same hEBs. The hematopoietic potential of the $CD45^-$PFV precursors was retained until day 22 of hEB development (unpublished observations).

When $CD45^-$PFV cells were plated in endo-culture conditions for 7 days, they became attached and spindle shaped, strongly expressed PECAM-1 and VE-cadherin, possessed higher Dil-LDL uptake capacity, expressed vWF and eNOS, and formed endothelial network in vitro. No $CD45^+$ cells nor hematopoietic CFU were detectable under these culture conditions. Clonal analysis demonstrated that a small number of $CD45^-$PFV cells were bipotent, possessing both hematopoietic and endothelial capacities. In addition to clones with either exclusively hematopoietic or endothelial differentiation capacity, 0.18% of the total wells seeded with single $CD45^-$PFV clones in a Hem:Endo culture medium (at a 50:50 ratio by volume) were capable of giving rise to both endothelial and hematopoietic progeny with a frequency of ~1:500. These results suggest that a proportion of $CD45^-$PFV cells possess human "hemangioblastic" properties.

Main interests and limitations

- Demonstrates that a unique population of cells within hEBs (named CD45-PFV hemogenic precursors) is uniquely responsible for the hematopoietic development from hESCs.
- First clonal demonstration that a small fraction of these precursors possess "hemangioblastic" capacities of differentiation and maturation toward both the hematopoietic and endothelial lineages. The frequency of 1:500 of these clones is similar to 1:300 frequency in mouse ESCs (Choi et al. 1998).

5.2 Hematopoietic Differentiation of Human Embryonic Stem Cells Progresses Through Sequential Hematoendothelial, Primitive, and Definitive Stages Resembling Human Yolk Sac Development (Zambidis et al. 2005)

Culture methods and media supplements: HEB cultures were performed in semisolid IMDM-based medium containing 1% methylcellulose (Stem Cell Technologies) supplemented with 15% FBS (Stem Cell Technologies), 50 μg/mL ascorbic acid (Sigma), 0.5% cholesterol/lipoprotein supplements (EX-CYTE), and 3.5% protein-free hybridoma medium-II PFHM-II (Invitrogen). After 4 days, hEBs are collected by gravity settling for 3–5 min followed by aspiration of the upper 2/3 of the hEB suspension to efficiently eliminate >90% of nonviable cells and replated (about 300–500/mL) in ultra nonadherent 6-well plates in "liquid differentiation medium" containing SFEM supplemented with 15% FBS, 50 μg/mL ascorbic acid, 0.5% insulin/transferrin/selenium supplements (Invitrogen), and 5% PFHM-II, and fed every 3–4 days with fresh medium.

CFU assays were performed in standard serum-free methylcellulose-based medium H4436 (Stem Cell Technologies), containing 50 ng/mL SCF, 50 ng/mL GM-CSF, 50 ng/mL G-CSF, 20 ng/mL IL-3, 20 ng/mL IL-6, and 3U/mL EPO, 0.5% EX-CYTE and 5% PFHM-II. The authors did not use bovine serum because it inhibits the expansion of primitive murine progenitors. Colonies were scored and picked up for cytospin or Q-RT-PCR 14–21 days later. BFU-Es were defined for both primitive and definitive colonies by standard definitions (three or more multiclustered erythroid colonies). For endothelial potential, plastic-adherent cells from mesodermal–hematoendothelial (MHE) colonies were replated after vigorous washing to eliminate nonadherent cells in EGM2 complete endothelial medium (Cambrex) on matrigel-coated plates.

Results: CD34 and CD31 expression both peaked at about 12–15 days of hEB development and were coexpressed on the same cells. CD45 was not expressed until about 1 week after the onset of CD34/CD31 expression (15–30 days) and only on 1–3% of hEBs. Expression of GATA-1, GATA-2, EKLF, SCL/Tal-1, CDX4, and PU.1 increased dramatically by >10- to 10,000-fold after 1 week of hEB development, coinciding with the emergence of CD31, CD34 and increase in Flk-1/KDR.

CFUs (mixed M, GM, and E) with morphologies similar to definitive colonies produced from somatic cells were generated from day 14 to 20 hEBs but not earlier. Semiadherent cluster colonies appeared at day 7 to 9 of hEB development, with a cellular architecture and phenotype highly reminiscent of human yolk sac blood islands. Indeed, these clusters contained cells with endothelial characteristics (50–60% expressed CD31 and VE-cadherin but not CD45 and had ability to incorporate Dil-LDL and to express vWF), that were intermixed with nonendothelial cells expressing the mesenchymal marker vimentin. Besides, cells expressing erythromyeloid markers (CD71, CD13, and CD45) budded from these adherent clusters (around 7–10 days after hEB replating). Wright-staining revealed that they contained primitive-type macrophages and nucleated primitive-type erythroblasts expressing embryonic ($\varepsilon 2\zeta 2$) and fetal (HbF, $\alpha 2\gamma 2$) but not adult (HbA, $\alpha 2\beta 2$) hemoglobins. Definitive CFU-Es (BFU-E and CFU-E) with a salmon red (as opposed to brilliant red) hemoglobinization were detected from day 12 to 20 hEBs and expressed both embryonic, fetal and adult globins. Definitive-type CFU-GM and CFU-M containing monocytes, macrophages and rare segmented neutrophils were also detected at this stage. Altogether, this suggests that the three main components of yolk sac blood islands (primitive-type erythromyeloid cells, endothelial cells, and mesenchymal stromal cells) were comprised within these clusters. In addition, hematopoiesis within hEBs arose through distinct hemato-endothelial, primitive, and definitive stages in a manner similar to human yolk sac development with predominance of multipotent primitive CFUs arising from day 7 to 12 of hEB development, followed by a wave of definitive multipotent CFUs from day 12 to 20, with no need for addition of exogenous HGFs or stromal cocultures.

Main interests and limitations

- Describes the developmental progression of human hematopoiesis during hEB differentiation and its analogy to mouse EB development in terms of hematopoietic surface markers and transcription factors.
- Characterization of two sequential waves of primitive, then definitive erythropoiesis.
- Similarly to our group (study summarized in section 5.1), this study reveals the existence of an endothelium-like intermediate (called MHE colonies here and $CD45^{-}$PFV in our study), which emerges within hEBs about 1 week after the initiation of hEB development and precedes the onset of hematopoiesis.

6. DERIVATION OF ERYTHROID LINEAGES

6.1 VEGF-A_{165} Augments Erythropoietic Development from Human Embryonic Stem Cells (Cerdan et al. 2004)

Culture methods and media supplements: HEB formation was performed as described in section 3.1, except that hEBs were treated with the same mixture of HGFs (SCF, Flt-3L, IL-3, IL-6, G-CSF, BMP-4) in the absence or presence of VEGF-A_{165} (5 ng/mL, R&D systems), and analyzed by flow cytometry, CFU assays, and semiquantitative RT-PCR at different time points between day 7 and 29. In some experiments, 3 U/mL EPO (Amgen) was added to the mixture of HGFs + VEGF. CFU assays were also performed as described in section 3.1, except that the erythroid colonies were considered as positive when composed of 8–50 cells and were scored every 3 days between 7 and 28 days of incubation.

Results: After 15 days of hEB differentiation in the presence of SCF, Flt-3L, IL-3, IL-6, G-CSF, and BMP-4, hESCs differentiated into hematopoietic progenitors as detected by multilineage CFU potential. Addition of VEGF at a concentration ranging between 1 and 20 ng/mL increased by tenfold the total number of erythroid colonies but not that of myeloid progenitors. Only in the presence of HGFs + BMP-4, was VEGF able to augment the generation of erythroid progenitors. Addition of EPO had no effect on hEBs differentiated in the presence of HGFs plus BMP-4, but enhanced by 2.5-fold the number of erythroid colonies derived from VEGF-treated hEBs. We suggest that both HGFs and BMP-4 are required for VEGF to augment erythroid development from hESCs, and that this effect can be augmented with EPO addition. Larger nucleated erythroblasts were detected among cells comprising erythroid colonies derived from VEGF-treated hEBs compared to control hEBs (treated with HGFs plus BMP-4). By day 15, VEGF-treated hEBs comprised ~3.5 ± 1.0% of $CD34^+/KDR^+$ cells compared with 0.8% ± 0.7 for control hEBs. Both populations comprised 86% ± 7.4 and 84% ± 5.0 $CD45^+$ cells, respectively, indicating their higher content in hematopoietic than endothelial cells. Fold increase in the percentage of $CD34^+KDR^+$ cells within VEGF-treated hEBs correlated with the increased number of erythroid colonies. Both embryonic (ε and ζ) globins were detected in VEGF-treated hEBs, whereas only ε globin was detected in control hEBs, at a twofold lower level. Both types of hEBs were devoid of detectable expression of the adult β globin at any time tested (up to day 15 of differentiation). Control hEBs expressed GATA-1 but not SCL/Tal-1 and PU-1 mRNAs, whereas VEGF-treated hEBs expressed both GATA-1 and SCL/Tal-1 mRNAs but not PU.1.

In erythroid colonies generated from VEGF-treated hEBs, the expression of ζ globin was no longer detectable, whereas the expression of ε persisted in colonies derived from both types of hEBs. This was associated with the appearance of the adult β globin at both the mRNA and protein (HbA) levels in colonies derived from both types of hEBs. Thus, a different pattern of globin expression was observed between hEBs and their derived erythroid colonies, consisting in the presence of embryonic ε and ζ globins and the absence of adult β globin in 15-day-differentiated hEBs followed by the disappearance of ζ globin and the appearance of β globin in 15-day-derived erythroid colonies.

Main interests and limitations

- This study indicates that hematopoietic composition derived from hESCs can be influenced by exogenous factors.
- That VEGF is one of these factors, by promoting erythropoietic development of cells expressing both ε and ζ embryonic globins.
- The erythroid cells produced undergo in vitro globin gene switching toward the adult program during colony formation.

6.2 Differentiation of Human Embryonic Stem Cells into Hematopoietic Cells by Coculture with Human Fetal Liver Cells Recapitulates the Globin Switch that Occurs Early in Development (Qiu et al. 2005)

Culture methods and media supplements: Two stromal cell layers, a human fetal liver-derived cell line FH-B-hTERT and the mouse BM stromal cell line S17, were used to differentiate hESCs into erythroid cells. HESCs were cocultured on either FH-B-hTERT or S17 for 8–21 days in DMEM supplemented with 20% FBS, 2 mM L-glutamine, and 1% nonessential amino acids. Media was changed every 2–3 days. CFUs were generated in methylcellulose (MethoCult GF media H4434, Stem Cell Technologies). Globin expression patterns were determined by quantitative real-time PCR in individual erythroid colonies.

Results: The frequency of CFUs (predominantly CFU-E and BFU-E and CFU-M, CFU-GM) was higher with FH-B-hTERT, first detected after 8 days coculture, and reached the highest number at day 14. The total number of erythroid colonies (both CFU-E and BFU-E) per 250,000 cells plated was about 200 for FH-B-hTERT and 75 for S17 at day 14. Between day 8 and 14, the ratio of erythroid/myeloid CFUs was greater than 3.5. After 17–21 days of coculture, this ratio was approximately equal to 1. Plating efficiency at day 14 for FH-B-hTERT was 1 in 1,000 and 1 in 2,500 for S17. Erythroid colonies appeared in small monoclusters similar to mouse 5-day CFU-Es. Cells within erythroid colonies resembled primitive erythroblasts found in 4–5 week human yolk sac. Analyzed individually by Q-RT-PCR after 8 days of coculture, the erythroid colonies (majority of CFU-E) expressed mainly ε globin, and with increased time in coculture produced more abundantly γ-globin, with a mean γ/ε globin mRNA ratio of 0.39 ± 0.06 which increased progressively to 4.22 ± 1.18 after coculture for up to 21 days, mimicking switch from ε to γ during in vivo erythroid development. Only traces of β globin expression (<0.1% of total globin expression) could be detected in the colonies at any time point examined.

Main interests and limitations

- The frequency of production of erythroid colonies is higher with FH-B-hTERT than S17.
- Individual analysis of erythroid colonies by Q-RT-PCR shows the occurrence of globin switching from ε to γ, but no significant expression of adult β globin. The authors propose that these cells do not advance to the fetal liver stage of differentiation and might be equivalent to yolk sac cells.
- The use of two different developmental stages of feeders indicates that it does not affect the developmental stage of the hematopoietic cells produced.

7. DERIVATION OF LYMPHOID LINEAGES AND IMMUNE CELLS

7.1 Functional Antigen-Presenting Leucocytes Derived from Human Embryonic Stem Cells in vitro (Zhan et al. 2004)

Culture methods and media supplements: A two-step hEB differentiation method was used. The first step was performed in ultra-low attachment plates using KO-DMEM, 20% FBS (Stem Cell Technologies), 2 mM L-glutamine, 0.1 mM nonessential amino acids (all from Invitrogen), and 0.1 mM β-mercaptoethanol (Sigma) for 14 days. Then hEBs were transferred to tissue culture plates using the same medium supplemented with 100 ng/mL SCF, 50 ng/mL Flt3L, 20 ng/mL TPO, 20 ng/mL IL-3, 100 ng/mL GM-CSF, and 20 ng/mL IL4 (all from Peprotech) for up to 6 weeks. Approximately $0.1–0.5 \times 10^6$ undifferentiated hESCs were plated per well of 6-well plates and formed about 20–30 hEBs. When harvested at day 10 to 20, on average every hEB contained about 10,000 cells. To use the differentiated hematopoietic cells obtained from hESC-derivatives in mixed leucocyte reaction (MLR) assays, the harvested cells were resuspended in RPMI 1640 medium with 10% FBS, and then activated for 4 h with 20 ng/mL TNF-α and 10 ng/mL prostaglandin E2, and then irradiated at 30 Gy to block cell proliferation. CFU assays were performed by plating up to 5×10^4 single cells in 35 mm plates, in methylcellulose media (Marrow-Grow, Quality Biological) supplemented with 100 ng/mL SCF, 10 ng/mL IL-3, 10 ng/mL IL-6, 10 ng/mL G-CSF, 10 ng/mL GM-CSF, and 5U/mL EPO. Colonies were scored after 14 days.

Results: Within 7–10 days after hEB plating, hematopoietic-like cells started to appear in suspension and were harvested weekly between week 2 and 6. Mean total number of harvested cells was 2.32×10^6 per well containing about 40 EBs. CFU assays revealed at all time points more (four- to fivefold) myeloid progenitors (CFU-GM) than erythroid. FACS analysis of cells harvested at week 2 showed that 96% of the nonadherent cells and 53.6% of the adherent cells were $CD45^+$, with 8.6% of $CD34^+CD45^+$ in the adherent cell fraction, and 2.8% in the nonadherent cell fraction. These frequencies fell to <1% in the nonadherent and adherent cell fractions at weeks 3 and 6, respectively. In both fractions, $CD33^+CD45^+$ (myeloid) cells were detected (about 69% and 38% for nonadherent and adherent, respectively) and about 5% of $CD14^+CD45^+$ cells. B lymphoid $CD19^+$ cells were not significantly detected in each fraction (<1.5%). Almost 27–32% of $CD2^+CD45^+$ (CD2 could be indicative of T, NK, monocytes, and dendritic cells (DCs)) cells were present in the nonadherent fraction and 50% of the $CD2^+$ subset coexpressed CD16. However, this fraction did not express other markers such as CD3, CD5, and CD7 (lymphoid) or CD56 and CD94 (NK). This is consistent with the notion that these cells are probably myeloid in origin. At weeks 3–6, MHC class II and the costimulatory molecules CD80 or CD86 were found more expressed in the nonadherent than adherent fraction. Wright–Giemsa stainings revealed the presence of cells similar to DCs, macrophages, and granulocytes with an immature morphology. The presence of macrophages was further confirmed by cytoplasmic expression of a naphthyl acetate esterase. Upon activation of the nonadherent fraction with TNF-α and prostaglandin E2, 25% of the cells expressed moderate to high amounts of HLA-DR and CD86 as well as CD80, CD40 (marker of antigen-presenting cells) and CD83 (marker of DCs). The nonadherent fraction (about 25% expressing MHC class II) was used as antigen-presenting cells in MLR reactions with allogeneic T lymphocytes. This activity was higher against purified $CD4^+$ than $CD8^+$ T cells or unfractionated mononuclear cells, suggesting that it involved MHC class II more than class I antigens.

Main interests and limitations

- This study shows that MHC Class II+ leucocytes resembling DCs and macrophages, capable of eliciting CD4 and CD8 T-cell responses, can be produced from hESCs. However, their antigen-presenting activities are two- to fivefold lower than those of adult blood leucocytes. Provides a foundation to investigate immune cell formation from hESCs.
- This study does not address whether the surface markers analyzed are shared by more than one type of cell.

7.2 Human Embryonic Stem Cell-Derived NK Cells Acquire Functional Receptors and Cytolytic Activity (Woll et al. 2005)

Culture methods and media supplements: Two-step coculture in vitro differentiation system was used. HESCs were cocultured on S17 in RPMI 1640 (Mediatech) supplemented with 15% FBS (Hyclone), 2 mM L-glutamine, 1% MEM-nonessential amino acids, and 0.1 mM β-mercaptoethanol. Medium was changed every 2–3 days. After 14–17 days, hESCs were sorted for $CD34^+$ or $CD34^+CD45^+$ hematopoietic progenitors either using EasySep CD34 selection kit (StemCell Tech) followed by CD45-PE labeling (BDPharmingen) or using FACSAria (BD Biosciences). Sorted $CD34^+$ or $CD34^+CD45^+$ progenitors were then transferred to wells with a confluent monolayer of irradiated mouse fetal liver cell line AFT024 in medium designed to maximize NK cell growth = NK cell conditions (DMEM:Ham's F-12, supplemented with 20% heat inactivated human AB serum (Nabi), 5 ng/mL sodium selenite (Sigma), 50 μM ethanolamine (MP Biomedicals), 20 mg/L ascorbic acid (Sigma), 25 μM β-mercaptoethanol, 10 ng/mL IL-15, 5 ng/mL IL-3, 20 ng/mL SCF, and 10 ng/mL Flt3L (all from Peprotech). Medium with fresh cytokines was changed weekly, with the exception of IL-3 which was only included for the first week of culture.

Results: In NK cell conditions, hESC-derived $CD34^+CD45^+$ cells expanded 40-fold and hESC-derived $CD34^+$ cells demonstrated almost no expansion, compared to 1,000-fold expansion from UCB-derived $CD34^+$ cells. After 21 days expansion, $CD34^+$ subset gave rise to 14.9% $CD56^+CD45^+$ cells, which increased to 37.5% after 28 days of culture. Similar results were obtained from $CD34^+CD45^+$ subset (20.7% after 21 days and 29% after 28 days). NK cell clonal frequency obtained by limiting dilution was 0.16% for the $CD34^+$ subset, and 2.4% for the $CD34^+$ $CD45^+$ subset. $CD56^+$ NK cells derived from $CD34^+CD45^+$ subset started to express KIRs after 18 days of culture: KIR2DL3 (CD158b), KIR3DL1 (CD158e1), KIR2DS4 (CD158i). After 50 days, 40% of the cells were $CD56^+KIR^+$ (KIR expression was found higher in hESC-derived NK cells compared to $CD34^+$ UCB-derived NK cells). However, hESC-derived NK cells did not express KIR2DL1/CD158a, while UCB-derived NK cells did not express CD158i. The expression of other KIRs was detected by Q-RT-PCR (KIR2DS1, KIR2DS5, KIR2DL4, KIR2DL5, KIR3DL2, KIR3DS1). HESC-derived NK cells also expressed CD94 (88% $CD56^+CD94^+$) and NKG2A (79.7%

$CD56^+NKG2A^+$) (upon dimerization interacts with HLA-E). Another group of activating receptors called natural cytotoxic receptors (NCR), including Nkp30 (49.9% $CD56^+Nkp30^+$), Nkp44 (72.3% $CD56^+Nkp44^+$), and Nkp46 (85.9% $CD56^+Nkp46^+$) were all expressed on $CD34^+CD45^+$ hESC-derived NK cells, as well as CD16 (17.4% $CD56^+CD16^+$), (FcγRIII) and the lymphoid associated markers CD2 (2.7% $CD56^+CD2^+$), and CD7 (59.2% $CD56^+CD7^+$). With the exception of CD2, the expression of all other markers was superior to that of $CD34^+$ UCB derived NK cells.

At day 32, hESC-derived $CD56^+CD45^+$ NK cells demonstrated cytolytic activity toward K562 target cells comparable to UCB-derived NK cells. The cytolytic activity resided in the $CD56^+$ population. As hESC-derived NK cells also expressed FcγRIII, that binds the Fc region of IgG molecules, antibody-dependent cell-mediated cytotoxicity (ADCC) against the NK-resistant Raji cell line in a CD20 dose-dependent manner. In response to overnight stimulation with IL-12/IL-18, sorted $CD34^+CD45^+$ hESC-derived NK cells also upregulated IFNγ production similar to what seen in UCB derived NK cells (35.2% $CD56^+IFN\gamma^+$ for hESC vs 20.2% for UCB).

Main interests and limitations

- Generation of functional NK cells from hESCs with a clonal frequency which is similar to that observed for similarly cultured UCB^-CD34^+ cells, but with a lower proliferation capability. Detailed characterization of phenotypic and functional properties of these hESC-derived NK cells that provides a foundation for comparison of NK cells generated from different ontogenic sources.
- Two pathways predominate NK cell maturation ($CD56^{bright}$ cells with low expression of CD16 and KIRs, poor cytolytic activity and high levels of cytokine production, and $CD56^{dim}$ cells with high expression of CD16 and KIRs, but most of the cytolytic activity). However, this study does not allow for discrimination between these pathways in hESCs.

7.3 Directed Differentiation of Human Embryonic Stem Cells into Functional Dendritic Cells Through the Myeloid Pathway (Slukvin et al. 2006)

Culture methods and media supplements: A three-step method was used with (1) the previously described coculture system on OP9 as described in section 2.2, followed by (2) expansion of myeloid cells with GM-CSF under feeder-free culture conditions and (3) maturation of the DCs generated with calcium ionophore A23187 treatment.

On day 9 and 10 of the hESC/OP9 cocultures, cells were harvested and resuspended in α-MEM supplemented with 10% FBS (Hyclone) and 100 ng/mL GM-CSF into tissue culture flasks coated with poly-2-hydroxyethyl methacrylate (Sigma) to prevent cell adherence. Cells were cultured for 8–10 days with a half-medium change every fourth day. Subsequently, cells were spun over 20% Percoll (Sigma). To induce differentiation of myeloid cells into DCs, the cells were then cultured again for 7–9 days in 2-hydroxyethyl methacrylate coated flasks in StemSpan SFEM (Stem Cell Technologies) supplemented with lipid mixture 1 (Sigma) and 100 ng/mL GM-CSF and 100 ng/mL IL-4. Half-medium was changed every fourth day. To further maturate DCs, cells were then cultured in SFEM with 400 ng/mL A23187 calcium ionophore (Sigma) for 48 h.

Results: After 9–10 days of culture with GM-CSF and removal of clumps and dead cells by Percoll separation, a cell population containing 90% $CD45^+$ cells was obtained. The majority of these cells expressed GM-CSFR/CD116 and the spectrum of myeloid markers (CD16, CD11b, CD11c, CD15, and weakly CD33). In a typical experiment with GM-CSF and IL-4, individual floating cells with well-defined dendrites could be seen after 7–10 days. DCs were identified by flow cytometry as expressing CD1a, DC-SIGN, CD4, CD11c, CD16, MHC class I and II, CD80 and CD86 as well as low levels of CD11b, CD123, and CD40. No expression of CD83, CD208 (DC-LAMP), CD207 (Langerin) nor Fascin, an actin-binding protein shown to be a highly selective DC marker was detected, suggesting that these DCs were immature. These cells also expressed CCL17, CCL13, and MMP-12 transcripts that are highly specific for DC genes and not monocytes or macrophages. In terms of cell yield, phenotypic, and functional properties, the addition of TNF-α (20 ng/mL) or IFN-α (10^4 U/mL) did not improve the generation of functional DCs from hESCs above the GM-CSF and IL4 combination. After treatment with A23187 calcium ionophore to further maturate DCs, cells began to express Fascin and CD83. These cells were able to uptake and process ovalbumin and induced proliferation of allogeneic adult lymphocytes in MLR as well as naïve UCB-derived T cells. This capacity was similar to that observed with DCs obtained from PB-derived monocytes but lower than that obtained from $CD34^+$-PB DCs. These hESC-derived DCs were also capable of presenting specific antigens to T cells through the MHC class I pathway but with a lower efficiency than both other populations. Subpopulations of immature monocytes expressing M-CSFR but lacking HLA-DR were also produced in this system.

Main interests and limitations

- This method provides functional dendritic precursors in numbers that are sufficient for functional studies and genetic manipulations (up to 4×10^7 DCs at a time from 10^7 hESCs initially plated).
- A distinct phenotype feature of hESC-derived DCs is the coexpression of CD14 with CD1a, which is not always observed on UCB-derived DCs.
- Requirements to be followed for their generation from hESCs:
  (i) Control the efficiency of the hESC/OP9 coculture system, as low numbers of $CD34^+CD45^+$ precursors fail to produce myeloid progenitors that differentiate to DCs.
  (ii) Use whole cell suspensions rather than isolated hematopoietic progenitors from hESC/OP9 cocultures.
  (iii) Culture the cells in nonadherent conditions.
  (iv) GM-CSF (compared to SCF or Flt3L) is the most critical factor for expansion of myeloid precursors.

8. DERIVATION OF HESC-DERIVED HEMATOPOIETIC CELLS CAPABLE OF REPOPULATING ANIMAL MODELS

In vitro studies do not demonstrate the development of "true" HSCs from hESCs. Indeed, the ability of HSCs to reconstitute the entire hematopoietic system in animal models such as the nonobese diabetic severe combined immunodeficiency (NOD/SCID) mouse provides the ultimate functional assay available so far to define mammalian HSCs. As detailed below, preliminary data from independent groups (Narayan et al. 2005; Wang et al. 2005b; Tian et al. 2006) already suggest that hESC-derived hematopoietic cells have the potential to give rise to HSCs.

8.1 Generation of Hematopoietic Repopulating Cells from Human Embryonic Stem Cells Independent Of Ectopic HOXB4 Expression (Wang et al. 2005b)

Culture methods and media supplements: HESCs-derived $CD45^{-}$PFV hemogenic precursors were generated as described in section 5.1, and transduced cells with HOXB4-expressing retrovirus, as described in section 3.4.

Results: We have observed that intravenous (IV) transplantation of high dose (5×10^5 to 1.6×10^7) of $CD45^{-}$PFV-derived hematopoietic cells caused early death in sub-lethally irradiated NOD/SCID recipient mice, partially due to emboli formed from rapid cellular aggregation in response to mouse serum. Less than 40% of the IV-transplanted mice survived 8 weeks after transplantation, in contrast to 100% survival of recipients receiving a similar dose of cultured primitive somatic hematopoietic cells. No human chimerism was detected in surviving recipients of hESC-derived hematopoietic cells. Bypassing the circulation by transplantation of $4–15 \times 10^4$ hESC-derived hematopoietic cells directly into the BM cavity of the femur (intra-femoral, IF injection) allowed recipient survival (>90% at 8 weeks). Detection of human hematopoietic engraftment 8 weeks posttransplantation was done by Flow cytometry and Southern blot/PCR analysis for human-specific α-satellite sequences. A representative example of multilineage human hematopoietic reconstitution of BM cells from the injected femur showed 3.87% $CD45^{+}$ cells that coexpressed CD19, or CD33, or glycophorin A and CD36, indicative of lymphoid, myeloid, and erythroid development. Southern blot analysis revealed that 11 out of 19 mice transplanted with hESC-derived hematopoietic cells by IF demonstrated SCID-repopulating cells, compared with 6 of 6 mice injected with purified UCB-derived cells. In contrast to somatic cells, human chimerism from injection of hESC-derived hematopoietic cells was barely detected in noninjected BM sites, indicating that very few transplanted cells were capable of mobilization and engraftment beyond the site of delivery. Retroviral-induced ectopic expression of HOXB4 did not improve the reconstituting ability into NOD/SCID recipients by IF transplantation (no chimerism detected by both Flow cytometry and PCR from HOXB4- and vector-transduced cells).

Main interests and limitations

- $CD45^{-}$PFV hemogenic precursors are capable of hematopoietic engraftment in NOD/SCID mice after intra-femoral but not IV injection, providing evidence of HSC function from hESCs. The levels of engraftment found are very low.
- Lentiviral based overexpression of HOXB4, the best-known candidate for conferring HSC function on mouse ESC-derived hematopoietic cells has no effect on HSC function of hESCs.
- Suggests that single-gene reconstitution strategies are unlikely to restore HSC function of hESC-derived hematopoietic cells.

8.2 Human Embryonic Stem Cell-derived Hematopoietic Cells are Capable of Engrafting Primary as Well as Secondary Fetal Sheep Recipients (Narayan et al. 2005)

Culture methods and media supplements: HESC differentiation was carried out on the mouse BM stromal cell line S17. On day 17, cocultured cells were harvested and $CD34^{+}$ cells concentrated with magnetic anti-CD34 microbeads (Miltenyi Biotech). $CD34^{+}/Lin^{-}$ or $CD34^{+}/CD38^{-}$ cells were purified on FACSVantage. Preimmune Dorset Merino sheep fetuses (65 days old, term gestation is 150 days) received transplants of 13,000–140,000 $CD34^{+}$/Lin- or $CD34^{+}/CD38^{-}$ cells. Cells were injected *in utero* into the fetal peritoneal cavity. Lambs were born at term and then animals were stimulated with human GM-CSF (hGM-CSF) for 5 days (only human cells respond to hGM-CSF).

Results: A maximum of 0.1% $CD34^{+}$ or $CD45^{+}$ human cells in BM and/or PB was detected by flow cytometry. Human CD4 and CD8 are absent in the sheep model, and CD19 was not detected. One sheep positive by PCR in the BM was sacrificed and 10^{6} cells were injected into a secondary fetal sheep recipient. At 26 months and after administration of hGM-CSF, the engraftment was confirmed by PCR for the human ß2-microglobulin gene. Differentiation of hematopoietic elements into both myeloid (0.1% CD15, 0.2% CD36) and lymphoid like (0.1% CD2) lineages was found. In addition, BM aspiration from the secondary recipient cultured in methylcellulose with cytokines (not defined) gave rise to 3 out of 24 myeloid colonies that were positive for human DNA.

Main interests and limitations

First report of a long-term reconstituted hematopoiesis in a xenotransplantation model different from the NOD/SCID mouse that provides a developmental age matched microenvironment (fetal sheep). However, levels of chimerism detected by PCR are extremely low.

8.3 Hematopoietic Engraftment of Human Embryonic Stem Cell-derived Cells is Regulated by Recipient Innate Immunity (Tian et al. 2006)

Culture methods and media supplements: HESCs allowed to differentiate on S17 cells for 7–24 days were used for IV and intra-BM injections. From 0.5×10^6 to 4×10^6 cells were injected into sub-lethally irradiated NOD/SCID mice. Some recipients were injected with anti-ASGM1 antibody in order to deplete NK (and possibly macrophages also) cell activity. Secondary transplants were done from mice originally injected with cells from 7 to 19 days of differentiation. In each case, BM from one primary recipient was IV injected to two or three NOD/SCID mice.

Results: Peaking at day 14, a population of $CD34^+CD31^+CD45^-$ cells developed, followed by a $CD34^+CD45^+$ cell population, that peaked at 17–21 days of coculture. CFU development (giving rise to myeloid–erythroid colonies) peaked during the same period. Nonsorted hematopoietic cells that had been allowed to differentiate for 7–10, 14–19, or 21–24 days were injected into primary NOD/SCID mice. The mean frequency of engraftment was 0.76% at day 7 to 10, 0.16% at day 14 to 19, and 0.24% at day 21 to 24. After treatment of the recipient mice with anti-ASGM1, the mean of engraftment was 0.9% (vs 0.3% in control recipients) at day 12 of differentiation, and 0.49% (vs 0.22%) at day 20. In secondary transplants, 13/28 recipients showed evidence of engraftment at 3–6 months post-transplant, ranging from 0.08 to 0.2% human $CD45^+$ cells detected in the BM.

Main interests and limitations

- Nonselected populations of differentiated derivatives of hESCs are capable of long-term primary and secondary engraftment into NOD/SCID mice but only low levels of engraftment are achieved.
- Time course analysis shows in vivo reconstituting ability of differentiated derivatives of hESCs at any time point tested.
- Both IV and intra-BM methods of transplantation are comparable in terms of level of engraftment. In contrast to the study summarized in section 8.1, IV transplantation of differentiated hESCs was successful in the same xenogenic model, suggesting that the methods of differentiation/selection of hESCs (coculture vs hEBs, nonselected populations vs $CD45^-$PFV-derived hematopoietic cells) might play a role in this process.
- Suggests a role for recipient NK cells as an immune barrier for hESC transplantation in this model.

9. OVERALL CONCLUSION

Current efforts are directed at improving hESC-derived hematopoiesis from hESCs in order to generate cells that are competent for repopulating adult hosts.

Although the preliminary data presented in section 8 suggest that hESCs have HSC properties, the transient nature of hematopoietic differentiation from hESCs

Table 2. Comparison between human EB- and co-culture-based hematopoietic differentiation systems

Expression/property	hEBs		Co-cultures	
CD45[a]	+		Low	
CD31/PECAM-1[a]	+		+	
CD34[a]	+		+	
VE-Cadherin[a]	+		+	
KDR/Flk1[a]	+		+	
SCL/Tal-1[b]	+		+	
GATA-1 and GATA-2[b]	+		+	
Timing of hematopoietic differentiation	CD34/CD31 around end of first week followed by CD45 around end of second week		CD34/CD31 around end of first week followed by CD45 around end of second week	
Bipotent hemogenic endothelium	+		ND	
Development of myeloid lineages	+		+	
Development of erythroid lineages	+		+	
Development of lymphoid lineages	T cells –	(MHC class II + cells)	T cells –	(NK + DC cells)
In vivo hematopoietic reconstitution	+	+	+	+
HOXB4-induced in vivo hematopoietic reconstitution	–		ND	

[a]Cell surface marker
[b]Transcription factor
PECAM-1 = platelet endothelial cell adhesion molecule-1
SCL = stem cell leukemia factor
ND = not determined

in both stroma- and hEB-based systems suggests that long-term self-renewal of HSCs is still not properly supported by these two methods. A comparison of several parameters reflecting the efficiency of hematopoietic differentiation achieved to date using these methods is presented in Table 2. Although the efficiency of hematopoietic differentiation is comparable between the methods, the hEB-based system may be preferable since it avoids the use of xenogenic or allogenic cells, and may be also more amenable to large-scale culture for clinical purposes. Preliminary studies presented in section 4 also suggest that combining methods may improve the hematopoietic differentiation from hESCs.

Further understanding of intrinsic and extrinsic factors affecting development of hESC-derived hematopoietic lineages is still required. In particular, standardized procedures for maintenance of the undifferentiated state of hESCs, controlled differentiation and genetic manipulation of hESCs and their hematopoietic derivatives need to be achieved. Future challenges will also include identification of reliable surrogate markers to distinguish hESC-derived HSCs from progenitors and/or design of new HSC in vivo assays based on human hematopoietic reconstitution.

REFERENCES

Bowles, K.M., Vallier, L., Smith, J.R., Alexander, M.R., and Pedersen, R.A. (2006) HOXB4 overexpression promotes hematopoietic development by human embryonic stem cells. Stem Cells, 24(5): 1359–1369.

Cameron, C.M., Hu, W.S., and Kaufman, D.S. (2006) Improved development of human embryonic stem cell-derived embryoid bodies by stirred vessel cultivation. Biotechnol. Bioeng., 17: 1654–7998.

Cerdan, C., Rouleau, A., and Bhatia, M. (2004) VEGF-A165 augments erythropoietic development from human embryonic stem cells. Blood, 103: 2504–2512. Epub 2003 Dec 4.

Chadwick, K. et al. (2003) Cytokines and BMP-4 promote hematopoietic differentiation of human embryonic stem cells. Blood, 102: 906–915.

Cho, S.K., Bourdeau, A., Letarte, M., and Zuniga-Pflucker, J.C. (2001) Expression and function of CD105 during the onset of hematopoiesis from Flk1(+) precursors. Blood, 98: 3635–3642.

Choi, K., Kennedy, M., Kazarov, A., Papadimitriou, J.C., and Keller, G. (1998) A common precursor for hematopoietic and endothelial cells. Development, 125: 725–732.

Chung, Y.S. et al. (2002) Lineage analysis of the hemangioblast as defined by FLK1 and SCL expression. Development, 129: 5511–5520.

Emambokus, N.R. and Frampton, J. (2003) The glycoprotein IIb molecule is expressed on early murine hematopoietic progenitors and regulates their numbers in sites of hematopoiesis. Immunity, 19: 33–45.

Kaufman, D.S., Hanson, E.T., Lewis, R.L., Auerbach, R., and Thomson, J.A. (2001) Hematopoietic colony-forming cells derived from human embryonic stem cells. Proc. Natl. Acad. Sci. USA, 98: 10716–10721.

Kim, S.J. et al. (2005) Hematopoietic differentiation of embryoid bodies derived from the human embryonic stem cell line SNUhES3 in co-culture with human bone marrow stromal cells. Yonsei Med. J., 46: 693–699.

Mikkola, H.K., Fujiwara, Y., Schlaeger, T.M., Traver, D., and Orkin, S.H. (2003) Expression of CD41 marks the initiation of definitive hematopoiesis in the mouse embryo. Blood, 101: 508–516.

Mitjavila-Garcia, M.T. et al. (2002) Expression of CD41 on hematopoietic progenitors derived from embryonic hematopoietic cells. Development, 129: 2003–2013.

Narayan, A.D. et al. (2005) Human embryonic stem cell-derived hematopoietic cells are capable of engrafting primary as well as secondary fetal sheep recipients. Blood, 107: 733.

Ng, E.S., Davis, R.P., Azzola, L., Stanley, E.G., and Elefanty, A.G. (2005) Forced aggregation of defined numbers of human embryonic stem cells into embryoid bodies fosters robust, reproducible hematopoietic differentiation. Blood, 106: 1601–1603.

Nishikawa, S.I., Nishikawa, S., Hirashima, M., Matsuyoshi, N., and Kodama, H. (1998) Progressive lineage analysis by cell sorting and culture identifies FLK1+VE-cadherin+ cells at a diverging point of endothelial and hemopoietic lineages. Development, 125: 1747–1757.

Oberlin, E., Tavian, M., Blazsek, I., and Peault, B. (2002) Blood-forming potential of vascular endothelium in the human embryo. Development, 129: 4147–4157.

Qiu, C., et al. (2005) Differentiation of human embryonic stem cells into hematopoietic cells by co-culture with human fetal liver cells recapitulates the globin switch that occurs early in development. Exp. Hematol., 33: 1450–1458.

Slukvin, I.I., Vodyanik, M.A., Thomson, J.A., Gumenyuk, M.E., and Choi, K.D. (2006) Directed differentiation of human embryonic stem cells into functional dendritic cells through the myeloid pathway. J. Immunol., 176: 2924–2932.

Tavian, M., Hallais, M.F., and Peault, B. (1999) Emergence of intraembryonic hematopoietic precursors in the pre-liver human embryo. Development, 126: 793–803.

Tavian, M., Robin, C., Coulombel, L., and Peault, B. (2001) The human embryo, but not its yolk sac, generates lympho-myeloid stem cells: mapping multipotent hematopoietic cell fate in intraembryonic mesoderm. Immunity, 15: 487–495.

Tian, X., Morris, J.K., Linehan, J.L., and Kaufman, D.S. (2004) Cytokine requirements differ for stroma and embryoid body-mediated hematopoiesis from human embryonic stem cells. Exp. Hematol., 32: 1000–1009.

Tian, X., Woll, P.S., Morris, J.K., Linehan, J.L., and Kaufman, D.S. (2006) Hematopoietic engraftment of human embryonic stem cell-derived cells is regulated by recipient innate immunity. Stem Cells, 24(5): 1370–1380.

Vodyanik, M.A., Bork, J.A., Thomson, J.A., and Slukvin, I.I. (2005) Human embryonic stem cell-derived CD34+ cells: efficient production in the co-culture with OP9 stromal cells and analysis of lymphohematopoietic potential. Blood, 105: 617–626. Epub 2004 Sep 16.

Wang, L. et al. (2004) Endothelial and hematopoietic cell fate of human embryonic stem cells originates from primitive endothelium with hemangioblastic properties. Immunity, 20: 31–41.

Wang, J. et al. (2005a) In vitro hematopoietic differentiation of human embryonic stem cells induced by co-culture with human bone marrow stromal cells and low dose cytokines. Cell Biol. Int., 29: 654–661.

Wang, L. et al. (2005b) Generation of hematopoietic repopulating cells from human embryonic stem cells independent of ectopic HOXB4 expression. J. Exp. Med., 201: 1603–1614.

Woll, P.S., Martin, C.H., Miller, J.S., and Kaufman, D.S. (2005) Human embryonic stem cell-derived NK cells acquire functional receptors and cytolytic activity. J. Immunol., 175: 5095–5103.

Zambidis, E.T., Peault, B., Park, T.S., Bunz, F., and Civin, C.I. (2005) Hematopoietic differentiation of human embryonic stem cells progresses through sequential hematoendothelial, primitive, and definitive stages resembling human yolk sac development. Blood, 106: 860–870. Online April 14, 2005; DOI 10.1182/blood-2004-11-4522.

Zhan, X., et al. (2004) Functional antigen-presenting leucocytes derived from human embryonic stem cells in vitro. Lancet, 364: 163–171.

CHAPTER 6

NEURAL DIFFERENTIATION

ZHI-JIAN ZHANG, JASON S. MEYER, AND SU-CHUN ZHANG

Department of Anatomy and Neurology, School of Medicine and Public Health, The Stem Cell Research Prorgram, The Waisman Center, The WiCell Institute, University of Wisconsin, Madison, WI 53705, USA

One of the keys to using human embryonic stem cells (hESCs) in brain research and their potential application in the treatment of neurological diseases is the directed differentiation of neuronal and glial subtypes. For potential future application in cellular therapy for neurological diseases, it is essential that hESCs can either be efficiently directed to a specific neural subtype or that the desired neural cells can be enriched or purified. Alternatively, as a model system to investigate early human brain development, it will be crucial to create hESC differentiation models that recapitulate *in vivo* development. Ideally, this system should be manipulated with defined components so that it will provide a dynamic tool for dissecting molecular mechanisms underlying early embryonic development that would otherwise not be readily obtainable. Regardless of the goals, the foundations for directed neural differentiation are the developmental principles learned from embryology studies. This requires a careful consideration of the intrinsic program of human precursor cells with necessary extrinsic instructive signals. It will be equally important to establish a rigorous set of criteria to define a target cell type derived from hESCs *in vitro*. In this chapter, we will summarize the success and shortcomings of attempts to direct hESCs to neurons and glial cells from the above perspectives and considerations, with a focus on a few extensively pursued cell types and differentiation systems.

1. NEURAL INDUCTION AND NEURAL SUBTYPE SPECIFICATION *IN VIVO*

The vertebrate nervous system has two major divisions, the central nervous system (CNS) consisting of the brain and the spinal cord, and the peripheral nervous system (PNS) consisting of the nervous tissues not included in the brain and spinal cord. The formation of the nervous system is a complex process that

J.R. Masters et al (eds.), Embryonic Stem Cells, 85–108.

begins with neural induction in which part of the ectoderm is specified to become the neural ectoderm, resulting in the formation of the neural plate, followed by the neural tube. Around the time of the neural tube closure, neural crest cells (the precursors of many cells within the PNS) emerge from the neural tube, migrate and contribute to the PNS as well as to several nonneural structures. The neuroepithelial cells within the neural tube give rise to neural progenitor cells in the CNS, producing neurons first, followed by the glial cell types astrocytes and oligodendrocytes at later stages. The cellular and molecular mechanisms underlying neural induction remain unclear. It has been suggested that inhibition of bone morphogenetic proteins (BMPs) by their antagonists noggin, follistatin, and chordin secreted from the organizer is involved, as well as activation of some positive instructive factors such as fibroblast growth factors (FGFs) (Wilson and Edlund 2001; Stern 2005).

Neural induction is followed by the patterning or regionalization of the neuroectoderm along the anterior–posterior (A–P) and dorsal–ventral (D–V) principal axes, requiring organizing centers that emit signaling molecules (Stern 2001). The A–P neural patterning occurs at open neural plate stages. Neural plate cells are induced to express position-specific genes along the A–P axis in broad domains corresponding to the forebrain, midbrain, hindbrain, and spinal cord by exposure to Wnts, FGFs, BMPs, and/or retinoic acid (RA) signals. Meanwhile, the neural tube is patterned along the D–V axis into more subdivisions by two opposing signals: sonic hedgehog (Shh) produced ventrally from the notochord and floor plate, and BMP produced dorsally from the roof plate. Through this patterning process, neuroectodermal cells in each subdivision along the A–P and D–V axes acquire their proper regional identity, thus becoming neural progenitors. Subsequently, these neural progenitors are differentiated into a large diversity of subtypes of neurons and glial cells by exposure to specific environmental cues such as a unique set of morphogens at precise concentrations according to a strict timeline (Lumsden and Krumlauf 1996; Rubenstein and Beachy 1998; Edlund and Jessell 1999; Jessell 2000; Osterfield et al. 2003).

During the generation of spinal cord motor neurons, neuroectodermal cells first obtain an initial rostral neural character through the regulation of BMP, FGF, and Wnt signaling. Then a spinal positional identity is acquired in response to caudalizing signals such as RA and finally, Shh secreted by the notochord and the floor plate specifies the pattern of generation of motor neurons and certain classes of ventral interneurons in a concentration-dependent manner (Jessell 2000; Briscoe and Ericson 2001).

To obtain a midbrain dopaminergic (DA) neuron cell fate after the formation of the midbrain–hindbrain boundary (MHB), neuroectodermal cells within the midbrain acquire a ventral midbrain DA progenitor identity in response to several secreted factors, including fibroblast growth factor 8 (FGF8), Wnt1 secreted by the MHB and Shh secreted by the notochord and the floor plate (Smits et al. 2006).

Multiple signaling cascades may be required to regulate these events at a different time and place for each neural cell type. Hence, in order to obtain a specific neural phenotype, neuroepithelial cells may need to simultaneously incorporate the signaling inputs from both A–P and D–V patterning factors and spatial morphogens to assume a positional identity and express a set of markers at the right time and in the right place. Thus, an understanding of the basic principles and mechanisms underlying neural development *in vivo* is essential to be able to direct neural differentiation from hESCs *in vitro*.

2. NEURAL LINEAGE DIFFERENTIATION FROM HUMAN ES CELLS

2.1 Neuroepithelial Differentiation

The differentiation of neural cell lineages from hESCs is attractive not only because of the unlimited supply of specific neural cells for potential cell therapy, but perhaps more importantly in the study of early human neural development. According to what has been learned from classical embryology studies, the first step in the neural differentiation of hESCs is the specification of the neuroectodermal fate, including the derivation of neuroepithelial cells.

Neuroepithelial differentiation of hESCs has been achieved by several different protocols to date (Table 1). The spontaneous differentiation of hESCs can be achieved by expanding the hESC cultures at a high density, which leads to overgrowth of the surviving hESCs and subsequent spontaneous differentiation (Reubinoff et al. 2000, 2001). Hence, the differentiation process is generally less controlled and the cultures obtained are heterogeneous, with modest efficiency of neural differentiation. This neural progenitor population can be further enriched under a neural cell culture condition containing the appropriate signals.

Highly enriched hESC-derived neural progenitors can also be attained through stromal cell derived inducing activity (SDIA) by coculturing hESCs on bone marrow-derived stromal cells (Perrier et al. 2004; Muotri et al. 2005; Tabar et al. 2005). The direct contact of hESCs with stromal cells has been interpreted in favor of an inductive mechanism for neural differentiation, although the molecular nature of the inducing signal(s) remains elusive. The coculture of hESCs with these cells for 4 weeks results in greater than 90% of the hESCs differentiating toward a neural precursor cell phenotype which express markers of the neuroectoderm such as Pax6, Sox1, nestin, and Musashi (Perrier et al. 2004; Tabar et al. 2005). Similarly, after 3–4 weeks of coculturing of hESCs with PA6 cells, most of the hESC colonies became positive for nestin (Muotri et al. 2005). It should be noted that while nestin is highly expressed in neural progenitors, it is occasionally found elsewhere outside of the nervous system. Hence, nestin expression alone is generally not sufficient to determine whether the differentiated cells are neural progenitors. Pax6 and Sox1, which are expressed by neuroectodermal cells at the earliest stage during embryonic development, are usually seen after 4 weeks of coculture with stromal cells. This is possibly due to a need for expansion of individual hESCs before these cells aggregate to a

Table 1. Summary of neuroepithelial and neural crest cell differentiation from human ESCs

Cell type	Reference	Cell line	Culture methods	Medium	Characterization			
					Morphology	Antibodies	*In vivo* tranplantation	Notes
Neuroepithelial cells	Zhang et al. 2001	H1, H9, H9.2	Floating EBs defined medium	DMEM/ F12/N2 FGF2	Neural tube-like rosette	Nestin PSA-NCAM Musashi-1	Neonatal mouse brain differentiated into neurons and glia	72–84% NEP of total cells 96% of NEP are nestin+
	Reubinoff et al. 2001	HES-1	On feeder cells then cell aggregates	DMEM/F12 knockout serum EGF, FGF2		Nestin PSA-NCAM	Newborn mouse brain differentiated into neurons and glia	54% NEP colonies among total colonies 97% of NEP cells are nestin+
	Carpenter et al. 2001	H1, H7, H9	Floating EBs defined medium	DMEM/F12/ N2/B27 FGF2, EGF, IGF-1 PDGF-AA, NT-3, BDNF, RA		Nestin, A2B5 PSA-NCAM	ND	56–87% A2B5 or PSA-NCAM+ cells of total cells
	Schulz et al. 2003	BG01 BG02	On feeder cells then adherent culture	DMEM/F12 N2,MEDII LIF, FGF2	Rosette	Nestin	ND	58% rosette cells of total cells
	Perrier et al. 2004	H1, H9, HES3	Coculturing with stromal cells (MS5, MS5-Wnt1, S2)	DMEM, N2 15% knockout serum	Rosette	Pax6, Sox1 Nestin, NCAM	ND	>90% neural rosettes cells of the total cells

Itsykson et al. 2005	HES1 HES2	Floating EBs defined medium	DMEM/F12/ B27 FGF2, Noggin	Rosette	Nestin PSA-NCAM Musashi-1	ND	At 3 weeks 78% nestin+ cells, 91.3% Musashi+ cells, 96.2% PSA-NCAM+ cells of the total cells
Li et al. 2005	H1, H9	Defined adherent colony culture floating EBs	DMEM/ F12/N2 FGF2	Rosette	Nestin, Otx2 Pax6 Sox1	ND	First report of sequential stages of neuroectodermal development
Gerrard et al. 2005	H1, H7 H1-T5	On matrigel or PLL/Laminin	N2 B27 medium Noggin, FGF2	Rosette	Nestin PSA-NCAM Musashi-1 Pax6, Sox1	ND	At 30 days 97.7% nestin+ cells, 96.3% Musashi+ cells, 92.3% PSA-NCAM+ cells of the total cells
Tabar et al. 2005	H1 HES3	Coculturing with stromal cells (MS5)	N2, FGF2, EGF, Noggin	Rosette	Nestin NCAM Pax6 Sox1	Adult (3-month-old) rat Striatum, differentiated into neurons and glia	<90% NEP cells of the total cells
Muotri et al. 2005	Cyth25	Coculturing with stromal cells (PA6)	DMEM/F12 10% knockout serum		Nestin	E14 mouse brain, differentiated into functional neural lineages, generated mature, active human neurons integrate into the adult mouse brain	Most of colonies are nestin+

(*Continued*)

Table 1. Summary of neuroepithelial and neural crest cell differentiation from human ESCs—Cont'd.

					Characterization			
Cell type	Reference	Cell line	Culture methods	Medium	Morphology	Antibodies	*In vivo* tranplantation	Notes
	Shin et al. 2005	BG01 BG02	On feeder cells then cells aggregates	DMEM/F12 15% FCS N2,MEDII FGF2	Rosette	Nestin Musashi-1	ND	58% rosette formation
	Lowell et al. 2006	HES 181	Coculturing with stromal cells (OP9-DI1) Delta1	N2 B27 FGF2		Pax6 Sox1	ND	15% PAX-6+ colonies
	Yao et al. 2006	H1 HSF6	On Matrigel defined medium	N2/B27 FGF2, Noggin	Rosette	Pax6 Sox1	ND	
Neural crest	Pomp et al. 2005	HES-1 HUES 7 HUES 1	Coculturing with stromal cells (PA6)	90% BHK-21/ GMEM 10% knockout serum	Bipolar, pseudounipolar, intermediate	Peripherin Brn3a p75 AP2 TH	ND	10–20% Brn3a+/ peripherin+ colonies

ND, not determined

sufficient density to be capable of differentiating into neural precursors. These neural precursors appear to be biased toward the mid- or hindbrain fate as evidenced by their preferential differentiation to dopaminergic neurons (Perrier et al. 2004; Brederlau et al. 2006; Martinat et al. 2006). Similar work using mouse ESCs indicates that SDIA-induced neural precursors express mid/hindbrain transcription factors but not forebrain markers (Watanabe et al. 2005). Thus, the stromal coculture method is very useful for differentiating hESCs to neural subtypes that are present in the mid/hindbrain regions. Nevertheless, this approach introduces unknown components into the system. If the differentiated cells are to be used for transplantation, the requirement of direct contact in the coculture system would create a need to remove the stromal cells which are often established tumorigenic cell lines.

Alternate strategies for neural differentiation from hESCs often involve a step in which the hESCs form free-floating aggregates, often referred to as embryoid bodies (EBs). This step serves at least two purposes. First, it removes self-renewing signals (e.g., following separation from mouse embryonic fibroblasts) and initiates cellular differentiation through cell–cell interactions. Human ESC aggregates form after hESC colonies are detached via enzymatic treatment (Zhang et al. 2001) or by mechanical scraping from the feeder cell and subsequent culture in suspension. Human ESCs within these aggregates differentiate spontaneously into heterogeneous cell types of all three embryonic germ layers. Hence, addition of signaling molecules is necessary at certain stages to bias the differentiation process toward a neural fate.

RA, a morphogen for multilineage differentiation, is one of the most commonly used chemicals for promoting neural differentiation. Treatment of differentiating cultures with RA yields reasonable neural differentiation from human ES cells (Carpenter et al. 2001). Within the differentiated neural cells, there is a wide range of developmental stages, from nestin and polysialylated neural cell adhesion molecule (PSA-NCAM)-expressing precursors to β-III tubulin positive neurons with a week of differentiation (Carpenter et al. 2001; Schuldiner et al. 2001). Perhaps more importantly, neural progenitors following RA treatment most likely are biased to a caudal fate, which will restrict the progenitors to neuronal and glial cell types within a more caudal region. It should be noted that some cell culture supplements such as the often used B27 may also contain RA.

According to the neural induction theory described above, inhibition of BMPs and Wnts or activation of FGF signaling promotes neuroectoderm specification (Wilson and Edlund 2001). Inhibition of BMP signaling by its antagonist noggin results in a robust differentiation of neuroepithelial-like cells from hESCs (Pera et al. 2004; Gerrard et al. 2005; Itsykson et al. 2005; Yao et al. 2006). It has been shown that a blockage of BMP signaling by noggin can direct the initial differentiation of hESCs into an intermediate cell type that lacked neural markers, but could be converted into neural progenitors upon culturing in basal medium supplemented with FGF2 (Pera et al. 2004). The initial noggin treatment on hESCs either in a suspension system or in a matrigel-adherent culture system resulted in a highly enriched neural progenitor cell population compared with the non-noggin treated cells, as more than 90% of the cells were positive for neural progenitor markers, including PSA-NCAM, Musashi, and nestin (Gerrard et al. 2005; Itsykson et al. 2005). In addition, these neural progenitors expressed Otx2, En1, and En2 whether in the presence or absence of noggin, indicating their identity as early anterior neuroectodermal cells not affected by noggin treatment (Itsykson et al. 2005). These observations seem to suggest that noggin is sufficient to block BMP signaling and enhance the neuroectodermal specification from hESCs. However, the possibility of other signaling pathways contributing to neural specification (such as FGFs) cannot be completely excluded from these studies. A recent study shows that coculturing hESCs with stromal cells secreting the Notch ligand Delta1 in the presence of FGF2 leads to a significant increase in the number of Pax6+ cells compared to the control group, suggesting that Notch signaling promotes neural differentiation in hESCs (Lowell et al. 2006).

Wnt signaling has been implicated in neural or epidermal fate determination through interactions with BMP and FGF signaling in chick and Xenopus embryos (Baker et al. 1999; Gomez-Skarmeta et al. 2001; Wilson et al. 2001). Several studies using mouse ESCs indicate that inhibition of Wnt signaling by the Wnt antagonist secreted frizzled-related protein 2 (Sfrp2) promotes neural epithelial differentiation (Aubert et al. 2002; Haegele et al. 2003; Bouhon et al. 2005). In contrast, another group has reported that an increase of Wnt/β-catenin signaling can stimulate neural differentiation from mouse ESCs (Otero et al. 2004). It will be useful to determine whether and how Wnt signing plays a role in neural induction using the hESC model, not only for a better understanding of early human neural development but also for obtaining neuroepithelial cells from hESCs with greater efficiency.

It has been shown that FGF signaling is required for neural induction by acting as a direct neural inducer (Kengaku and Okamoto 1993; Lamb and Harland 1995; Alvarez et al. 1998; Wilson et al. 2000; Linker and Stern 2004; Delaune et al. 2005). Based on this theory, we have established a chemically defined culture system for neuroectoderm differentiation from hESCs using FGF2. A chemically defined culture system will provide ultimate control over the extrinsic signaling environment for systematic manipulation of the cell fates (Zhang et al. 2001). The initial step of this process is the formation of ESC aggregates in suspension with medium containing serum replacement for 4 days, followed by transferring the ESC aggregates to a serum-free neural differentiation medium (DMEM/F12 medium plus N2) in the presence of FGF2 for 3 days. Subsequently, the aggregates are plated onto an adhesive substrate at a low density. Under this condition, columnar neuroepithelial cells are observable after ~10 days of differentiation from the hESC stage. These columnar cells further form neural tube-like rosette structures in the center of individual colonies after 14–16 days of differentiation. The neuroectodermal identity of these rosette cells is confirmed by their expression of neuroepithelial markers such as nestin, Musashi-1, Pax6, Sox1, Otx2 and CD-133 (Zhang et al. 2001; Li et al. 2005). The formation of neural tube-like rosettes has also been observed under various culture conditions using other hESC lines (Schulz et al. 2003; Tabar et al. 2005; Yao et al. 2006). Hence, the neural tube-like rosette is a useful and readily identifiable sign of neural induction in live cultures. This system results in consistent and robust neural differentiation, as 70–90% of the differentiated progeny are neuroepithelial cells. Cells at this stage do not express mature phenotypes of neurons and glial cells, indicating that the neuroepithelial cells are at a relatively synchronized developmental stage. An important aspect of this system is that the formation of neural rosette structures by the hESCs after 2 weeks of culture mirrors neural plate/tube formation at 3 weeks of human gestation (O'Rahilly and Muller 1994) considering that hESCs are derived from a 5- to 6-day-old embryo. Hence, the culture system can provide a useful platform for the dissection of molecular interactions underlying the early phase of neuroectoderm specification in humans.

2.2 Neural Crest Differentiation

Neurons and glial cells of the PNS are derived from the neural crest. The neural crest is induced at the lateral edge of the neural plate through interactions with surrounding tissues. Although the precise nature of the neural crest-inducing signals is not yet fully understood, it is likely that the combination of an intermediate level of BMP signaling together with the action of Wnt, FGF, RA, and Notch activates a genetic program in the ectoderm that defines the prospective neural crest cells (Morales et al. 2005). Around the time of neural tube closure and as they initiate their migration into the periphery, neural crest cells progressively adopt specific fates as a result of both intrinsic and extrinsic influences. Differentiation of a neural crest lineage from hESCS has not been systematically investigated although cells with phenotypes of neural crest derivatives have been observed in various culture conditions. Mouse and monkey ES cells can be differentiated into neural crest derivatives such as the sensory lineage (Brn3a+/Peripherin+ neurons) and autonomic lineage (TH+/Phox2b+/Peripherin+ neurons) when cocultured with PA6 stromal cells together with BMP treatment (Mizuseki et al. 2003). Using a similar coculture system but without BMP treatment, peripheral sensory, and sympathetic-like neurons were generated from hESCs which were characterized by the coexpression of Brn3.0/peripherin and TH/peripherin, respectively (Pomp et al. 2005). Nevertheless, the efficiency of deriving neural crest lineage cells from hESCs is low and only a limited number of cell types have been examined. This is likely due to the fact that the approach is not specific for the induction of the neural crest cells, since SDIA mainly promotes the differentiation of other neural subtypes such as midbrain DAergic-like neurons (Zeng et al. 2004; Brederlau et al. 2006). Therefore, an optimal protocol for the differentiation of neural crest cells from hESCs remains to be developed.

2.3 Directed Differentiation of Neural Subtypes

Of specific importance with regard to possible hESC-based cell therapies for neurodegenerative disorders is the directed differentiation of desired neuronal subtypes and glial cells. The keys to directing hESCs to a particular neural subtype have been found within the developmental principles of the nervous system. Developmentally, a specific neural cell fate is determined by the interplay between the intrinsic program of precursor cells and temporally and spatially available extracellular signals. Therefore, to achieve directed differentiation of subclasses of neurons from hESCs, one would select a set of morphogens that program precursors at a particular stage toward a specific neuronal type.

Another important issue for generating neural subtypes from stem cells is how these cells produced *in vitro* can be identified. In the brain and spinal cord, each type of neural cell, particularly the neuron, carries a unique set of identifying markers representing its regional, genetic, functional, electrochemical, and morphological properties, which can be used as a standard for characterizing a specific cell type *in vitro*. Cells under unusual culture environments or stress conditions may aberrantly express some genes and may exhibit altered morphologies. Thus, the mere expression of a single gene or morphological criterion by itself is not sufficient to define a cell type *in vitro*. Specification and determination of a neural cell type depends on sequentially regulated gene expression. It thus requires an exhaustive set of molecular markers in combination with positional, morphological, and functional indicators to define a cell type (Svendsen et al. 2001; Zhang 2001), while the absence of other markers is equally important. For identification of neuronal subtypes, in addition to the requirements described above, an additional set of criteria is needed to define the transmitter phenotypes such as those involved in the synthesis of the transmitter, metabolizing enzymes as well as transporters.

2.3.1 Midbrain dopaminergic neurons

Among neuronal cell populations, midbrain dopaminergic (DA) neurons in the substantia nigra pars compacta and in the ventral tegmental area are involved in the control of movement and emotional behavior, respectively, and their degeneration or functional impairment causes Parkinson's disease and other neurological disorders. Midbrain DA neurons are generated in MHB of the developing embryo. Although the detailed mechanisms underlying the development of midbrain DA neurons are not yet fully understood, it has been shown that signaling molecules such as FGF8, Shh, and Wnts can activate the transcription of Otx2, En1, Pax2, Lmx1a, Lmx1b, Nurr1, and Pitx3, which coordinate to specify the midbrain dopaminergic fate (Andersson et al. 2006; Smits et al. 2006).

In order to determine the differentiated progeny of hESCs as midbrain DA neurons, the cells should possess a variety of characteristics. First, they should possess the basic neuronal properties, as outlined above. Secondly, the cells should possess the biochemical machinery to metabolize the transmitter DA such as tyrosine hydroxylase (TH), aromatic L-amino acid decarboxylase (AADC), dopamine transporter (DAT), and vesicular monoamine transporter-2 (VMAT2), but not gamma-aminobutyric acid (GABA), serotonin, dopamine beta hydroxylase (DβH), and phenylethanolamine N-methyltransferase (PNMT). Additionally, the cells should express midbrain regional characteristics by expressing En1, Lmx1a, Lmx1b, Nurr1,and Pitx3, but not characteristics of other neural regions such as Bf1 and Hox genes. Finally, the cells should be able to secrete and reuptake DA in an activity-dependent manner and potentially reverse the functional deficit in a Parkinson's animal model.

The differentiation of hESCs to dopaminergic-like neurons has been achieved using several protocols, involving the use of coculturing with stromal cells and/or the patterning molecules FGF8 and Shh (Table 2). Perrier and colleagues (Perrier et al. 2004) showed that the coculture of hESCs with mouse bone marrow mesenchymal cell lines (MS5, MS5-Wnt1, and S2 stromal cells) for 4 weeks led to the efficient differentiation of neuroepithelial cells. Extended propagation of these neural progenitor cells in the presence of FGF8, Shh, and related differentiation factors such as TGF-β3 resulted in significant numbers of TH-positive neurons (up to 40% of the total cells, ~70% of the total neurons). Some of the TH-positive cells coexpressed En1, 50% of these cells coexpressed AADC, while 100% coexpressed VMAT2. The presence of midbrain DA neurons was also confirmed by the expression of Pax2 and Pax5, evoked DA release, the presence of tetrodotoxin-sensitive action potentials and the electron-microscopic visualization of TH-positive synaptic terminals. This study provides sufficient characterization of a dopaminergic phenotype and thus, it provides an efficient protocol for obtaining high yields of midbrain DA neurons from hESCs.

A similar coculture approach for generating DA neurons was also utilized by other groups using different hESC lines, but these studies resulted in a lower efficiency of DA neuron derivation (Buytaert-Hoefen et al. 2004; Zeng et al. 2004; Park et al. 2005). One of the advantages of the above approach is that it is a simple and relatively efficient technique for generating DA neurons from hESCs. However, the coculture with stromal cells may introduce unknown and potential tumorigenic factors into the system, which will be a particular burden for future clinical applications of hESC-derived DA neurons.

We have established a chemically defined culture protocol for the directed differentiation of DA neurons from hESCs (Yan et al. 2005). The neuroepithelial cells generated using this method initially carry a forebrain identity (Zhang et al. 2001; Li et al. 2005). Exposure to FGF8, followed by Shh treatment, resulted in the differentiation of neuroepithelial cells to DA neurons that express TH and AADC but not DβH. The DA identity is further confirmed by the activity-dependent release of DA. In this study, we have discovered that, depending on the intrinsic properties of neuroepithelial cells, exposure to the same set of

Table 2. Summary of differentiation of midbrain dopaminergic neurons and motor neurons from human ES cells

					Characterization						
Cell type	Reference	Cell line	Culture Methods	Medium	Morphology	Anti-bodies	*In vitro* electro phsiology	*In vitro* release	*In vitro* uptake	*In vivo* tranplan-tation	Notes
Midbrain DA neurons	Yan et al. 2005	H9, H1	Defined medium	DMEM/ F12/N2 FGF8, Shh	10–20 μm in diameter multipolar with axons and dend-rites	TH, En1 AADC VMAT2 c-RET	Functional	Yes	ND	ND	About 30% TH of total cells
	Perrier et al. 2004	H9, H1, HES-3	Coculturing with stromal cells (MS5) (MS5-Wnt1)	DMEM/ N2 FGF8, Shh TGF-beta3		TH, En1 AADC VMAT2 Lmx	Functional	Yes	ND	ND	Up to 40% TH of total cells
	Buytaert-Hoefen et al. 2004	BG01	Coculturing with stromal cells (PA6)	GMEM 10% knockout serum		TH	ND	ND	ND	ND	13 TH+/ well (12-well plate)
	Park et al. 2004	MB03	Defined medium	N2, bFGF, TGF-a		TH	ND	Yes	ND	ND	20% TH of total cells
	Ben-Hur et al. 2004	HES-1	DMEM/ F12/N2	DMEM/ F12/B27 EGF, bFGF		TH	ND	ND	ND	102–630 TH+ cells per brain with partial behavioral recovery (12 weeks)	0.56% TH of total cells

Schulz et al. 2004	BG01 BG03	Defined medium	DMEM/ F12/N2	TH, DAT VMAT2 AADC	Functional	Yes	ND	Some TH+ survived (8 weeks)	60–70% TH of total neurons
Zeng et al. 2004	BG01	Coculturing with stromal cells (PA6)	GMEM 10% knockout serum	TH	ND	Yes	ND	Few TH+ survived (5 weeks)	87% TH–containing colonies
Park et al. 2005	HSF-6, SNU-hES-3 Miz-hES-1	Coculturing with stromal cells (PA6-Shh)	ITS/N2/ AA, FGF8	TH, Pax2	Functional	Yes	Yes	No clear TH+ survived (6 weeks)	41.1% TH of total neurons
Martinat et al. 2006	H9	Coculturing with stromal cells (MS5) (MS5-Wnt1)	DMEM/ N2, FGF8, Shh TGF-beta3	TH	Functional	Yes	ND	Low level of TH immunoreactivity in graft with fuctional recovery (6 weeks)	Over-expression of Nurr1 and Pitx3
Brederlau et al. 2006	SA002.5	Coculturing with stromal cells (PA6)	GMEM 8% knockout serum	TH	Functional	Yes	ND	Few TH+ survived no behavioral recovery (13 weeks)	7.4% TH of total cells 37.1% of total neurons

(Continued)

Table 2. Summary of differentiation of midbrain dopaminergic neurons and motor neurons from human ES cells—Cont'd.

					Characterization						
Cell type	Reference	Cell line	Culture Methods	Medium	Morphology	Anti-bodies	*In vitro* electro phsiology	*In vitro* release	*In vitro* uptake	*In vivo* tranplan-tation	Notes
Motor neurons	Li et al. 2005	H1, H9	Defined medium	DMEM/ F12/N2 FGF2, RA Shh	Neuronal	Olig 2, HB9 Islet 1 HoxC8 ChAT VAChT Synapsin	Functional	ND	ND	ND	24% HB9+ cells of total cells
	Singh-Roy et al. 2005	H1	Defined medium	N2 RA, Shh	Neuronal	Olig 2, HB9 Islet 1 ChAT	Functional	ND	ND	ND	Cell sorting, up to 1% HB9+ cells of total cells
	Shin et al. 2005	BG01, BG02	Defined medium	B27 RA, Shh	Neuronal	Olig 2 Islet 1 ChAT	ND	ND	ND	ND	No definitive demons-tration of motor neu-rons, in vivo application

morphogens, namely Shh and FGF8, generate different types of DA neurons. When the early neuroepithelial cells (differentiated from hESCs for 10 days) were treated with Shh and FGF8, some of the DA neurons express the midbrain transcription factor En1. In contrast, most of the DA neurons differentiated from late neuroepithelial cells (differentiated for 15–17 days from hES cells) do not express En1. Instead, some of them express Bf1, a forebrain transcription factor, suggesting that many of the DA neurons may be a forebrain type of cell. Indeed, many of them coexpress GABA, a phenotype of the forebrain, especially olfactory DA neurons (Gall et al. 1987; Max et al. 1996). This finding illustrates the importance of coordinating the intrinsic program of a precursor cell with extracellular morphogens in specifying a particular subtype of neuron. It also emphasizes the need of multiple markers to define a type of neuron, such as a subtype of DA neurons.

Both the stromal cell coculture method (Buytaert-Hoefen et al. 2004; Perrier et al. 2004; Zeng et al. 2004; Park et al. 2005) and the chemically defined induction culture system (Schulz et al. 2004; Yan et al. 2005) described above can result in a robust differentiation of DA neurons. However, neither method appears to be sophisticated enough to produce DA neurons that carry all the midbrain dopaminergic traits such as expression of En1, Nurr1, Lmx1b, Pitx3, and DAT. The problem appears to be the lack of coordination between ventral midbrain patterning and the induction of the dopaminergic pathway. By overexpressing Nurr1 (Chung et al. 2002; Kim et al. 2002; Sonntag et al. 2004) or Pitx3 (Chung et al. 2005) in mouse ESCs, differentiated DA neurons appear to possess some (but not a whole set of) midbrain DA neuronal markers. Mouse ESCs overexpressing Nurr1 generate more TH/En1 double positive DA neurons in the presence of SHH and FGF8 (Kim et al. 2002).

Expression of Pitx3 in mouse ESCs increases the number of ADH2 + DA neurons, while the total number of DA neurons remains unchanged after *in vitro* differentiation, suggesting an important role of Pitx3 for specification of certain subgroups of midbrain DA neurons (Chung et al. 2005). Overexpression of both Nurr1 and Pitx3 in mouse and human ESC-derived neural precursors while cocultured with PA6 stromal cells resulted in an increase in the number of TH-positive cells and gene expression of some midbrain DA markers such as DAT (Martinat et al. 2006). Recently, it has been shown that overexpression of Lmx1a in mouse ESCs can efficiently promote the differentiation of midbrain DA neurons in the presence of Shh and FGF8 (Andersson et al. 2006). Cells generated in this way display the correct phenotype of ventral midbrain DA neurons as they possess the whole complement of markers including Lmx1a, Lmx1b, En1, Nurr1, Pitx3, and DAT in the same TH-expressing neurons. Together, these findings indicate that multiple intracellular signaling events as well as their coordination with extracellular signals need to be in place in order to specify bona fide midbrain DA neurons. The chemically defined differentiation system will likely allow the delineation of environmental factors that make cell-fate decision at each step along the differentiation process.

2.3.2 Spinal motor neurons

Spinal motor neurons are generated within a specific region (pMN domain) in the ventral half of the developing neural tube (Jessell 2000). Motor neurons at varying levels of the spinal cord innervate different groups of muscles. Hence, signaling molecules that instruct motor neuron specification in different segments of the spinal cord also vary (Liu et al. 2001). The best known signaling pathway is mediated by Shh and RA for the specification of cervical spinal motor neurons by activating the transcription of Olig2 in the progenitors and HB9 in postmitotic motor neurons.

To characterize the progeny of hESCs as spinal motor neurons, they should meet most, if not all of the following criteria. First and foremost, they should exhibit general neuronal properties as described above. Secondly, since spinal motor neurons utilize the neurotransmitter acetylcholine, they should also possess related properties such as the expression of choline acetyltransferase (ChAT) and vesicular acetylcholine transferase (VAChT), and the release of acetylcholine in an activity-dependent manner. Thirdly, spinal motor neurons are specified through transcription of Olig2 and HB9. Hence, expression of the transcription factors Olig2 in the progenitors and HB9 and related factors such as Hox genes, Islet1, and Lim3 is critical to distinguish them from other cholinergic neurons. Finally, the ability to induce acetylcholine receptor clustering in myocytes and to induce muscle contraction is the hallmark of a functional motor neuron.

Spinal motor neurons have been generated from mouse ESCs as demonstrated in a variety of studies (Wichterle et al. 2002; Harper et al. 2004; Ikeda et al. 2004; Miles et al. 2004; Soundararajan et al. 2006). More recently, a few groups have reported differentiation of motor neurons or motor neuron-like cells from hES cells (Li et al. 2005; Shin et al. 2005; Singh-Roy et al. 2005). In each example, known important signaling molecules such as RA and Shh were used to guide motor neuron differentiation (Table 2). In the first reported case of successful hESC-derived motor neuron differentiation from Li et al. (2005), early neuroepithelial cells were generated as neural rosettes *in vitro* (Zhang et al. 2001) in the presence of RA to caudalize the cells to a spinal fate. Isolation of these caudalized neuroepithelia in the form of rosettes was followed by growth in suspension culture as cell aggregates in the presence of Shh to direct differentiation toward the ventral spinal cord fate. After about 4 weeks of differentiation from hESCs, many neural precursors express Olig2, the transcription factor expressed by motor neuron progenitors. Further differentiation for another week yields ~20% of all cells expressing the motor neuron-specific transcription factor HB9.

Refinements of this protocol have increased the yield of HB9-positive motor neurons to nearly 50% of the total population. In addition to expression of HB9, these cells have also been shown to express a number of other motor neuron-related markers including ChAT, VAChT, and Islet 1/2. Importantly, the hESC-generated motor neurons induce acetylcholine receptor clustering on myocytes after the motor neurons innervate the muscle cells and stimulate muscle contraction. Thus, the motor neurons generated from hESCs possess most of the hallmarks of spinal cord motor neurons. Analysis of the expression of Hox genes suggests that the majority of motor neurons resemble cervical spinal motor neurons as they express HoxC8. These findings suggest that signaling pathways involved in the specification of cervical spinal motor neurons is very similar to that in animal embryos. Additionally, this study has identified a relatively early stage of neuroectoderm development that is responsive to morphogens for motor neuron specification, which has important implications in the generation of other neuronal subtypes including different types of DA neurons described above.

Singh-Roy and colleagues (2005) have differentiated hESCs to motor neurons in order to isolate the target cells. Human ESCs were differentiated to motor neurons by growing them to nearly 90% confluency, followed by transient transfection with a green fluorescent protein (GFP) construct under the control of a HB9 enhancer. These highly confluent cells were then grown as free-floating EBs in the presence of RA and Shh for nearly a week until GFP expression was observed. The cells were sorted based on their expression of GFP and plated in coculture with skeletal myoblasts to allow for survival and maturation. Although the differentiation culture itself generated ~1% of HB9-expressing motor neurons among the total population, it can be enriched to a nearly pure population of motor neurons, as the cells can be sorted based on the HB9-regulated GFP expression.

2.3.3 Oligodendrocytes

In addition to neurons, the glial cells of the CNS are important. Oligodendrocytes are a particular type of glial cell found in the CNS which function to ensheath axons, and through this insulating feature they assist in the conduction of a neural impulse down the length of an axon. Defects in oligodendrocytes have been implicated in diseases such as multiple sclerosis (MS) in which oligodendrocytes are lost, and thus the propagation of neural impulses down the length of the axon is severely reduced.

Oligodendrocytes within the spinal cord traditionally were thought to be generated within the same region as motor neurons, but they are not generated until later in development once the motor neurons have been generated. Like motor neurons, oligodendrocytes arise from progenitor cells that express the transcription factor Olig2, although it is still unclear whether or not motor neurons and oligodendrocytes share a common progenitor (Noble et al. 2004; Richardson et al. 2006; Wu et al. 2006). Several signaling molecules have been implicated as being instrumental for oligodendrocyte differentiation, including Shh, RA, FGF-2, and EGF, as well as the transcription factor Olig2.

To characterize the progeny of hESCs as oligodendrocytes they should meet most, if not all of the following criteria. Morphologically, oligodendrocyte progenitors exhibit a bipolar morphology. They differ from bipolar neuronal progenitors in that the processes of oligodendrocyte progenitors are similar and they are generally shorter than neurites found on neuronal progenitors. Oligodendrocyte progenitors are extremely motile, and they often migrate to areas where there are few cells such as in the periphery of a culture. In contrast, neuronal progenitors in culture tend to migrate in chains and their neurites connect to each other. More mature oligodendrocytes are generally easily distinguishable from neurons and astrocytes given their small cell bodies with little cytoplasm barely surrounding the nucleus and its typical highly branched thin processes often forming web-like structures. Available antibodies are highly specific to the oligodendrocyte lineage including O4, GalC, CNP, MBP, PLP, etc. Nevertheless, attention should be paid to the subcellular localization of the antigens as most of them are specifically and almost exclusively localized to the cell membrane. Formation of myelin sheaths by oligodendrocytes *in vitro* or *in vivo* can be unequivocally demonstrated by electron microscopy.

Oligodendrocyte differentiation from hESCs has been observed along neural differentiation (Zhang 2001; Itsykson et al. 2005; Nistor et al. 2005). The derivation of a large proportion of oligodendrocytes from hESCs has recently been reported by Keirstead and colleagues (Faulkner and Keirstead 2005; Keirstead et al. 2005; Nistor et al. 2005). This has been achieved with a relatively simple procedure. Human ESCs were differentiated as cell aggregates in a "glial restricted medium" in the presence of FGF2 and EGF for 2 days, followed by the exposure to RA (10 μM) for 8 days. This treatment results in the formation of "yellow spheres". The yellow spheres were mechanically selected and plated onto matrigel to grow a more homogenous population again in the presence of FGF2 and EGF. Within a few weeks, the growth factors were removed and the cells were allowed to differentiate to multipolar cells with branched processes *in vitro*. These cells adopt phenotypes similar to that of oligodendrocytes, including the expression of related markers such as O4, GalC, RIP, NG2, and PDGFRα. Based on expression of these markers, at least 80% of the differentiated progeny appear to be oligodendrocytes. Morphologically, the oligodendrocytes generated in this way appear quite different from those of primary cultures from brain tissues of many species including humans (Zhang et al. 2000; Windrem et al. 2002). Most of the oligodendrocyte markers such as PDGFRα, NG2, O4, GalC stained the cells diffusely instead of being localized to cell membranes of primary oligodendrocytes as described above. In the future, it will be very useful and important for other laboratories to reproduce the results and to confirm that the hESC-generated oligodendrocytes differ from primary oligodendrocytes in morphology and antigenic expression.

2.3.4 Astrocytes

Astrocytes are the most abundant cell type and are distributed throughout the brain and spinal cord. They participate in almost every aspect of physiology and pathology of the CNS. Astrocytes are also often seen in neural differentiation cultures from hESCs, but usually after several weeks of differentiation (Carpenter et al. 2001; Reubinoff et al. 2001; Zhang et al. 2001; Gerrard et al. 2005). This delay at least partially corresponds to the intrinsic program of human neuroepithelial cells producing neurons followed by the generation of astrocytes. To date, there is no report describing the directed differentiation of astrocytes from hESCs, at least under defined conditions. Yet, astrocytes may also be critical for the determination/maturation of neuronal subtypes. For instance, astrocytes in the ventral mesencephalon, but not the dorsal mesencephalon or other parts of the brain, play an instructive role in the specification of neural progenitors to the midbrain DA neuronal fate and/or survival of the differentiated neurons (Wagner et al. 1999). The functional differences of astrocytes from different regions of the brain may be attributed to the molecular profiles produced by regionally specific astrocytes. Ventral mesencephalic astrocytes express a high level of Wnts (Castelo-Branco et al. 2006), which has also been shown to be important in the specification of midbrain DA neurons (Castelo-Branco et al. 2003). DA neurons differentiated from hESCs survived poorly following transplantation into the brain of animal models of Parkinson's disease. One of the reasons could be the lack of astrocytes in the culture system as most of the DA differentiation cultures, when used for transplantation, contain few, if any, astrocytes. Hence, directed differentiation of astrocytes, particularly those possessing appropriate regionally defined characteristics, will likely have significant implications in our understanding of glial development as well as their potential use in cell therapy.

3. CONCLUDING REMARKS AND FUTURE DIRECTIONS

Neuroectodermal differentiation from hESCs is generally robust under various differentiation conditions described above. Further differentiation to neuronal subtypes has been achieved to varying degrees. Spinal motor neurons can now be efficiently and reproducibly differentiated from hESCs under a defined condition. These *in vitro* produced motor neurons possess almost all of the hallmarks of a motor neuron in the spinal cord. Still, this is limited to a subset of motor neurons, mainly cervical motor neurons. Dopaminergic neurons can also be efficiently generated from hESCs. However, these DA neurons generated by current protocols are by no means authentic as none of the cells possess all of the hallmarks of a midbrain DA neuron. Many other neural subtypes such as serotonergic and GABAergic neurons, although commonly seen in general neural differentiation cultures, have not yet been achieved through directed differentiation. Therefore, directed differentiation of neural subtypes from hESCs will remain a major focus of efforts in the next few years.

To date, most of the neural differentiation protocols are based on direct contact coculture with stromal cells or morphogen-producing cells with an aim to achieving an efficient production of target cell types. This type of approach has substantial weaknesses from the standpoint of both basic research and potential future clinical applications. For mechanistic studies, the coculture approach brings in unknown factors. For potential cell therapy, it brings potentially dangerous elements into the system as most of the cell lines are established tumorigenic cells. Therefore, future work needs to identify signals the stroma cells have provided and to devise a defined system for guided differentiation. In this regard, creative and more sophisticated approaches that take into consideration the need of stage-specific progenitors will be necessary for the production of certain types of neurons and glia such as midbrain dopaminergic neurons.

In general, analysis of hESC-derived neural cell types has not been sufficiently rigorous. Dopaminergic phenotypes have been well demonstrated in some of the studies by expression of DA metabolism-related enzymes but lack of other monoamine metabolizing proteins together with activity-dependent release of DA. However, additional phenotypes of midbrain DA neurons such as En1, Nurr1, Lmx1b, Pitx3, and DAT have either not been looked at or examined only by RT-PCR. As neural progenitors with various regional identities and transmitter properties are present in most of the differentiation culture conditions, the mere expression of midbrain related transcription factor mRNA in mixed cultures is not sufficient to define that TH-positive neurons are ventral midbrain DA neurons. It will be necessary to demonstrate colocalization of TH with a complete set of nuclear midbrain transcription factors, as well as in combination with other midbrain DA neuronal properties to confirm the cell's authentication as a midbrain DA neuron. Given the mixed nature of most differentiation cultures, a mere look at the target cells may not be sufficient. Some other cell types, at least related cell types such as serotonergic and GABAergic neurons that may be produced under the dopaminergic cultures should be investigated. This is important as the presence of these contaminating cells may interfere with or mask the function of the target cell type.

Acknowledgments

Studies in our laboratory have been supported by the NIH-NCRR (RR016588), NIH-NINDS (NS045926, NS046587), the Michael J. Fox Foundation, the National ALS Association, and the Myelin Project.

REFERENCES

Alvarez, I.S., Araujo, M., et al. (1998) Neural induction in whole chick embryo cultures by FGF. Dev. Biol., 199(1): 42–54.

Andersson, E., Tryggvason, U., et al. (2006) Identification of intrinsic determinants of midbrain dopamine neurons. Cell, 124: 393–405.

Aubert, J., Dunstan, H., et al. (2002) Functional gene screening in embryonic stem cells implicates Wnt antagonism in neural differentiation. Nat. Biotechnol., 20(12): 1240–1245.

Baker, J.C., Beddington, R.S., et al. (1999) Wnt signaling in Xenopus embryos inhibits bmp4 expression and activates neural development. Genes Dev., 13(23): 3149–3159.

Ben-Hur, T., Idelson, H., et al. (2004) Transplantation of human embryonic stem cell-derived neural progenitors improves behavioral deficit in Parkinsonian rats. Stem Cells, 22(7): 1246–1255.

Bouhon, I.A., Kato, H., et al. (2005) Neural differentiation of mouse embryonic stem cells in chemically defined medium. Brain Res. Bull., 68(1–2): 62–75.

Brederlau, A., Correia, A.S., et al. (2006) Transplantation of human embryonic stem cell-derived cells to a rat model of Parkinson's disease: effect of in vitro differentiation on graft survival and teratoma formation. Stem Cells. 24: 1433–1440.

Briscoe, J. and Ericson, J. (2001) Specification of neuronal fates in the ventral neural tube. Curr. Opin. Neurobiol., 11(1): 43–49.

Buytaert-Hoefen, K.A., Alvarez, E., et al. (2004) Generation of tyrosine hydroxylase positive neurons from human embryonic stem cells after coculture with cellular substrates and exposure to GDNF. Stem Cells 22(5): 669–674.

Carpenter, M.K., Inokuma, M.S., et al. (2001). Enrichment of neurons and neural precursors from human embryonic stem cells. Exp. Neurol., 172(2): 383–397.

Castelo-Branco, G., Sousa, K.M., et al. (2006) Ventral midbrain glia express region-specific transcription factors and regulate dopaminergic neurogenesis through Wnt-5a secretion. Mol. Cell Neurosci., 31(2): 251–262.

Castelo-Branco, G., Wagner, J., et al. (2003) Differential regulation of midbrain dopaminergic neuron development by Wnt-1, Wnt-3a, and Wnt-5a. Proc. Natl. Acad. Sci. USA, 100(22): 12747–12752.

Chung, S., Hedlund, E., et al. (2005) The homeodomain transcription factor Pitx3 facilitates differentiation of mouse embryonic stem cells into AHD2-expressing dopaminergic neurons. Mol. Cell Neurosci., 28(2): 241–252.

Chung, S., Sonntag, K.C., et al. (2002) Genetic engineering of mouse embryonic stem cells by Nurr1 enhances differentiation and maturation into dopaminergic neurons. Eur. J. Neurosci., 16(10): 1829–1838.

Delaune, E., Lemaire, P., et al. (2005) Neural induction in Xenopus requires early FGF signalling in addition to BMP inhibition. Development, 132(2): 299–310.

Edlund, T. and Jessell, T.M. (1999) Progression from extrinsic to intrinsic signaling in cell fate specification: a view from the nervous system. Cell, 96(2): 211–224.

Faulkner, J. and Keirstead, H.S. (2005) Human embryonic stem cell-derived oligodendrocyte progenitors for the treatment of spinal cord injury. Transpl. Immunol., 15(2): 131–142.

Gall, C.M., Hendry, S.H., et al. (1987) Evidence for coexistence of GABA and dopamine in neurons of the rat olfactory bulb. J. Comp. Neurol., 266(3): 307–318.

Gerrard, L., Rodgers, L., et al. (2005) Differentiation of human embryonic stem cells to neural lineages in adherent culture by blocking bone morphogenetic protein signaling. Stem Cells, 23(9): 1234–1241.

Gomez-Skarmeta, J., de La Calle-Mustienes, E., et al. (2001) The Wnt-activated Xiro1 gene encodes a repressor that is essential for neural development and downregulates Bmp4. Development, 128(4): 551–560.

Haegele, L., Ingold, B., et al. (2003) Wnt signalling inhibits neural differentiation of embryonic stem cells by controlling bone morphogenetic protein expression. Mol. Cell. Neurosci., 24(3): 696–708.

Harper, J.M., Krishnan, C., et al. (2004) Axonal growth of embryonic stem cell-derived motoneurons in vitro and in motoneuron-injured adult rats. Proc. Natl. Acad. Sci. USA, 101(18): 7123–7128.

Ikeda, R., Kurokawa, M.S., et al. (2004) Transplantation of motoneurons derived from MASH1-transfected mouse ES cells reconstitutes neural networks and improves motor function in hemiplegic mice. Exp. Neurol. 189(2): 280–292.

Itsykson, P., Ilouz, N., et al. (2005) Derivation of neural precursors from human embryonic stem cells in the presence of noggin. Mol. Cell. Neurosci., 30(1): 24–36.

Jessell, T.M. (2000). Neuronal specification in the spinal cord: inductive signals and transcriptional codes. Nat. Rev. Genet., 1(1): 20–29.

Keirstead, H.S., Nistor, G., et al. (2005) Human embryonic stem cell-derived oligodendrocyte progenitor cell transplants remyelinate and restore locomotion after spinal cord injury. J. Neurosci., 25(19): 4694–4705.

Kengaku, M. and Okamoto, H. (1993) Basic fibroblast growth factor induces differentiation of neural tube and neural crest lineages of cultured ectoderm cells from Xenopus gastrula. Development, 119(4): 1067–1078.

Kim, J.H., Auerbach, J.M., et al. (2002) Dopamine neurons derived from embryonic stem cells function in an animal model of Parkinson's disease. Nature, 418(6893): 50–56.

Lamb, T.M. and Harland, R.M. (1995) Fibroblast growth factor is a direct neural inducer, which combined with noggin generates anterior–posterior neural pattern. Development, 121(11): 3627–3636.

Li, X.J., Du, Z.W., et al. (2005) Specification of motoneurons from human embryonic stem cells. Nat. Biotechnol., 23(2): 215–221.

Linker, C. and Stern, C.D. (2004) Neural induction requires BMP inhibition only as a late step, and involves signals other than FGF and Wnt antagonists. Development, 131(22): 5671–5681.

Liu, J.P., Laufer, E., et al. (2001) Assigning the positional identity of spinal motor neurons: rostrocaudal patterning of Hox-c expression by FGFs, Gdf11, and retinoids. Neuron, 32(6): 997–1012.

Lowell, S., Benchoua, A., et al. (2006) Notch promotes neural lineage entry by pluripotent embryonic stem cells. PLoS Biol., 4(5): e121.

Lumsden, A. and Krumlauf, R. (1996) Patterning the vertebrate neuraxis. Science, 274(5290): 1109–1115.

Martinat, C., Bacci, J.J., et al. (2006). Cooperative transcription activation by Nurr1 and Pitx3 induces embryonic stem cell maturation to the midbrain dopamine neuron phenotype. Proc. Natl. Acad. Sci. USA, 103(8): 2874–2879.

Max, S.R., Bossio, A., et al. (1996). Co-expression of tyrosine hydroxylase and glutamic acid decarboxylase in dopamine differentiation factor-treated striatal neurons in culture. Brain Res. Dev. Brain Res., 91(1): 140–142.

Miles, G.B., Yohn, D.C., et al. (2004) Functional properties of motoneurons derived from mouse embryonic stem cells. J. Neurosci., 24(36): 7848–7858.

Mizuseki, K., Sakamoto, T., et al. (2003) Generation of neural crest-derived peripheral neurons and floor plate cells from mouse and primate embryonic stem cells. Proc. Natl. Acad. Sci. USA, 100(10): 5828–5833.

Morales, A.V., Barbas, J.A., et al. (2005) How to become neural crest: from segregation to delamination. Semin. Cell. Dev. Biol., 16(6): 655–662.

Muotri, A.R., Nakashima, K., et al. (2005) Development of functional human embryonic stem cell-derived neurons in mouse brain. Proc. Natl. Acad. Sci. USA, 102(51): 18644–18648.

Nistor, G.I., Totoiu, M.O., et al. (2005) Human embryonic stem cells differentiate into oligodendrocytes in high purity and myelinate after spinal cord transplantation. Glia, 49(3): 385–396.

Noble, M., Proschel, C., et al. (2004) Getting a GR(i)P on oligodendrocyte development. Dev. Biol., 265(1): 33–52.

O'Rahilly, R. and Muller, F. (1994) Neurulation in the normal human embryo. Ciba Found. Symp., 181: 70–82; discussion 82–89.

Osterfield, M., Kirschner, M.W., et al. (2003) Graded positional information: interpretation for both fate and guidance. Cell, 113(4): 425–428.

Otero, J.J., Fu, W., et al. (2004) Beta-catenin signaling is required for neural differentiation of embryonic stem cells. Development, 131(15): 3545–3557.

Park, C.H., Minn, Y.K., et al. (2005) In vitro and in vivo analyses of human embryonic stem cell-derived dopamine neurons. J. Neurochem., 92(5): 1265–1276.

Pera, M.F., Andrade, J., et al. (2004) Regulation of human embryonic stem cell differentiation by BMP-2 and its antagonist noggin. J. Cell. Sci., 117(Pt 7): 1269–1280.

Perrier, A.L., Tabar, V., et al. (2004) Derivation of midbrain dopamine neurons from human embryonic stem cells. Proc. Natl. Acad. Sci. USA, 101(34): 12543–12548.

Pomp, O., Brokhman, I., et al. (2005) Generation of peripheral sensory and sympathetic neurons and neural crest cells from human embryonic stem cells. Stem Cells 23(7): 923–930.

Reubinoff, B.E., Itsykson, P., et al. (2001) Neural progenitors from human embryonic stem cells. Nat. Biotechnol., 19(12): 1134–1140.

Reubinoff, B.E., Pera, M.F., et al. (2000) Embryonic stem cell lines from human blastocysts: somatic differentiation in vitro. Nat. Biotechnol., 18(4): 399–404.

Richardson, W.D., Kessaris, N., et al. (2006) Oligodendrocyte wars. Nat. Rev. Neurosci., 7(1): 11–18.

Rubenstein, J.L. and Beachy, P.A. (1998) Patterning of the embryonic forebrain. Curr. Opin. Neurobiol., 8(1): 18–26.

Schuldiner, M., Eiges, R., et al. (2001) Induced neuronal differentiation of human embryonic stem cells. Brain Res., 913(2): 201–205.

Schulz, T.C., Noggle, S.A., et al. (2004) Differentiation of human embryonic stem cells to dopaminergic neurons in serum-free suspension culture. Stem Cells, 22(7): 1218–1238.

Schulz, T.C., Palmarini, G.M., et al. (2003) Directed neuronal differentiation of human embryonic stem cells. BMC Neurosci., 4: 27.

Shin, S., Dalton, S., et al. (2005) Human motor neuron differentiation from human embryonic stem cells. Stem Cells Dev., 14(3): 266–269.

Singh-Roy, N., Nakano, T., et al. (2005) Enhancer-specified GFP-based FACS purification of human spinal motor neurons from embryonic stem cells. Exp. Neurol., 196(2): 224–234.

Smits, S.M., Burbach, J.P., et al. (2006) Developmental origin and fate of meso-diencephalic dopamine neurons. Prog. Neurobiol., 78(1): 1–16.

Sonntag, K.C., Simantov, R., et al. (2004) Temporally induced Nurr1 can induce a non-neuronal dopaminergic cell type in embryonic stem cell differentiation. Eur. J. Neurosci., 19(5): 1141–1152.

Soundararajan, P., Miles, G.B., et al. (2006) Motoneurons derived from embryonic stem cells express transcription factors and develop phenotypes characteristic of medial motor column neurons. J. Neurosci., 26(12): 3256–3268.

Stern, C.D. (2001) Initial patterning of the central nervous system: how many organizers? Nat. Rev. Neurosci., 2(2): 92–98.

Stern, C.D. (2005) Neural induction: old problem, new findings, yet more questions. Development, 132(9): 2007–2021.

Svendsen, C.N., Bhattacharyya, A., et al. (2001) Neurons from stem cells: preventing an identity crisis. Nat. Rev. Neurosci., 2(11): 831–834.

Tabar, V., Panagiotakos, G., et al. (2005) Migration and differentiation of neural precursors derived from human embryonic stem cells in the rat brain. Nat. Biotechnol., 23(5): 601–606.

Wagner, J., Akerud, P., et al. (1999) Induction of a midbrain dopaminergic phenotype in Nurr1-overexpressing neural stem cells by type 1 astrocytes. Nat. Biotechnol., 17(7): 653–659.

Watanabe, K., Kamiya, D., et al. (2005) Directed differentiation of telencephalic precursors from embryonic stem cells. Nat. Neurosci., 8(3): 288–296.

Wichterle, H., Lieberam, I., et al. (2002) Directed differentiation of embryonic stem cells into motor neurons. Cell, 110(3): 385–397.

Wilson, S.I. and Edlund, T. (2001) Neural induction: toward a unifying mechanism. Nat. Neurosci., 4 Suppl: 1161–1168.

Wilson, S.I., Graziano, E., et al. (2000) An early requirement for FGF signalling in the acquisition of neural cell fate in the chick embryo. Curr. Biol., 10(8): 421–429.

Wilson, S.I., Rydstrom, A., et al. (2001) The status of Wnt signalling regulates neural and epidermal fates in the chick embryo. Nature, 411(6835): 325–330.

Windrem, M.S., Roy, N.S., et al. (2002) Progenitor cells derived from the adult human subcortical white matter disperse and differentiate as oligodendrocytes within demyelinated lesions of the rat brain. J. Neurosci. Res., 69(6): 966–975.

Wu, S., Wu, Y., et al. (2006) Motoneurons and oligodendrocytes are sequentially generated from neural stem cells but do not appear to share common lineage-restricted progenitors *in vivo*. Development, 133(4): 581–590.

Yan, Y., Yang, D., et al. (2005) Directed differentiation of dopaminergic neuronal subtypes from human embryonic stem cells. Stem Cells, 23(6): 781–790.

Yao, S., Chen, S., et al. (2006) Long-term self-renewal and directed differentiation of human embryonic stem cells in chemically defined conditions. Proc. Natl. Acad. Sci. USA, 103(18): 6907–6912.

Zeng, X., Cai, J., et al. (2004) Dopaminergic differentiation of human embryonic stem cells. Stem Cells, 22(6): 925–940.
Zhang, S.C. (2001) Defining glial cells during CNS development. Nat. Rev. Neurosci. 2(11): 840–843.
Zhang, S.C., Ge, B., et al. (2000) Tracing human oligodendroglial development in vitro. J. Neurosci. Res., 59(3): 421–429.
Zhang, S.C., Wernig, M., et al. (2001) In vitro differentiation of transplantable neural precursors from human embryonic stem cells. Nat. Biotechnol., 19(12): 1129–1133.

CHAPTER 7

GERM CELL DIFFERENTIATION

VANESSA T. ANGELES AND RENEE A. REIJO PERA
Human Embryonic Stem Cell Center; Center for Reproductive Sciences; Department of Obstetrics, Gynecology, and Reproductive Sciences; Institute for Stem Cell and Tissue Biology; Institute for Human Genetics; University of California at San Francisco, San Francisco, CA 94143, USA

1. GERM CELL DEVELOPMENT

Germ cells possess a unique distinction: they are the only cells required for the transmission of genetic material from generation to generation in sexually reproducing organisms. Amazingly, germ cells routinely and consistently reproduce a cell's totipotency, or the ability to differentiate into every cell type in the organism. Thus, germ cells are required for the survival of a species and ultimately for the propagation of life.

The term germ cells collectively refers to multiple stages of gametes including primordial germ cells, gonocytes, oogonia, and spermatogonia. The mature cell types are included as well, although these cells are more commonly referred to as sperm and oocytes (or eggs). All other cells that comprise the body, whether they are neurons, cardiomyocytes, blood cells, or epithelial cells, are incapable of dividing and differentiating into cells, which can propagate the species. By definition then, all non-germline cells are known as somatic cells, a term derived from the Latin word *soma*, meaning body.

1.1 Germ Cell Formation

Two divergent methods of germ cell development have evolved (Saffman and Lasko 1999; Houston and King 2000). First, in nonmammalian species, inheritance of germ plasm determines the cells which will transmit the genetic material of the organism. Germ plasm is microscopically distinct oocyte cytoplasm that is particularly rich in RNAs and RNA-binding proteins and segregates with cells destined to become germ cells (Saffman and Lasko 1999;

J.R. Masters et al (eds.), Embryonic Stem Cells, 109–128.

Houston and King 2000). In mammalian species, however, male and female germ cells are specified independently of germ plasm via inductive signaling from neighboring cells (Tam and Zhou 1996; McLaren 1999; Lawson et al. 1999; Ying et al. 2000; Ying and Zhao 2001; Ying et al. 2001; Yoshimizu et al. 2001).

Despite the differences between the two processes, a number of factors that retain their function in germ cell development are highly conserved. For example, in *Drosophila,* the disruption of genes such as *Oskar*, *Vasa, Tudor*, *Germ cell-less*, and *Aubergine* results in the lack of a germ line (Santos and Lehmann 2004). These genes function to assemble the germ plasm, where the highly conserved interacting RNA-binding proteins Pumilio and Nanos can be found. These proteins repress translation, thus indirectly silencing gene transcription in nascent germ cells (Lin and Spradling 1997; Forbes and Lehmann 1998; Parisi and Lin 1999; Santos and Lehmann 2004). In *Pumilio* and *Nanos* mutants, nascent germ cells may divide prematurely, migrate abnormally, and subsequently die during early embryonic development (Jaruzelska et al. 2003; Tsuda et al. 2003; Santos and Lehmann 2004). Recently, the homologues of these and other germ plasm components have been identified in mammalian germ cells, including those of humans.

Another gene whose function is highly conserved from model organisms to humans is the *DAZ* gene. In humans, deletions and variants of *DAZ* homologs are associated with the production of very few or no germ cells and in diverse model organisms, these genes are required solely for the development of the germ cell lineage (Reijo et al. 1995; Eberhart et al. 1996; Ruggiu et al. 1997; Maegawa et al. 1999; Houston and King 2000; Karashima et al. 2000; Tung et al. 2006). In particular, in *Xenopus*, *Xdazl* RNA is localized to germ plasm and depletion studies have confirmed that it is required for primordial germ cell (PGC) development while, in mice, loss of function of *Dazl (Daz-like)* leads to loss of the fetal germ cell populations in both sexes (Ruggiu et al. 1997; Houston and King 2000; Lin and Page 2005).

While the components of germ plasm are conserved in mammalian species, the mechanism of germ cell development is not. Outside the embryo proper, cells in the extraembryonic ectoderm actively secrete factors, namely bone morphogenetic protein 4 (BMP4) and BMP8b (Lawson et al. 1999; Ying et al. 2000). These molecules act as signals for neighboring cells within the proximal epiblast to enter into a program of germ cell development at approximately embryonic day 6–6.5 (E6–6.5). This effect is non-cell autonomous, as evidenced when the cells in the proximal epiblast were replaced with cells from the distal epiblast: the transplanted cells still assumed a germ cell fate, when placed in contact with the extraembryonic ectoderm (Tam and Zhou 1996).

In mice, a founder population is established and is comprised of approximately 45 primordial germ cells, which are first detected at E7.25 as a cluster of cells in the proximal epiblast which stains positively for tissue nonspecific alkaline phosphatase (TNAP) (Chiquoine 1954; Ginsburg et al. 1990). Prior to gastrulation, these primordial germ cells migrate out of the embryo proper and reside in the extraembryonic tissues until gastrulation is complete. Once the three germ layers have formed, the cells reenter the embryo, migrate into and invade the genital ridges, where they begin to colonize, proliferate mitotically to increase germ cell number, and erase genomic imprints (E9.5–11.5) (Gomperts et al. 1994; Hajkova et al. 2002). The genital ridges differentiate into either the testes or ovaries, and this signals the germ cells to assume either a male or female identity and differentiate into sperm or oocytes, respectively.

1.2 Meiosis

A major hallmark of oogenesis and spermatogenesis is the completion of meiosis, where DNA replication is followed by two subsequent divisions that result in haploid cells with 1C DNA content. Germ cells must be haploid, since the sperm and oocyte pronuclei will eventually fuse to restore 2C DNA content. In females, oogenesis arrests before the first meiotic division is complete, whereas spermatogenesis is halted during mitotic proliferation.

1.3 Genomic Imprinting

Genomic imprinting is another fundamental property of mammalian germ cells. Epigenetic modifications to the genome, typically by DNA methylation, result in the expression of genes from only one of the two parental chromosomes. The "instructions" regarding gene expression are established in the parental germ cells via differential methylation of the DNA. Methylation predominantly occurs on the cytosine residue of CpG dinucleotides which typically cluster together to form "CpG Islands" (Murphy and Jirtle 2003).

Interestingly, genomic imprints are altered throughout the life cycle of the organism (Reik et al. 2001; Hajkova et al. 2002). Imprinting is established in germ cells as they mature into sperm or eggs. Upon fertilization, imprinting is maintained through the replication and segregation of chromosomes during development. Then, as germ cells develop in the new organism, genomic imprints are erased and are eventually re-established during maturation of new germ cells, thereby completing the cycle.

Each of the processes described (namely germ cell specification, gene and protein expression, differentiation, meiosis, and erasure and establishment of genomic imprinting) must be precisely executed to create a functional germ cell.

2. *IN VITRO* GAMETOGENESIS

Scientists have begun to recapitulate this complex and intricate series of events *in vitro* using embryonic stem cells (ESCs). To date, four groups have differentiated mouse embryonic stem cells (mESCs) along the germ cell lineage, to varying degrees of development (Hubner et al. 2003; Toyooka et al. 2003; Geijsen et al. 2004; Lacham-Kaplan 2006). Scientists have also differentiated human embryonic stem cells (hESCs) into putative *in vitro*-derived germ cells (Clark et al.

2004a). Isolation and analysis of these cells would enable researchers to probe the mechanisms of human germ cell development—a field that is hindered due to the inability to study its progression *in vivo*. Thus, the ability to derive germ cells from ESCs would provide a long-awaited system with which to study the genetics of germ cell development and the mechanics of genomic imprinting. This system has implications in the fields of somatic cell nuclear transfer and infertility studies and will provide insight into potential treatments.

2.1 Mouse Embryonic Stem Cells can Differentiate along the Germ Cell Lineage

Initially, it was thought that mESCs were pluripotent (capable of giving rise to multiple, but not all cell lineages) rather than totipotent, as there was no evidence that these cells differentiated into germ cells (Figure 1). In reality, the germ cells were in fact present although the means to identify them were not.

The first evidence that mESCs possessed the ability to differentiate along the germ cell lineage was published in 2003 (Hubner et al. 2003). In this study, from the Hans Scholer laboratory, Hubner et al. engineered a fluorescent germ cell-specific reporter to identify PGCs *in vitro*. Expression of Oct4, a transcription factor expressed in both ES and germ cells, was restricted to germ cells by deleting two conserved regions of the promoter. The promoter was also engineered to drive expression of a green fluorescent protein (GFP) instead of Oct4 (*gcOct4-GFP*). This construct was transfected into mESCs, followed by characterization of expression in germ cells in transgenic mice. Of the three lines constructed, two showed germ cell-specific expression.

The *gcOct4-GFP* ESCs were then differentiated in a monolayer *in vitro*, in ESC media lacking growth factors other than those contributed by serum. After

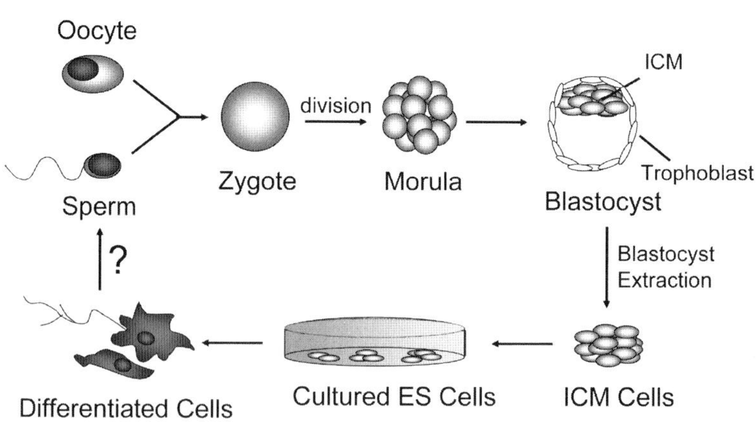

Figure 1. Germ cell fusion leads to zygote and eventual blastocyst formation. The inner cell mass is extracted from blastocysts and maintained in culture as embryonic stem cells which possess the capability of differentiating into multiple cell types. Some scientists questioned whether ESCs possessed the ability to differentiate into mature germ cells, namely the sperm and oocyte.

several days in culture, approximately 40% of the cells were GFP positive and were later isolated via flow cytometry. To characterize the isolated cells, expression of the germ cell markers Oct4, C-kit, and Vasa were analyzed and found to be expressed in a subset of the population.

During differentiation, clusters of Vasa-positive cells detached and formed small aggregates in the supernatant. These cells were collected via centrifugation, replated and further differentiated. In these cultures, the aggregates became increasingly organized and began to resemble early ovarian follicles. Within 2 weeks, the aggregates appeared similar to advanced follicle-like structures, 20% of which had oocytes approximately 40μm in diameter.

In vivo, supporting cells in the ovaries secrete factors necessary for oocyte development. Similarly, the supernatant of the cells grown *in vitro* had increased levels of steroidogenic enzymes, indicating that the supporting somatic cells secreted estradiol as they would in the endogenous niche.

At day 26 of differentiation, putative oocytes were released from their follicle-like structures, resembling ovulation. These putative oocytes had a fragile zona pellucida and most were within the normal size range at 50–70 μm. After 43 days of differentiation, the oocyte morphology began to resemble that of pre-implanted embryos, indicating that spontaneous activation had occurred. Morphologically, the blastocysts looked similar to normally occurring blastocysts.

Although this research provided the first evidence that ESCs were capable of differentiating into germ cells, it offers no insight into the function of the putative germ cells. There was evidence of expression of the meiotic marker Dmc1, though the authors did not show evidence of a haploid chromosome complement. Additionally, analysis of imprinting and ability of the putative oocytes to be fertilized and give rise to pups remains to be completed before these cells can accurately be defined as germ cells.

Soon after the work from the Scholer laboratory was published, the Noce laboratory revealed that they were also able to differentiate mESCs into germ cells, namely mature sperm (Toyooka et al. 2003). Again, the struggle here was to accurately identify putative germ cells *in vitro*. Scientists constructed two reporters with either GFP or LacZ placed under control of the mouse Vasa homologue (MVH) promoter. Neither of these reporters generated a positive signal in mESCs that were differentiated in a monolayer. Next, a three-dimensional differentiation strategy was attempted, in which mESCs were differentiated in suspension where they could form structures known as embryoid bodies (EBs). These EBs are thought to more likely represent the endogenous niche in which germ cells normally arise. After 3–5 days of differentiation as EBs, approximately one-tenth of the aggregates became either GFP or LacZ positive, with clusters of cells strongly expressing the reporters at the periphery of EBs after 5–7 days. At day 5, the EBs were dissociated and sorted via flow cytometry. The GFP and LacZ-positive populations were assayed for and tested positively for expression of known germ cell markers, namely Oct3/4, E-cadherin, Ssea1, C-kit, Gcna1, and Scyp3.

Since mammalian germ cells are induced by neighboring cells in the extraembryonic ectoderm (a trophoblast precursor), Toyooka et al. hypothesized that exogenous signals are also required in culture. Thus, mESCs were cocultured with D7.5 trophoblast cells that expressed either BMP4 or BMP8b. After a single day, the number of PGCs in culture increased significantly when cells were exposed to Bmp4; these enriched putative germ cells were sorted via flow cytometry to yield a more pure population.

To further reconstruct the endogenous niche, germ cells were co-aggregated with E12.5–E13.5 male gonadal cells, followed by transplantation into testicular tubules of male *nude* mice. Following 6–8 weeks of differentiation *in vivo*, the recipient testes were analyzed, revealing LacZ-positive germ cells in the tubules and mature sperm in the lumen of several tubules. The tubules contained cells which stained positively for β-gal and Hsc70t, to detect LacZ-positive cells and elongated spermatids respectively, indicating that the *in vitro*-derived germ cells were competent to participate in spermatogenesis. Although the differentiation procedure yielded mature sperm, evidence of meiosis, erasure of genomic imprints or function were not assessed in this study.

The third group to report successful differentiation of germ cells from mESCs came from the George Daley laboratory (Geijsen et al. 2004). Here, the PGC population was hypothesized to be a subset of the population that was positive for both Oct4 (as indicated by an Oct4-GFP reporter) and stage-specific early antigen-1 (SSEA1). Since these markers are also expressed in undifferentiated cells, mESCs were differentiated as EBs in the presence of retinoic acid, a molecule which quickly differentiates mESCs while sustaining a PGC population.

EBs were plated on mouse embryonic fibroblasts (MEFs) and grown for 7 days in the presence of retinoic acid. Under these conditions a small subset of the population remained SSEA1 positive. These cells, upon further analysis, formed colonies which stained positively for alkaline phosphatase and were surrounded by cells which resembled PGCs that had begun to migrate.

Next, scientists assayed for erasure of genomic imprints, a major hallmark of germ cell development. Geijsen et al. differentiated mEBs in the presence of retinoic acid then assessed the methylation status of several clones. After 10 days of differentiation, all clones surveyed were unmethylated, indicating the successful erasure of imprints. This study provided the first evidence that the biological properties of germ cells were maintained as the cells developed *in vitro*.

The putative germ cells were then isolated via immunomagnetic sorting of the SSEA1-positive population and the expression of germ cell markers was assayed. The findings indicated that the developing EB effectively mimics the endogenous environment in which PGCs naturally form, at least to some extent. Accordingly, both luteinizing hormone receptor (LHR) and Mullerian inhibiting substance (MIS) were present in the supernatant, indicating that Leydig cells and Sertoli cells respectively produced appropriate secretions. Additionally, it was determined that sex-determining region on Y (*SRY*), a gene which promotes male germ cell development, was expressed in the putative germ cells.

The Fe-J1 antibody was used to assay for the presence of male meiotic germ cells, of which only 0.01% of the population stained positively. This indicated that meiotic progression was inconsistent *in vitro* and future studies should investigate this problem further. The few haploid cells identified were isolated nonetheless and used in functional studies to determine their ability to fertilize mature oocytes. Intracytoplasmic sperm injection (ICSI) was used to inject a single sperm into a recipient oocyte. Fifty percent of the oocytes injected began to cleave, then arrested at the 2-cell stage while 20% progressed to the blastocyst stage. This evidence alludes to the functional competence of *in vitro*-derived sperm.

Recently, an additional report was published demonstrating differentiation of ESCs to putative germ cells (Lacham-Kaplan et al. 2006). Lacham-Kaplan et al. differentiated mESCs in the presence of medium conditioned by fetal testicular cell cultures (TCC). The ESCs were differentiated in a hanging drop, and after 48 h, 72 h, and 120 h, stained positively for Oct3/4, Mvh, and C-kit. Strikingly, after 72–120 h of culture in TCC media, ovarian-like structures appeared in approximately 81% of the hanging drops. After 6–7 days of differentiation, follicle-like structures appeared, which, when dissociated, revealed putative oocytes ranging in size from 15 to 35 μm. No zona pellucida was detected around the "oocytes," which is likely a result of the lack of expression of Zp1 and Zp2, as assayed by RT-PCR. The oocytes did express some oocyte-specific markers, namely Fig-α, Zp3, and Stra8, but also incorrectly expressed SRY, a marker of male germ cells. No assessment of meiosis, imprinting or function was made in this study.

2.2 Human Embryonic Stem Cells can also Differentiate into Putative Germ Cells

In 2004, Clark et al. (2004a) provided the first evidence that hESCs were also capable of differentiating along the germ cell lineage . Again, the limitation in the human system is the inability to isolate these cells upon differentiation. Given this shortcoming, this report focused on characterization of putative germ cells through analysis of mRNA and protein expression of germ cell-specific and germ cell-enriched markers; a thorough profile of markers was compiled and used throughout the manuscript.

hESCs differentiated spontaneously when cultured in suspension and in the absence of FGF2 or other growth factors. Based on mRNA and protein levels, it was determined that undifferentiated hESCs express markers of early germ cell development, but not those of late development. To confirm these findings in single cells, immunohistochemistry was used to assay expression of STELLAR, DAZL (markers of early germ cells), and VASA (which is expressed later by migratory germ cells). Both STELLAR and DAZL were present in undifferentiated hESCs, while VASA was not, which signified that hESCs may be similar to PGCs.

Because hESCs are inner cell mass (ICM) explants, Clark et al. sought to compare these two cell populations, specifically assaying for expression of germ cell-specific genes. The two populations were found to be closely related, although *NCAM1* and *DAZL* expression had been turned on in ESCs. This indicated that ICM extraction from blastocysts may have induced a spontaneous differentiation of hESCs into PGCs, although this differentiation is limited to early stages of germ cell development since expression of *VASA* was not detected.

ESCs were cultured in suspension as EBs for 14 and 21 days to allow for further progression into the germ cell lineage, sectioned and analyzed via immunohistochemistry. Again, expression patterns of STELLAR, DAZL, and VASA proteins were analyzed. All three germ cell-specific proteins were present in EBs, although, as expected, not every cell was STELLAR, DAZL, or VASA positive since somatic differentiation likely occurred in parallel. Given the counts of VASA-positive cells at D14 and D21, and comparing these to the percentage of STELLAR and DAZL positive cells at D0, the researchers concluded that a cell that expresses STELLAR or DAZL at day 0 does not necessarily continue to later stages of germ cell formation, as assessed by VASA expression.

Meiotic progression of the putative germ cells was also surveyed. PGCs were stained with synaptonemal complex protein 3 (SCP3) and MutL homologue 1 (MLH1) to determine the fidelity of meiosis. Although at D14, SCP3-positive cells were identified, the staining was cytoplasmic and sometimes punctate within the nucleus, rather than aligned on the chromosomes as it is in normal meiotic progression. MLH1 expression was never seen, even after 22 days of differentiation, indicating that recombination nodules had not formed. It appeared that the cells had begun to enter into meiosis, although external signals required for completion of this process may have been lacking.

In total, the five research studies described provide strong evidence that germ cell development can be recapitulated *in vitro*. Thus, we now turn our focus to the methodology used to differentiate hESCs into germ cells *in vitro*.

3. METHODS

hESCs are commonly cultured on mouse or human embryonic fibroblasts (MEFs) in the presence of FGF2 to maintain their undifferentiated state. To induce differentiation of hESCs, serum is added to the medium and the cells are removed from the feeder layer and moved into suspension culture. This induces the formation of EBs and promotes differentiation in an environment that may closely resemble the endogenous niche (Figure 2).

3.1 Enrichment of the Germ Cell Population With BMPs

Evidence has been provided that bone morphogenetic proteins (BMPs), namely BMP4, BMP7, and BMP8b, when added to ESC-differentiation media can enhance germ cell differentiation, as assessed by *VASA* expression (Kee et al. 2006).

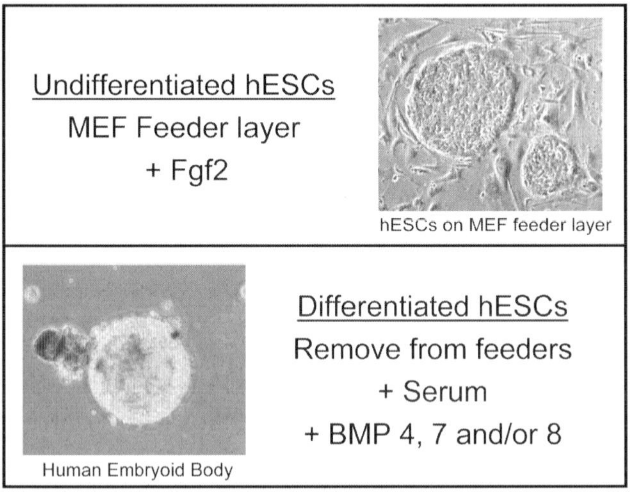

Figure 2. Culture requirements for undifferentiated and differentiated hESCs. Undifferentiated hESC are grown on a feeder layer of MEFs in media supplemented with FGF2. To differentiate, feeders and FGF2 are removed and serum is added. To enrich the germ cell population, a cocktail of BMPs can be supplemented.

BMP4 was added to ESC-culture medium at 1, 10 and 100ng/mL. After a single day of differentiation, *VASA* expression increased in increments ranging from 1.3- to 3.4-fold. Expression of SYCP3, a marker that is expressed upon entry into meiosis, also increased in BMP4-treated cultures, although to a lesser extent. Additionally, it was shown that BMP7 and BMP8b also act to induce germ cell differentiation from hESCs, but only when combined with BMP4 in ES-differentiation medium.

To enrich for germ cells *in vitro*, differentiate hESCs to EBs in suspension culture by transferring approximately 3×10^5 undifferentiated ESCs to a single well of a 6-well low-adhesion plate. Culture the EBs in differentiation medium containing 100ng/mL each of BMP4, BMP7, and BMP8b (R&D Systems, Inc). EBs derived from hESCs can be harvested after 1, 3, 7, or the appropriate number of days in culture with or without BMPS (as a negative control) by transferring the contents of each well to a 15-ml conical tube and allowing EBs to settle by gravity or via centrifugation at 1,000 rpm for 5 minutes. Aspirate the supernatant and store EBs at –80°C until analysis. To determine the effects of BMP, fluorescent-activated cell sorting (FACS) can be used to identify the nascent hESC-derived germ cells, followed by analysis of *VASA* expression via quantitative PCR (see below).

3.3 Markers and Reporters

The major limitation of this *in vitro* differentiation system is the inability to isolate putative germ cells from neighboring somatic cells in culture. Currently, two markers are available to potentially distinguish the germ cell population from the somatic cells of EBs. Placental alkaline phosphatase (PLAP) and SSEA1 can be used to identify germ cell populations in mouse and human EBs respectively although the purity of the isolated populations is uncertain. Using these antibodies, the germ cell populations can then be sorted via FACS and isolated.

Ideally, fluorescent reporters that take advantage of the germ cell-specific expression of *DAZL* or *VASA* could be used to identify PGC populations in human EBs. When expression of GFP is driven by the *DAZL* or *VASA* promoters, it can be used to identify germ cell populations and to track them during development.

The T-Rex lentiviral (LV) technology (Invitrogen) allows for constitutive or regulated gene expression and can be used to construct genetically modified clonal hESC sublines. Currently, a vector that directs constitutive expression of eGFP under control of the CMV promoter has been constructed and H9 (WA09; XX karyotype) control lines have been established (personal communication). eGFP recombinant lentiviruses are produced by transient transfection into 293T cells using a commercial packaging mix (Invitrogen). Harvest infectious lentiviruses at 48 and 72 hours, concentrate by ultracentrifugation, and purify on a sucrose gradient. Concentration can be determined via plating assays. For hESCs, infection requires seeding approximately 1×10^6 cells in a 6-well plate on irradiated CF-1 feeders, followed by growth for 4–7 days in hESC medium. LV concentrations to infect cells cover a range, according to instructions (Invitrogen). Although it is a common dogma that hESCs do not tolerate clonal growth, infected cells can be trypsinized and pipetted to make a single cell suspension, passed through a 22 gauge needle, centrifuged, and washed. Cells can then be sorted singly by FACS on a MoFlo cell sorter and collected into knockout serum replacement (KSR) medium with FGF2 into 12-well plates seeded with feeders (60,000 feeder cells/well). Optimally, 1/3 of the wells will have a single colony after 7 days. These clonal colonies are then expanded, analyzed for pluripotency and karyotyped as per standard protocol. DAZL-GFP and VASA-GFP reporters can be constructed in this manner, followed by sub-cloning and expansion.

Once germ cells have been enriched and isolated, it is important to assess the following characteristics: morphology, gene and protein expression, evidence of meiosis, erasure and establishment of genomic imprints, and function (Figure 3).

3.4 Morphology

Morphologically, it is difficult to identify PGCs *in vitro*, although there are some guidelines. Cells that form small aggregates or clusters and that detach from the colony may be similar to migratory PGCs. More easily distinguishable, however, are the mature germ cells. Oocytes are considerably larger than their somatic counterparts and can reach sizes of 120 μm. *In vivo*, oocytes are surrounded by follicles, which are composed of 1–2 layers of flattened granulosa cells at the primordial follicle phase. As the oocyte grows and matures, the supporting

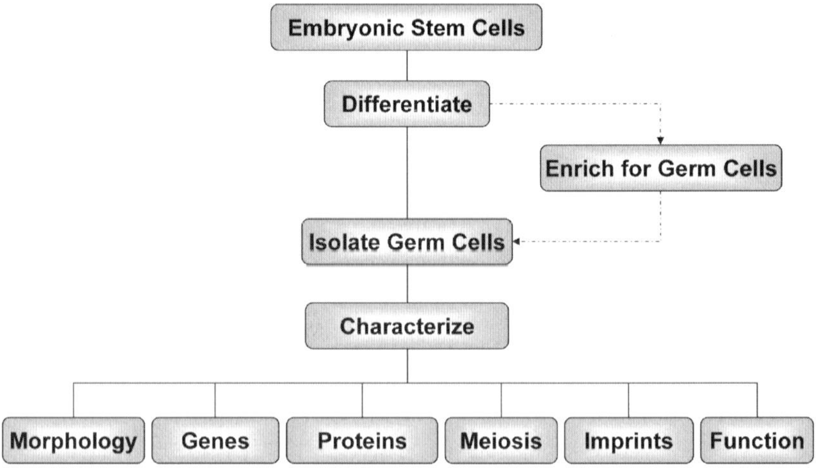

Figure 3. In vitro gametogenesis. Embryonic stem cells are differentiated in suspension as EBs. To promote germ cell development, BMPs can be added to differentiation medium, followed by subsequent isolation of putative germ cells. Several criteria must be fulfilled before the isolated cells can be characterized as true germ cells.

somatic cells proliferate to accommodate the increasing oocyte size. Male germ cell development is composed of multiple stages, of which the more recognizable are spermatogonial stem cells, round spermatids and mature sperm.

3.5 Sorting Protocol for Putative Germ Cells

EBs are cultured in suspension for a defined differentiation period, collected and centrifuged at 1,000 rpm prior to removing the supernatant. On the day of FACS, undifferentiated ESCs (to be used as a negative control) are removed from the feeder layer via digestion with 1 mg/mL collagenase type IV/1 mg/mL dispase (Gibco BRL) for 5 minutes, collected and centrifuged. EBs and ESCs are then incubated in 0.25% Trypsin/0.1% EDTA for 5 minutes and the suspension is pipetted to reduce cell clumps. Cells are centrifuged and resuspended in cold 1% bovine serum albumin (BSA) in PBS (PBS-B). The cell suspension is then passed through a 40 μm cell strainer to ensure single cells can be sorted; filtered cell suspensions are incubated with a 1/150 dilution of PLAP or no primary antibody. To wash, cells are collected by centrifugation and resuspended in cold PBS-B. Cells are recentrifuged, resuspended in Texas-red anti-rabbit IgG (1:200) for 20 minutes and then diluted with cold PBS-B to be centrifuged, and resuspended in PBS-B with propidium iodide (PI; 0.5 mg/ml in FACS buffer). The entire cell suspension is again passed through a cell strainer and analyzed on a MoFlo sorter. Propidium iodide (PI)-positive cells are discarded while those positive for Texas-red are collected singly or as populations into 96-well plates in hESC media onto feeder cells.

3.6 Quantitative PCR to Assess Germ Cell Differentiation Transcriptionally

Quantitative PCR (QPCR) is as described (Clark et al. 2004a, b). Extract total RNA using the RNeasy RNA extraction kit (Qiagen). Prepare cDNA using SuperScript III reverse transcriptase according to the manufacturer's protocol (Invitrogen). PCR is done using 50 ng cDNA with 2 μM primers in standard buffer and conditions using either a SYBR Green PCR Master Mix (Applied Biosystems) or Taqman Mastermix (Applied Biosystems) (Clark et al. 2004a, b). Results are analyzed using an iCycler iQ PCR system (Biorad). Expression of markers diagnostic of germ cells (particularly *VASA*) is normalized to *GAPDH* using REST XL (relative expression software tool) (Pfaffl et al. 2002). Controls with no cDNA or the absence of reverse transcriptase in preparation of cDNAs are included to distinguish products which may arise from amplification of genomic DNA.

3.7 Quantitative PCR to Assess Somatic Differentiation, Transcriptionally

Somatic development is dominant in differentiating EBs and is assessed in each experiment via standard analysis, as outlined (Thomson et al. 1998; Bodnar et al. 2004; Clark et al. 2004a, b). Somatic markers used in QPCR include *NCAM1*, *AFP*, and *KDR*. Although this set of markers does not cover all somatic fates, it serves as a reference that: (1) somatic differentiation occurred and (2) ectoderm, endoderm, and mesoderm derivatives were differentiated. Histology to distinguish somatic cell types is also described (Shamblott et al. 1998, 2001). Where necessary, additional marker panels for somatic differentiation are established (Shamblott et al. 1998, 2001). These panels include PCR assays for neural markers that include nestin, vimentin, sox1, sox2, Nfl, Map2c, tau, Smi32, Nse, Tyrh, Gfap, Cnp, Galc, and O4; for muscle that include Myf-5, Myf-6, MyoD, MyoG, Mhca, and Mlc2V; for vascular/hematopoietic systems that include CD34, Flk1, and Ac133; and for endoderm that include Afp, Gata4, Hnf3b, Hnf4a, Aldb, Lpk, and Alb (Shamblott et al. 1998, 2001). Antibodies for many of these markers are available (Abeyta et al. 2004; Clark et al. 2004a, b).

3.8 Western blot and Immunohistochemical Analysis to Assess Germ Cell Development Translationally

Western blot protocols and antibody dilutions for use on tissue sections, hESCs, mESCs, and EBs are described (Dorfman et al. 1999; Reijo et al. 2000; Xu et al. 2001; Jaruzelska et al. 2003; Moore et al. 2003; Clark et al. 2004a). Antibodies available currently include anti-DAZ, anti-DAZL, anti-DAZ/DAZL, anti-VASA, anti-PUM2/PUM1, anti-PUM2, anti-PUM1, anti-OCT4, anti-BOULE, anti-SCP3, anti-MLH1, and anti-GDF9. OCT4, MLH1, and GDF9 antisera are purchased (Active Motif); anti-SCP3 are available from Santa Cruz

Antibodies. Other antibodies have been generated against target-specific peptide sequences (Invitrogen Antibody Services) and characterized as reported (Dorfman et al. 1999; Reijo et al. 2000; Xu et al. 2001; Jaruzelska et al. 2003; Moore et al. 2003; Clark et al. 2004a). All antibodies recognize both mouse and human proteins (except human Y chromosome specific DAZ-antisera).

Immunohistochemical techniques are standard and as described (Reijo et al. 2000; Jaruzelska et al. 2003; Moore et al. 2003; Clark et al. 2004a, b). Human EBs are fixed briefly in 4% paraformaldehyde, dehydrated, and paraffin-embedded. Serial sections are de-paraffinized rehydrated, rinsed, blocked and prepared for immunofluorescence or immunohistochemistry. Sections are generally incubated overnight with primary antibodies. For immunofluorescence, incubate sections for 1 hour at room temperature, with primary and secondary antibodies, then rinse and mount with anti-fade. Undifferentiated hESCs are prepared for immunofluorescence on whole mounts by growing the cells on Matrigel (to eliminate the need for a MEF feeder layer) for at least 4 days. Mounts are collected and fixed in 4% paraformaldehyde and then stained as outlined; parallel techniques are used for histology and immunohistochemistry for somatic cells (Shamblott et al. 2001; Clark et al. 2004a, b; Shamblott et al. 1998; Thomson et al. 1998).

3.9 Hypotonic Immunohistochemistry for Meiotic Markers and FACS of Haploid Cells

In some reports on germ cell differentiation from mESCs, chromosome spreads suitable for analysis of meiosis were not reported. In contrast, in the report on human germ cell differentiation from hESCs, meiosis was analyzed via chromosome spreads (Clark et al. 2004a). Procedures for production of chromosome spreads via hypotonic immunohistochemistry of meiotic markers in mESCs, hESCs, and EBs are as described in previous publications and assay the coating of meiotic chromosomes with SCP3 protein and establishment of recombination nodules, as detected by MLH1 (Clark et al. 2004a; Gonsalves et al. 2004). hESCs can be removed from the feeder layer via digestion with 1 mg/mL collagenase Type IV/1 mg/mL dispase (Gibco BRL) for 5 minutes. hESC colonies and EBs are gently mechanically dissociated, prior to resuspension in hypoextraction buffer (30 mM Tris pH 8.2, 50 mM sucrose, 17 mM citric acid, 5 mM EDTA, 0.5 mM DTT, 0.5 mM Pefabloc) (Clark et al. 2004a) for 30 minutes. Collect cells in 100 mM sucrose, then dissociate to single cells using a 20 gauge needle. Pretreat glass slides with 1% paraformaldehyde in PBS (pH9.2) which contains 0.25% Tween20. Place slides in 0.04% photoflo (KODAK) in distilled water then incubate for 30 minutes in antibody dilution buffer (ADB). ADB is comprised of 10% normal donkey serum, 3% BSA and 0.5% Tween 20. Incubate slides overnight at 37°C with rabbit anti-human SCP3 (1/500) and mouse anti-rat MLH (1/25) antibodies, diluted in ADB. Wash slides in ADB for 10 minutes and follow with an overnight incubation in ADB at 4°C. Incubate with secondary antibodies (MLH: rhodamine-conjugated anti-mouse, SCP3: FITC-conjugated anti-rabbit) for 45 minutes at 37°C. Wash 4 times in PBS and seal and mount with anti-fade mounting media (Molecular Probes). Control slides that contain human spermatogenic cell spreads can be included in each experiment as a positive control (Gonsalves et al. 2004).

FACS is as described (Feng et al. 2002). EBs or control testis tissues (from human or mouse, minced with a scalpel and suspended in PBS) can be trypsinized, collected, centrifuged, and resuspended in PBS (pH 8). Cells are rinsed three times, suspended in PBS-B and then treated with RNAse in FACS buffer and 0.2% Triton X-100, prior to addition of PI solution. Cells are sorted on a MoFlo to quantify and isolate cells with 1C, 2C, and 4C DNA content.

3.10 Imprinting Analysis

Bisulfite genomic sequencing (Figure 4) can be used to assay imprinting in PLAP- or SSEA1-sorted, differentiated hESC-derived germ cells. In this procedure, cells are harvested and DNA extracted using a ZR Genomic DNA II Kit (Zymo Research). 2 μg of DNA are methylated using the EZ DNA Methylation Kit (Zymo Research), in which the DNA is bisulfite-treated at 50°C overnight followed by on-column desulfonation and elution. Differentially methylated regions (DMRs) of imprinted genes such as H19, KCNQ1, and Peg1 are amplified by PCR from bisulfite-treated DNA (Judson et al. 2002); products are then gel purified and cloned into the TOPO vector (Invitrogen) before transforming into *Escherichia coli*. Approximately 20 colonies are selected and lysed. PCR products are then sequenced at each DMR to determine the methylation status of each clone.

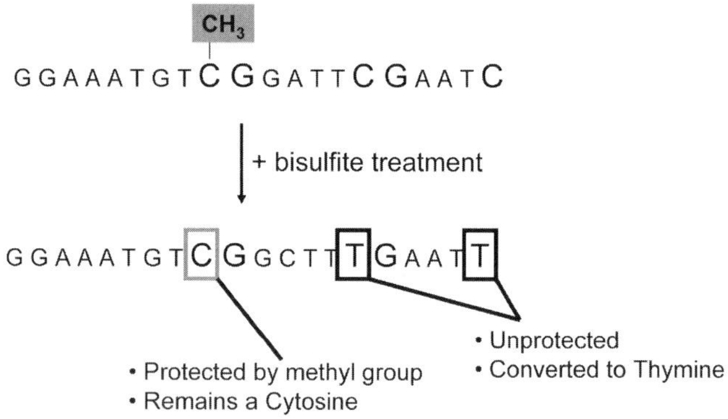

Figure 4. Bisulfite genomic sequencing. Treatment of DNA with bisulfite allows for analysis of genomic imprints. Methylated cytosines are protected whereas unmethylated cytosines are converted to thymine residues. DNA sequencing reveals these changes and the original methylation pattern can be interpreted.

Methylation-sensitive enzymes can be used to verify sequencing data (Kelsey and Reik 1998; Geijsen et al. 2004).

3.10.1 Function

Once germ cell populations have been established *in vitro*, it is important to determine if the biological function has been maintained. This can be assayed via transplantation experiments into mouse testes, which possess a well-characterized spermatogenic environment (Brinster and Zimmermann 1994; Nagano et al. 2001; Nagano et al. 2002). Transplantation studies may provide a more appropriate niche than that which is provided by the EB. hESCs at different stages of differentiation can be transplanted into mouse testes and the development into germ cells assayed. Co-culturing hESCs with human fetal testis tissue prior to transplantation experiments may further influence germ cell development.

3.11 Assess Germ Cell Development Through Transplantation

The ability for germ cells to colonize and expand upon transplantation to spermatogenic tubules is a functional test of their inherent biological properties. Thus, to assess the functional status of ESC-derived germ cells, three transplantation assays can be used, including tests of the ability of putative spermatogonia to colonize adult spermatogenic tubules, of putative PGCs to colonize prepubertal spermatogenic tubules and of coaggregated, putative fetal germ cells to colonize embryonic somatic gonad transplants to the adult testis. In all cases the *nude* mouse is used to avoid any immunological rejection that might occur with xenotransplantation even though the testis is immunologically privileged. Protocols for spermatogonial transplantation are well-documented (Boettger-Tong et al. 2000; Johnston et al. 2001; Nagano et al. 2001; Nagano et al. 2002; McLean et al. 2003) and protocols for transplantation of PGCs and fetal germ cells have been described recently but are straightforward (Toyooka et al. 2003; Chuma et al. 2005). One half of each sample can be transplanted to each testis and then harvested and analyzed at 60 days post-transplantation, as described below.

3.11.1 Protocol I: Standard germ cell transplantation to adult spermatogenic tubules

For germ cell transplantation, use total human testis cell preparations from biopsies, total testis cell preparations from GFP-positive mice and GFP-positive hESC-derived germ cell preparations. Samples are treated essentially as published (McLean et al. 2003; Kubota et al. 2004). For positive controls (mouse and human testes), samples are enzymatically digested in Hanks buffer containing collagenase Type IV, trypsin and DNAse as outlined. Cells are then transferred to ice and tubules are allowed to settle and fresh digestion medium is added for a second incubation. Pipette the cell suspension to break up clumps, centrifuge and resuspend in EKRB medium (Enriched Krebs-Ringers Bicarbonate medium) containing 0.03% trypan blue at a concentration of 10^7 cells/mL (approximately 1% or fewer are spermatogonia). In the case of hESC-derived germ cells, differentiate for 0, 7, and 14 days followed by FACS for PLAP to enrich for nascent germ cells. Cells to be transplanted are resuspended in EKRB.

Recipient mice are prepared for transplantation, as detailed. Treat recipients with 40 mg/kg Busulphan (subcutaneous injection) to deplete germ cells, 4 weeks prior to transplantation. At the time of transplantation, mice should be approximately 5–7 weeks old and anesthetized with Avertin. Open the body wall to locate the rete testis. Donor cells are loaded into an injection needle and then transplanted with 10^7 total testicular cells from mice or humans and dilutions of hESC-derived germ cells (0, 10^3, 10^4). Analyze recipients 60 days following transplantation. Analysis includes direct visualization of GFP fluorescence and FACS selection of germ cells from homogenates of one testis, to count the number of cells present in each transplant and to analyze development of transplanted germ cells further. The other testis can be stained for germ-cell specific marker proteins and analyzed for cell types; an aliquot of the second testis should also be frozen for molecular analyses. Cells obtained via FACS from the transplanted testis can be used for immunohistochemistry, meiotic spreads, and QPCR. A positive control of mouse total testicular cells is included in each transplantation experiment. The purpose of these transplantation experiments is to assess: (1) qualitative ability of mESC- and hESC-derived germ cells to colonize adult spermatogenic tubules; (2) optimum day of differentiation (0, 7, and 14 days) and cell number for adult colonization; and (3) quantitative parameters of germ cell transplantation with wildtype cells to adult tubules. Note that this protocol measures differentiation of germ cells to spermatogonia.

3.11.2 Protocol II: Transplantation to prepubertal spermatogenic tubules

Recently, a report was published of spermatogenesis following transplantation of epiblast and primordial germ cells into postnatal mouse testis (Chuma et al. 2005). Remarkably, in this work, the authors report that PGCs, which are derived from the epiblast, can establish colonies of spermatogenesis after transfer to the 5–10 day postnatal testis. In addition, the authors demonstrate that the epiblast itself can initiate spermatogenesis (as well as teratoma formation) in 5–10 day old mice, upon transplantation. Finally, the report documents the production of normal fertile offspring by IVF using spermatozoa derived from PGCs as early as 8.5 days post coitum. Control mouse cell preparations and hESC-derived germ cells are transplanted into mice at 5–10 days of age, as outlined below. For a positive control, one can transplant the germ cells from E12.5 embryos carrying a germ cell-specific GFP reporter. Tissues are digested as above and resuspended in DMEM as described. Recipient mice in this protocol are not treated with Busulfan. Analysis is done following gonadectomy at 60 days post-transplantation. Analysis mirrors that above, including direct visualization of GFP fluorescence and FACS selection of germ cells from homogenates of one testis, to count the number of cells present after each differentiation time period and to analyze development of isolated germ cells further. The other testis can be stained for germ cell-specific marker proteins and analyzed for cell types; an aliquot of the second testis can also be frozen for molecular analyses. Cells obtained via FACS from the transplanted testis are used for immunohistochemistry, meiotic spreads, and quantitative PCR. The purpose of this transplantation experiment again assesses: (1) qualitative ability of mESC- and hESC-derived germ cells to colonize prepubertal spermatogenic tubules; (2) optimum day of differentiation (0, 7, and 14 days) and cell number for colonization of prepubertal spermatogenic tubules; and (3) quantitative parameters of germ cell transplantation with wildtype cells to prepubertal tubules. Note that this protocol measures differentiation of PGCs to mature germ cells (in mouse preparations) and to the spermatogonial stage in humans.

3.11.3 Protocol III: Germ cell transplantation to the testis capsule after coaggregation

An underlying assumption of this protocol, used by Toyooka and colleagues with mESC-derived germ cells, is that differentiated ESC-derived germ cells are too immature to populate either adult or prepubertal spermatogenic tubules. Thus, this transplantation relies upon coaggregation with fetal testis and subsequent transplantation to the adult testis capsule (Toyooka et al. 2003). For this procedure, EBs are dissociated by incubation with 0.01% Type IV collagenase and collected for transplantation after sorting by FACS. Control donor cells are from E13.5 fetal testis and carry a germ cell specific reporter such as the germ cell specific OCT4-GFP. Gonadal cells are obtained from E13.5 embryos; testes are morphologically distinguishable from ovaries and are disaggregated as above in Hanks buffered saline solution (HBSS) containing collagenase, trypsin, and DNAse. Mix dilutions of approximately 0, 10^3, and 10^4 mESC- or hESC-derived germ cells or control donor cells with 10^4 gonadal cells and culture overnight in 96-well plates in human EB medium. Tightly adherent aggregates are transplanted to testis capsules of mice.

As above, recipient *nude* mice are also prepared for transplantation in this protocol but again are not treated with Busulphan. At the time of transplantation, adult mice are approximately 5–7 weeks old. In this procedure, the testis capsule membrane is lifted and a small excision produced in order to push the aggregated transplant under the capsule. Recipients are gonadectomized at 60 days post-transplantation. Analyses are as above after removal of the implant. The purpose of the aggregate transplantation experiments is again to assess: (1) qualitative ability of ESC-derived germ cells to colonize spermatogenic tubules after coaggregation with fetal testis; (2) optimum day of differentiation (0, 7, and 14 days) and cell number for colonization after coaggregation with fetal testis; and (3) quantitative parameters of germ cell transplantation with wild-type cells after coaggregation with fetal testis. Note that this protocol measures differentiation of germ cells to spermatogonia and provides a fetal somatic environment by coaggregation.

3.12 Analysis of Results of Transplantation Experiments

Harvested tissue can be analyzed as outlined above beginning with analysis of germ cell numbers via FACS and subsequent immunohistochemistry. Somatic development may be assayed by histology, immunohistochemistry and QPCR for NCAM1, AFP, and KDR or other markers of choice. Premeiotic germ cell development is assayed by QPCR for mRNA markers as described (Clark et al. 2004a, b). Additionally, germ cell development can be assayed via protein markers, immunohistochemistry, erasure of imprinting, and establishment of sex-specific imprinting. Meiotic and postmeiotic differentiation may be assayed as described above. Measurements are compared across the three transplantation protocols and across species using quantitative measures and statistical analysis appropriate for data sets expected.

REFERENCES

Abeyta, M.J. et al. (2004) Unique gene expression signatures of independently derived human embryonic stem cell lines. Hum. Mol. Genet., 13: 601–608.

Bodnar, M.S. et al. (2004) Propagation and maintenance of undifferentiated human embryonic stem cells. Stem Cells Dev., 13: 243–253.

Boettger-Tong, H.L. et al. (2000) Juvenile spermatogonial depletion (jsd) mutant seminiferous tubules are capable of supporting transplanted spermatogenesis. Biol. Reprod., 63: 1185–119.

Brinster, R.L. and Zimmermann, J.W. (1994) Spermatogenesis following male germ-cell transplantation. Proc. Natl. Acad. Sci. USA, 91: 11303–11307.

Chiquoine, A.D. (1954) The identification, origin, and migration of the primordial germ cells in the mouse embryo. Anat. Rec., 118: 135–146.

Chuma, S. et al. (2005) Spermatogenesis from epiblast and primordial germ cells following transplantation into postnatal mouse testis. Development, 132: 117–122.

Clark, A.T. et al. (2004a) Spontaneous differentiation of germ cells from human embryonic stem cells in vitro. Hum. Mol. Genet., 13: 727–739.

Clark, A.T. et al. (2004b) Human STELLAR, NANOG, and GDF3 genes are expressed in pluripotent cells and map to chromosome 12p13, a hotspot for teratocarcinoma. Stem Cells, 22: 169–179.

Dorfman, D.M., Genest, D.R., and Reijo Pera, R.A. (1999) Human DAZL1 encodes a candidate fertility factor in women that localizes to the prenatal and postnatal germ cells. Hum. Reprod., 14: 2531–2536.

Eberhart, C.G., Maines, J.Z., and Wasserman, S.A. (1996) Meiotic cell cycle requirement for a fly homologue of human deleted in Azoospermia. Nature, 381: 783–785.

Feng, L.X. et al. (2002) Generation and in vitro differentiation of a spermatogonial cell line. Science, 297: 392–395.

Forbes, A. and Lehmann, R. (1998) Nanos and Pumilio have critical roles in the development and function of Drosophila germline stem cells. Development, 125: 679–690.

Geijsen, N. et al. (2004) Derivation of embryonic germ cells and male gametes from embryonic stem cells. Nature, 427: 148–154.

Ginsburg, M., Snow, M.H., and McLaren, A. (1990) Primordial germ cells in the mouse embryo during gastrulation. Development, 110: 521–528.

Gomperts, M., et al. (1994) Interactions between primordial germ cells play a role in their migration in mouse embryos. Development, 120: 135–141.

Gonsalves, J. et al. (2004) Defective recombination in infertile men. Hum. Mol. Genet., 13: 2875–2883.

Hajkova, P. et al. (2002) Epigenetic reprogramming in mouse primordial germ cells. Mech. Dev., 117: 15–23.

Houston, D.W. and King, M.L. (2000a) Germ plasm and molecular determinants of germ cell fate. Curr. Top Dev. Biol., 50: 155–182.

Houston, D.W. and King, M.L. (2000b) A critical role for Xdazl, a germ plasm-localized RNA, in the differentiation of primordial germ cells in *Xenopus*. Development, 127: 447–56.

Hubner, K. et al. (2003) Derivation of oocytes from mouse embryonic stem cells. Science, 300: 1251–1256.

Jaruzelska, J. et al. (2003) Conservation of a Pumilio-Nanos complex from Drosophila germ plasm to human germ cells. Dev. Genes Evol., 213: 120–126.

Johnston, D.S. et al. (2001) Murine germ cells do not require functional androgen receptors to complete spermatogenesis following spermatogonial stem cell transplantation. Endocrinology, 142: 2405–2408.

Judson, H. et al. (2002) A global disorder of imprinting in the human female germ line. Nature, 416: 539–542.

Karashima, T., Sugimoto, A., and Yamamoto, M. (2000) Caenorhabditis elegans homologue of the human azoospermia factor DAZ is required for oogenesis but not for spermatogenesis. Development, 127: 1069–1079.

Kee, K. et al. (2006) Bone morphogenetic proteins induce germ cell differentiation from human embryonic stem cells. Stem Cells Dev., 15: 831–837.

Kelsey, G. and Reik, W. (1998) Analysis and identification of imprinted genes. Meth. Enzymol., 14: 211–235.

Kubota, H., Avarbock, M.R., and Brinster, R.L. (2004) Culture conditions and single growth factors affect fate determination of mouse spermatogonial stem cells. Biol. Reprod., 71: 722–731.

Lacham-Kaplan, O., Chy, H., and Trounson, A. (2006) Testicular cell conditioned medium supports differentiation of embryonic stem cells into ovarian structures containing oocytes. Stem Cells, 24: 266–273.

Lawson, K.A. et al. (1999) Bmp4 is required for the generation of primordial germ cells in the mouse embryo. Genes Dev., 13: 424–436.

Lin, H. and Spradling, A.C. (1997) A novel group of pumilio mutations affects the asymmetric division of germline stem cells in the *Drosophila* ovary. Development, 124: 2463–2476.

Lin, Y. and Page, D.C. (2005) Dazl deficiency leads to embryonic arrest of germ cell development in XY C57BL/6 mice. Dev. Biol., 288: 309–316.

Maegawa, S., Yasuda, K., and Inoue, K. (1999) Maternal mRNA localization of zebrafish DAZ-like gene. Mech. Dev., 81: 223–226.

McLaren, A. (1999) Signaling for germ cells. Genes Dev., 13: 373–376.

McLean, D.J. et al. (2003) Characterization of spermatogonial stem cell maturation and differentiation in neonatal mice. Biol. Reprod., 69: 2085–2091.

Moore, F.L. et al. (2003) Human Pumilio-2 is expressed in embryonic stem cells and germ cells and interacts with DAZ (Deleted in AZoospermia) and DAZ-like proteins. Proc. Natl. Acad. Sci. USA, 100: 538–543.

Murphy, S.K. and Jirtle, R.L. (2003) Imprinting evolution and the price of silence. Bioessays, 25: 577–588.

Nagano, M., McCarrey, J.R., and Brinster, R.L. (2001) Primate spermatogonial stem cells colonize mouse testes. Biol. Reprod., 64: 1409–1416.

Nagano, M., Patrizio, P., and Brinster, R.L. (2002) Long-term survival of human spermatogonial stem cells in mouse testes. Fertil. Steril., 78: 1225–1233.

Parisi, M. and Lin, H. (1999). The *Drosophila pumilio* gene encodes two functional protein isoforms that play multiple roles in germline development, gonadogenesis, oogenesis and embryogenesis. Genetics, 153: 235–250.

Pfaffl, M.W., Horgan, G.W., and Dempfle, L. (2002) Relative expression software tool (REST) for group-wise comparison and statistical analysis of relative expression results in real-time PCR. Nucleic Acids Res., 32: 1372–1379.

Reijo, R. et al. (1995) Diverse spermatogenic defects in humans caused by Y chromosome deletions encompassing a novel RNA-binding protein gene. Nat. Genet., 10: 383–393.

Reijo, R.A. et al. (2000) DAZ family proteins exist throughout male germ cell development and transit from nucleus to cytoplasm at meiosis in humans and mice. Biol. Reprod., 63: 1490.

Reik, W., Dean, W., and Walter, J. (2001) Epigenetic reprogramming in mammalian development. Science, 293: 1093–1098.

Ruggiu, M. et al. (1997) The mouse Dazla gene encodes a cytoplasmic protein essential for gametogenesis. Nature, 389: 73–77.

Saffman, E.E. and Lasko, P. (1999) Germline development in vertebrates and invertebrates. Cell Mol. Life Sci., 55: 1141–1163.

Santos, A.C. and Lehmann, R. (2004) Germ cell specification and migration in *Drosophila* and beyond. Curr. Biol., 14: R578–R589.

Shamblott, M.J. et al. (1998) Derivation of pluripotent stem cells from cultured human primordial germ cells. Proc. Natl. Acad. Sci. USA, 95: 13726–13731.

Shamblott, M.J. et al. (2001) Human embryonic germ cell derivatives express a broad range of developmentally distinct markers and proliferate extensively in vitro. Proc. Natl. Acad. Sci. USA, 95: 13726–13731.

Tam, P.P. and Zhou, S.X. (1996) The allocation of epiblast cells to ectodermal and germ-line lineages is influenced by the position of the cells in the gastrulating mouse embryo. Dev. Biol., 178: 124–132.

Thomson, J.A. et al. (1998) Embryonic stem cell lines derived from human blastocysts. Science, 282: 1145–1147.

Toyooka, Y. et al. (2003) Embryonic stem cells can form germ cells in vitro. Proc. Natl. Acad. Sci. USA., 100: 11457–11462.

Tsuda, M. et al. (2003) Conserved role of nanos proteins in germ cell development. Science, 301: 1239–1241.

Tung, J.Y., Nelson, L.M., Turek, P.J., Witte, J.S., Cramer, D.W., Cedars, M.I., Pera, R.A. (2006) Variants in Deleted in AZoospermia-Like (DAZL) are correlated with reproductive parameters in men and women. Hum. Genet., 118: 730–740.

Xu, E.Y., Moore, F.L., and Pera, R.A. (2001) A gene family required for human germ cell development evolved from an ancient meiotic gene conserved in metazoans. Proc. Natl. Acad. Sci. USA, 98: 7414–7419.

Ying, Y. and Zhao, G.Q. (2001) Cooperation of endoderm-derived BMP2 and extraembryonic ectoderm-derived BMP4 in primordial germ cell generation in the mouse. Dev. Biol., 232: 484–492.

Ying, Y. et al. (2000) Requirement of Bmp8b for the generation of primordial germ cells in the mouse. Mol. Endocrinol., 14: 1053–1063

Ying, Y., Qi, X., and Zhao, G.Q. (2001) Induction of primordial germ cells from murine epiblasts by synergistic action of BMP4 and BMP8B signaling pathways. Proc. Natl. Acad. Sci. USA, 98: 7858–7862.

Yoshimizu, T., Obinata, M., and Matsui, Y. (2001) Stage-specific tissue and cell interactions play key roles in mouse germ cell specification. Development, 128: 481–490.

CHAPTER 8

MESODERMAL DIFFERENTIATION

NADAV SHARON AND NISSIM BENVENISTY
Department of Genetics, Institute of Life Sciences, The Hebrew University, Jerusalem, Israel

1. INTRODUCTION

Human embryonic stem cells (hESCs) are self-renewing cells derived from the inner cell mass (ICM) of human embryos (Thomson et al. 1998). Since the ICM gives rise to all the cells designated to proliferate and evolve into the complete embryo, it is believed that hESCs are pluripotent, capable of differentiating to all the human tissues (Schuldiner et al. 2000).

During *in vitro* differentiation of hESCs, the cells may recapitulate *in utero* embryogenesis to some extent (Dvash et al. 2004). One of the first and foremost stages of this natural process is the formation of the three embryonic germ layers during gastrulation. Cells migrating through the primitive streak form the intra-embryonal layers of *mesoderm* and *endoderm*, whereas the remainder outside layer becomes *ectoderm*. This division dictates the formation of the major body axes, and the first acquirement of specificity by the cells forming the embryo. The interactions between the different layers will promote further development, until organogenesis will mold the designated organs from the cells in each of the embryonic germ layers.

Due to the scarcity of experimental material, the study of the first stages of human embryogenesis is very difficult. Especially limited is the knowledge regarding gastrulation, as this elusive stage occurs during the first weeks of pregnancy. The recent isolation of hESCs (Thomson et al. 1998), with their ability to differentiate into progenies of the three embryonic germ layers (Itskovitz-Eldor et al. 2000), opened a new window on the study of this topic.

We hereby review the progress achieved in the study of differentiation of mesoderm-derived cells through the research of hESCs. Special attention will be given to the methods used for the direction of hESCs differentiation into tissues derived from the mesodermal lineage.

J.R. Masters et al (eds.), Embryonic Stem Cells, 129–148.

1.1 Mammalian Mesoderm and its Derivatives

The first process during embryogenesis to initiate the formation of the embryo is gastrulation, during which the epiblast differentiates into the three embryonic germ layers. Following gastrulation and the establishment of the mesoderm between the ectoderm and the endoderm, the mesoderm further differentiates into five cell groups (Figure 1) (for a review see Carlson 1988).The *chordamesoderm* forms the *notochord*, a transient organ which defines the anterior-posterior axis of the embryo, and induces differentiation of adjacent tissues. The *head mesenchyme* will participate in the formation of the skull and face, including the outer layers of the eye. The three other mesoderm derivatives will comprise much of the remaining body. The *dorsal*, or *paraxial mesoderm*, which lines the sides of the notochord, synchronously segments to form the somites, which will later compose most of the body skeleton and its muscles, and the connective tissue layers of the skin. Further away from the center of the embryo marked by the notochord, lies the *intermediate mesoderm* which will become the kidney and most of the genitalia. More to the lateral edges of the developing embryo is the *lateral mesoderm*. This will turn in part to the extra embryonic organs, and in part to the *somatic* and *splanchnic mesoderms*. The first will develop into the

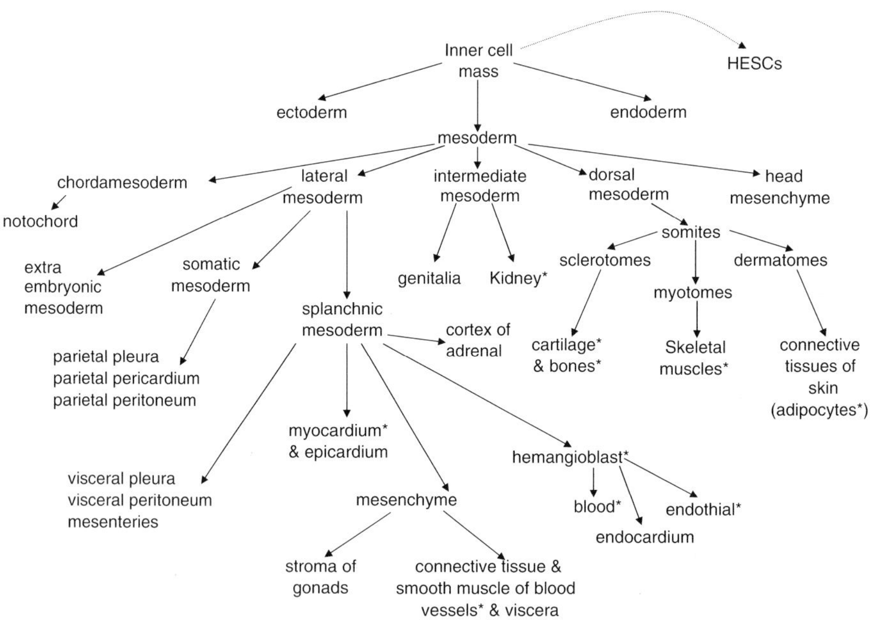

Figure 1. Major differentiation pathways into mesodermal lineages, based on Carlson (1998). Tissues marked by a star have been derived from human embryonic stem cells, as discussed in the chapter.

parietal membranes of the peritoneum, the heart and the lungs; whereas the latter will form the mesenteries and the membranes lining the inner cavities of the lungs and the heart, along with the visceral membranes encapsulating the abdominal organs or surrounding the heart. The circulatory system including the heart, blood, and blood vessels, together with the smooth muscle surrounding the viscera and the blood vessels, are also of splanchnic mesoderm origin, and so is the cortex of the adrenals and the stroma of the gonads. (based on Carlson 1988; Gilbert 2000).

1.2 The Study of Early Human Development with hESCs

Investigation into the early stages of human embryo development poses great difficulties, as the only source available to study the processes following implantation into the uterus are aborted embryos. We therefore relied mainly on model organisms, which may differ in their development to that of man. hESCs, with their pluripotency, may therefore provide unique insights into embryogenesis.

The importance of hESCs derives also from their potential for clinical tissue repair, due to their immense proliferative ability and the relative ease with which they may be genetically manipulated (Eiges et al. 2001). Future hopes for the transplantation of hESC-derived tissues requires comprehensive knowledge as to the processes of embryology, which will allow the establishment of protocols for directing hESC differentiation to the desired cell type.

Since hESCs are known to differentiate into progeny of the three embryonic germ layers (Itskovitz-Eldor et al. 2000), it is believed that they recapitulate the embryonal formation of these three primal cell types, which is the hallmark of gastrulation. In order for hESCs to initiate such a process, they have to be grown under strict conditions which allow for their proliferation and differentiation.

To allow for their ongoing proliferation while maintaining their self-renewal potential, hESCs are grown as monolayers plated on feeder cells such as mouse embryonic fibroblasts (MEF). Factors secreted by these cells prevent stem cell differentiation, and supplementation with medium conditioned by feeders produces similar results (Thomson et al. 1998; Xu et al. 2001). Spontaneous differentiation of hESCs begins with the removal of the feeder cell influence by spreading the stem cells directly on gelatine-coated plates. In order to promote cell differentiation in a manner that will simulate intracellular interactions, hESCs are spread on a nonadhesive plate. This promotes aggregation into embryoid bodies (EBs)—spherical cell clusters with a cavitated center (Itskovitz-Eldor et al. 2000; Schuldiner et al. 2000). Another simulation of *in utero* development is provided by promoting the *in vivo* differentiation of the cells. This is achieved by injecting hESCs into murine organs such as the kidney capsule or the testis, where they form benign tumors named teratomas (Thomson et al. 1998).

Directing the differentiation of hESCs to particular lineages involves their exposure to various exogenous factors (Schuldiner et al. 2000). This may be achieved by plating the cells in the presence of other more differentiated cell lines, or by supplementing the growth medium with auxiliary molecules. A combination of methods may also be used. For instance, it is possible to aggregate the cells into EBs first, later disaggregating them to give differentiated embryonic stem cells (DES). These may be plated in the presence of specific growth factors, thus allowing both intracellular interactions during the primal stages of differentiation and maximal exposure to effector molecules later on (Schuldiner et al. 2000).

2. MESODERM DIFFERENTIATION

Very little is known about the genes involved in human mesoderm formation, and most of our knowledge is derived from the mouse and lower vertebrates.

By conducting a large-scale transcription analysis, Dvash et al. (2004) showed that hESCs aggregated to EBs may simulate the gradual changes in gene expression accompanying early embryogenesis. In this framework, it was shown that within 30 days of culture it is possible to cluster different genes according to several discernable gene expression profiles. Some of these genes are transiently expressed during the first days following EB formation, which is thought to model the early cell differentiation that occurs during gastrulation. Within this group of genes the transitory upregulation of *lefty-A* and its related genes was notable (Dvash et al. 2004).

2.1 Lateral Splanchnic Mesoderm

2.1.1 Cardiomyocytes

Itzkovitz-Eldor et al. (2000) reported the spontaneous differentiation of hESCs aggregated in EBs to cardiomyocytes, after observing their synchronous rhythmic contraction (Table 1). Their authenticity was later verified through the examination of the structural components of the pulsating cells, showing myofibrils in consecutive stages of arrangement into sarcomeres. Analysis of various molecular markers further supported the observation, and both pharmacological and electrophysiological surveys proved that these cells function in accordance with cardiac muscle (Kehat et al. 2001). Recent studies distinguished the three cardiomyocyte groups within differentiated EBs, functioning in a manner characteristic of either nodal cells, embryonic atrial cells, or embryonic ventricular cells (He et al. 2003; Mummery et al. 2003). These and other studies pointed to the fact that hESC derived cardiomyocytes do not necessarily mature completely, and tend to retain the hallmarks of fetal heart even after prolonged incubation (2 months) (Snir et al. 2003). Accumulating evidence suggests that the gradual progress towards maturation provides a good representation of embryonal cardiac development, and attempts were made to describe stage-specific markers (Segev et al. 2005). Lately, grafting experiments further emphasized the

Table 1. Summary of mesodermal tissues derived from human embryonic stem cells, showing method of differentiation, culture conditions and methods of characterization

Cell lineage	Differentiation method	Culture conditions	Cell type	Characterization method			References
				mRNA markers	Protein markers	Function and morphology	
Mesendoderm/ primitive streak (hypothesized)	EB			Mixl1	Mixl1		(Mossman et al. 2005)
Mesoderm (hypothesized)	EB			Lefty			(Dvash et al. 2004)
Splanchnic Mesoderm							
Cardiomyocytes	EB DES Monolayer	spontaneous/ 5-aza-dc Culture with HGF, EGF, RA, TGFβ, bFGF Coculture with VE-like cells	Sarcomeres, nodal/ pacemaker, fetal ventricular, fetal atrial	α- cardiac actin, cTnI/T, MLC-2A/V, α-myosin heavy chain, GATA4, NKX2.5, ANF, Cardiac L- type calcium channel (α1c), Kv4.3, Isl1, Cav1.2, Nav1.5, HCN2	Cardiac α/β myosin heavy chain, α actinin, cTnI, desmin, Cx43, CX45, GATA4, NKX2.5, MEF2, MLC-2A, MLC-2V, tropomyosin, ryanodine receptors, Cardiac L-type calcium channel (α1c), Isl1	Synchronous rhythmic pulsation, electrophysiological, pharmacological	(Itskovitz-Eldor et al. 2000); (Kehat et al. 2001); (Kehat et al. 2002). (Segev et al. 2005). (Xu et al. 2002); (Schuldiner et al. 2000), (Mummery et al. 2003); (Passier et al. 2005); (He et al. 2003); (Satin et al. 2004)
Hemangioblast	EB	Culture with G-CSF, SCF, BMP4, Flt3L, IL3/6			CD45-, VE-cadherin+, CD31+, Flk1+; vWF-, eNOS-	Ac-LDL uptake, no CFU ability	(Wang et al. 2004)

(*Continued*)

Table 1. Summary of mesodermal tissues derived from human embryonic stem cells, showing method of differentiation, culture conditions and methods of characterization—Cont'd.

Cell lineage	Differentiation method	Culture conditions	Cell type	Characterization method			References
				mRNA markers	Protein markers	Function and morphology	
Hematopoietic	EB	Spontaneous/ adhesion to plate/coculture with bone marrow cells/ culture with G-CSF, GM-CSF , SCF, BMP4, VEGF, Flt3L, Thrombopoietin, erythropoietin, IL3/4/6, RPMI1640 medium/ methylcellulose/ transfection of hESCs with HOXB4	Macrophage, Granulocytes, Erythrocyte, Megakaryocyte, Eosinophils, Basophils, Neutrophils, NK cells, T cells, B cells	CD3δ/3ε/3ξ/ 31/34/41a/ 43/45, α-β-γ-δ- ξ-globin [Indications of Gradual switch from ε to γ globin], GATA1/2, PU1, Tal1, Flk1, Flt3, VpreB, Igα, KIR2DL3/L4/ L5, KIR2DS1/ S4/S5, KIR3D/ S1/L1/L2, CDX4, HoxB4	CD2/7/10/13/14/ 15/16/19/31/33/ 34/36/38/40/41/ 41a/ 42b/43/ 45/56/66b/71/ 80/ 83/86/90/ 94/117/164, ε-ξ-β-globin, HbF, HbA, glycophorinA, , Ep-CAM, Flk1, MHC-I/II, HLA-DR, Flk1, vWF, KIR2DL3/ S4, KIR3DL1, NKG2A, NKp30/44/46	Staining, mixed lymphocyte reaction, presence of Rhodamin-extruding cells and ALDH expression, cytolytic activity of NK cells, typical reaction to exogenous proteins, methylcellulose assay	(Itskovitz-Eldor et al. 2000); (Schuldiner et al. 2000); (Chadwick et al. 2003); (Cerdan et al. 2004); (Wang et al. 2005a); (Kim et al. 2005); (Zhan et al. 2004); (Bowles et al. 2006); (Kaufman et al. 2001); (Qiu et al. 2005); (Tian et al. 2006); (Tian et al. 2004); (Vodyanik et al. 2005); (Gaur et al. 2006); (Woll et al. 2005); (Wang et al. 2004); (Zambidis et al. 2005); (Wang et al. 2005b) (Narayan et al. 2006)
	DES	(a) Isolation of CD31+Flk1+ VE-Cad+ CD45- cells from EBs. (b) Culture with G-CSF, SCF, Flt3, IL3, IL6/methylcellulose					

	Monolayer	Coculture with bone marrow, stromal cells, OP9 bone marrow stromal cells (M-CSF$^-$) yolk sac cells or fetal liver/culture with GM-CSF, G-CSF, SCF, Flt3L, thrombopoirtin, erythropoietin, IL3/6/7/15/ methylcellulose		
	In vivo	(a) Isolation of CD31+/Flk1+/ VE-cad+/CD45- cells from EBs. (b) Injection to bone marrow of mouse femur: (a) Coculture with murine bone marrow stroma. (b) CD 34+/38- injected *in utero* to fetal liver (c) Induction with human GM-CSF		Succesful engraftment to secondary recipient, methylcellulose assay

(Continued)

Table 1. Summary of mesodermal tissues derived from human embryonic stem cells, showing method of differentiation, culture conditions and methods of characterization—Cont'd.

Cell lineage	Differentiation method	Culture conditions	Cell type	Characterization method			References
				mRNA markers	Protein markers	Function and morphology	
Endothel	EB	Spontaneous/ formation in Alginate scaffold		CD31/34/133, VE-cad, GATA 2/3, Vcam1, PCDH12, CDH5, VEGF, VEGFC/D, EPAS1, Flt1/4, ANGPT1/2, vWF, HoxB4,	CD31/34, VE-cad, vWF, calponin, eNOS	Uptake of ac-LDL, formation of microvesicles with murine blood cells in lumen, positive for Ulex europaeus agglutinin, no CFU ability, tube-like structure by CD31/34 cells, depth organization of vessel-like structures by CD34 cells	(Levenberg et al. 2002, Levenberg et al. 2003); (Laflamme et al. 2005); (Kaufman et al. 2001); (Vodyanik et al. 2005); (Gerecht-Nir et al. 2004a); (Gerecht-Nir et al. 2004b); (Gerecht-Nir et al. 2005); (Tzukerman et al. 2003); (Wang et al. 2004); (Zambidis et al. 2005)
	DES	Seeding on PLLA/PLGA scaffold/ CD31+ cells on Matrigel: (a) Isolation of CD31 + Flk1 + VE-Cad + CD45- cells from EBs. (b) Culture with pituitary extracts and VEGF/ seeding on methylcellulose, later on GEM2					
	Monolayer	Coculture with murine bone marrow or yolk sac cells					
	Teratoma	Ovarian carcinoma cells injected into teratoma					

	In vivo	(a) Isolation of CD31+ cells from EBs. (b) Seeding on PLLA/PLGA polymer scaffolds. (c) Engrafment to mouse/ injection of cells from EBs enriched for cardiomyocytes to rat heart					
Vascular smooth muscle	EB	Spontaneous		SM-MHC, caldesmon, LMOD1, PDGFB, PDGFRB, TGFB3, TGFBR2/3	SMA, SM-MHC	Electrophysiological, elongated cells around lumens, SM-MHC cells forming voids	(Mummery et al. 2003); (Levenberg et al. 2003); (Gerecht-Nir et al. 2004b); (Gerecht-Nir et al. 2005)
	DES	Seeding on PLLA/PLGA scaffold					
	Monolayer	Coculture with VE-like cells					
	Teratoma						
Paraxial mesoderm							
Paraxial mesoderm (mesenchyme)	Monolayer	Coculture with murine bone marrow stromal cells, isolation of $CD73^{+}$ cells and culture in normal medium		DSC54, neuropilin1, HGF, forkhead box D1, notch homolog 2	CD29/44/73/105, STRO1, VCAM, ICAM1, ALCAM, vimentin, αSMA	Differentiation to fat, cartilage, bone, muscle	(Barberi et al. 2005)
Mesenchyme (towards bone formation)	EB	Culture with ascorbic acid, β-glycerophosphate, dexamethasone			STRO-1		(Cao et al. 2005)

(*Continued*)

Table 1. Summary of mesodermal tissues derived from human embryonic stem cells, showing method of differentiation, culture conditions and methods of characterization—Cont'd.

Cell lineage	Differentiation method	Culture conditions	Cell type	Characterization method: mRNA markers	Characterization method: Protein markers	Characterization method: Function and morphology	References
Cartilage	DES	Spontaneous/ seeding on PLLA/PLGA scaffold, possible: further supplement of TGFβ1		CMP (matrilin1), collagenII, aggrecan		Staining	(Schuldiner et al. 2000); (Goldstein et al. 2002); (Levenberg et al. 2003); (Barberi et al. 2005)
	In vivo	ES transplantation into chick somites*					
	Pellet culture	ES-derived mesenchyme cultured with TGFβ3, ascorbic acid					
Osteoblasts	DES monolayer EB	Culture with ascorbic acid phosphate, β-glycerophosphate, dexamethasone		Cbfa1, coll1, osteocalcin, osteopontin (OPN), bone sialoprotein (BSP), bone-specific ALP, runx2,	Osteocalcin, Col1, bone specific ALP, BSP	Nodule/spicule formation, staining, X ray diffraction, SEM, FTIR	(Sottile et al. 2003); (Bielby et al. 2004); (Ahn et al. 2006); (Karp et al. 2005); (Barberi et al. 2005); (Cao et al. 2005)
	monolayer	ES-derived mesenchyme cultured with dexamethasone, β-glycerol phosphate, ascorbic acid					

	In vivo	(a) DES supplemented with ascorbate 2-phosphate, β-glycerophosphate, and later dexamethasone. (b) Spread on PDLLA scaffold and engrafment to SCID mouse				
	EB	Culture on human primary bone-derived cells				
Skeletal muscle	Monolayer	ES-derived mesenchyme, possible: medium conditioned by murine myoblasts	MyoD, myosin heavy chain IIa, myogenin	MyoD, fast-switch/ sarcomeric myosin,	Multinucleated myotubes	(Barberi et al. 2005)
Adipocytes	EB	Culture with Rosiglitazone	ADD1, PPARγ, aP2, adiponectin	Leptin in medium	Lipid droplets in cytoplasm	(Xiong et al. 2005); (Barberi et al. 2005)
	Monolayer	ES-derived mesenchyme cultured with dexamethasone, insulin, isobutyl-xanthine				
Intermediate mesoderm						
Kidney	EB DES	Spontaneous Culture with NGF	Rennin, kallikrein			(Schuldiner et al. 2000)
Urogenital	DES	Culture with NGF or HGF	Wt1			(Schuldiner et al. 2000)

* human cells localized to chick perichondrium of vertebral arch.

functional similarity of hESC-derived cardiomyocytes and heart tissue. In two recent papers, Xue et al. (2004) and Kehat et al. (2004) reported the transplantation of EB-derived pulsating tissue into animal hearts (guinea pig and swine, respectively) whose pacemaking activity was ablated. In both cases, the engrafted human cells integrated with the host myocardium and induced partial rhythmic activity (Kehat et al. 2004; Xue et al. 2005). In another study, the injection of EB-derived cells enriched for cardiomyocytes into the healthy heart of an immunocompromised rat supported human cardiomyocyte proliferation. Functional integration of the engrafted human cells with the animal heart was not shown, but the xenograft did form vascular connections with the host (Laflamme et al. 2005).

Directed differentiation of hESCs towards the myocardial lineage was apparently obtained by Schuldiner et al. (2000) through the addition of various growth factors to cells derived from EBs. Factors which upregulated the expression of cardiac actin, a prominent cardiomyocyte marker, included bFGF and TGFβ (Schuldiner et al. 2000). The time-dependent addition of 5-aza-dC was also reported to enrich for cardiac muscle populations (Xu et al. 2002). Previous studies indicate that the formation of cardiac cells in the developing vertebrate embryo is strongly dependent on induction by endodermal tissues. Indeed, coculture of HESCs with visceral-endoderm-like cells resulted in their differentiation into ventricular, atrial, and pacemaker-like cardiomyocytes, even without aggregating into EBs (Mummery et al. 2003). Further investigation of the cocultures revealed an increase in cardiomyocyte populations when fetal calf serum (FCS) was removed from the medium, and supplementation with ascorbic acid further increased cell numbers (Passier et al. 2005).

2.1.2 Blood and blood vessels

hESCs can differentiate into the progeny of both hematopoietic and endothelial lineages. There still remains the question, however, as to whether this differentiation recapitulates embryonal development. Genome analysis showed that within differentiating EBs, temporal changes in gene expression correlate substantially with data concerning embryonic hematopoietic and endothelial differentiation (Gerecht-Nir et al. 2005). However, such studies do not address the processes at the level of the individual cell. Within the mammalian embryo, both cell types are formed in designated foci termed "blood islands", leading to the hypothesis of the "hemangioblast", a common progenitor of hematocytes and endothelial cells.

It was suspected that hESCs go through this progenitor stage (Kaufman et al. 2001). Wang et al. (2004) provided further evidence in support when they isolated a group of cells which evolve within differentiating EBs and possess the ability to differentiate into both hematopoietic and endothelial lineages, depending on the culture conditions. These cells, expressing CD31, CD34, FLK1, and VE-cadherin, but not CD45, were shown to become either characteristic $CD45^+$ $CD34^+$ hematopoietic cells capable of colony formation under permissive

hematopoietic conditions, or VE-cadherin^{+} vWF^{+} eNOS^{+} Cd45^{-} endothelial cells (Table 1). Their differentiation to either lineage was shown to be affected by the addition of cytokines or other factors (Wang et al. 2004). Zambidis et al. (2005) showed that after a possible hemangioblastic stage, hESCs follow two consecutive waves of differentiation within the second and third weeks from EB formation. During this phase, the stem cells give rise to primitive and later to definite hematopoietic cells. These two appearances coincide with the typical gradual development of blood cells in the yolk sac of the early embryo (Zambidis et al. 2005). Evidence for recapitulation comes also from later differentiation stages, as the specific maturation pathway of hESCs into natural killer (NK) cells seems to follow the familiar developmental stages of this lineage (Woll et al. 2005). On the other hand, when a wide-genome expression analysis juxtaposed hESC-derived CD34^{+} CD38^{-} hematopoietic progenitors with similar cells from the bone marrow or the umbilical cord, substantial differences were observed. Furthermore, transplantation of hESC-derived hematopoietic cells to mice showed low efficiency in comparison to cord blood cell engraftment.

This incompatibility may be attributed to differences between primary and later hematopoietic progenitors. Indeed, it seems that use of hESCs as an *in vitro* model of hematopoiesis has partly recapitulated only the first stages of fetal hematopoiesis in the yolk sac. Further research is needed to reliably promote hESC differentiation in a manner analogous to the later stages of blood development (Lu et al. 2004; Qiu et al. 2005; Wang et al. 2005b).

2.1.2.1 Blood: The first experiments to differentiate hESCs *in vitro* via EBs showed expression of globin family mRNA, pointing to the presence of hematopoietic progenitors within the differentiated stem cells (Itskovitz-Eldor et al. 2000; Schuldiner et al. 2000). Later studies used special culture methods and more markers to show that hESCs can differentiate into cells with characteristics similar to those of embryonic and mature blood cells derived from erythroid and various myeloid lineages (Kaufman et al. 2001; Chadwick et al. 2003), including functional antigen-presenting cells, capable of arousing a T-lymphocyte reaction (Zhan et al. 2004). As to the lymphocytic lineage, differentiation of hESCs into B-cells and NK cells was also obtained, but a method for their differentiation into T-cells remains to be found (Vodyanik et al. 2005). During their differentiation to the myeloid lineage, hESCs pass through an early stage of an hematopoietic precursor, and can even express proteins shared by both hematopoietic and endothelial lineages (Kaufman et al. 2001).

A common way of directing hESC differentiation to blood cells and endothelium is coculture with yolk sac, fetal liver, or the bone marrow (both adult and fetal) cells of murine or human origin (Table 1) (Kaufman et al. 2001; Kim et al. 2005; Qiu et al. 2005; Vodyanik et al. 2005; Wang et al. 2005a). Isolating these progenitor cells and transferring them to methylcellulose enriched with cytokines, further allows for their differentiation, which culminates in a resemblance to cells of myeloid and erythroid origin (Kaufman et al. 2001). Addition of cytokines with or without growth factors and morphogen to hESCs or EBs cocultured with bone marrow stromal cells in EB medium, prior to culture of the differentiating cells on methylcellulose, was also shown to facilitate differentiation and production of larger blood cell populations (Chadwick et al. 2003; Lu et al. 2004; Wang et al. 2005a). To obtain lymphoid differentiation, the isolated progenitors were further cocultured with stromal cells, supplemented with various cytokines (Vodyanik et al. 2005). Induction of hESC differentiation to blood cell lineages was also obtained by transfecting the cells with HOXB4—a transcription factor known to have a role in the self-renewal of hematopoietic stem cells. When aggregated to EBs, the transfected cells were shown to yield larger hematopoietic populations than wild-type hESCs, and addition of cytokines further expanded their numbers (Bowles et al. 2006).

The extent to which the differentiation of hESCs into blood cells may be effectively used in medical procedures was evaluated in grafting experiments. The culture of human stem cells with murine bone marrow stromal cells allowed for the initiation of their differentiation in the required direction. The hESC-derived hematopoietic progenitors obtained by this protocol were injected into fetal sheep liver, and their progeny were found in the recipient's bone marrow and peripheral blood, albeit in low numbers. Bone marrow from the primary recipient was later engrafted into another sheep, which was also found to have human blood cells in bone marrow and peripheral blood (Narayan et al. 2006). hESC-derived hematopoietic precursors showed some engraftment ability in murine bone marrow as well. Such engraftment experiments, however, proved more fruitful when conducted with hematopoietic progenitors from cord blood origin (Wang et al. 2005b).

2.1.2.2 Endothelium and vasculature: Levenberg et al. (2002) observed the increased expression of endothelial genes within hESCs differentiating spontaneously *in vitro* as EBs (Table 1). This increase correlated with the gradual formation of complex networks of vascular-like structures within the aggregated cells, and so the researchers moved on to isolate endothelial cells derived from hESCs. Such cells, expressing the endothelial marker CD31, were shown to resemble human vein endothelial cells (HUVEC) in their protein expression, and possessed the expected structure both internally and externally (Levenberg et al. 2002).

Some vasculogenesis was also seen in hESC-derived teratomas (Tzukerman et al. 2003; Gerecht-Nir et al. 2004b). A more specific method for *in vitro* differentiation of hESCs to endothelium or endothelial precursor cells was obtained by coculturing them with murine yolk sac or bone marrow cells (Kaufman et al. 2001). Other, more innovative techniques encouraged such a process by the use of artificial polymeric scaffolds. Applying the cells onto porous alginate constructs allowed the formation of EBs with elaborate vascular structures (Gerecht-Nir et al. 2004a), whereas seeding CD31-positive cells on Matrigel suggested they may differentiate and organize into tubular structures.

PLLA/PLGA scaffolds also supported the *in vitro* vascular endothelial differentiation of either $CD31^+$ cells or hESCs within heterogeneously differentiating stem cells, and allowed for the engraftment of such cells into mice. This facilitated the formation of human microvessels-containing murine blood cells in their hollows, suggesting an integration with the host vascular system (Levenberg et al. 2002; Levenberg et al. 2003). *In vivo* differentiation of hESCs to blood vessels was also reported when a heterogeneous population of partially differentiated hESCs enriched for cardiomyocyte-like cells was injected into a rat heart (Laflamme et al. 2005).

2.1.3 Smooth muscle

In blood vessels, the endothelial cells are encapsulated within a sheath of smooth muscle. Differentiation of hESCs to muscle may have occurred during their coculture with murine visceral endoderm cells, as this produced a small group of differentiated cells with the electrophysiological properties of vascular smooth muscle (Mummery et al. 2003). Stronger evidence came from seeding of differentiating hESCs on polymeric structures, as elongated smooth muscle actin (SMA) expressing cells were located around lumens (Levenberg et al. 2003).

2.2 Dorsal (Paraxial) Mesoderm

During embryogenesis, the neural tube is lodged between two stripes of mesodermal cells, which segment synchronously to become the somites. The cells in the somites differentiate into three distinct groups. The *Sclerotome* will differentiate further to form the cartilage and skeleton, The *Myotome* will develop into the skeletal muscles, and the *Dermatome* will become the dermis and the adipocytes.

A recapitulation of this developmental pathway was achieved when hESCs differentiated into mesenchymal like cells, and later cultured in three separate methods to form progeny of each of the three groups (Barberi et al. 2005). Most studies, however, skipped investigation of the intermediate stages, and went directly to prove differentiation into dorsal (paraxial) mesoderm (Table 1).

2.2.1 Cartilage

The ability of hESCs to differentiate into cartilage was first shown by expression of CMP (matrilin1), a cartilage-specific gene (Schuldiner et al. 2000). Addition of TGFβ to cells derived from human EBs and grown on biodegradable scaffold seemed to induce chondrocyte formation (Levenberg et al. 2003). TGFβ and ascorbic acid were also shown to facilitate differentiation of mesenchymal-like cells derived from hESCs to chondrocytes (Barberi et al. 2005). *In ovo* implantation of human undifferentiated embryonic stem cells to chick embryo somites did not result in large-scale dorsal (paraxial) mesoderm progeny, as would be expected. However, some of the human cells did seem to integrate into the avian perichondrium of the vertebral arch (Goldstein et al. 2002).

2.2.2 Bone

Osteoblasts may derive from two embryonic germ layers. Whereas the bones comprising most of the skull originate from the ectodermal neural crest, the remainder of the skeleton is of mesodermal origin. The progenitor embryonic germ layer also dictates the mode of bone formation. The ectodermal bones form directly by intramembranous ossification, whereas the mesodermal bones require an intermediate cartilage tissue which serves as a mold (Gilbert 2000). However, studies of bone formation by hESCs referred only to the derivation of osteoblasts. Since the process which led to this point can only be inferred, it is not certain whether the osteoblast-like cells formed are of mesodermal origin. Since the majority of the human skeleton is of mesodermal origin, and as hESCs can differentiate into cartilage, it is plausible that *in vitro* osteogenesis from hESCs is of mesodermal origin.

The presence of bone-forming cells can be deduced from the precipitation of the minerals comprising the bone (Bielby et al. 2004; Ahn et al. 2006). Such precipitates are visible by chemical staining or by physical methods such as x-ray crystallography or electron microscopy (Karp et al. 2005).

Bone-forming cells can differentiate spontaneously by plating hESCs without MEFs (Barberi et al. 2005; Karp et al. 2005). However, large-scale *in vitro* differentiation of hESCs into osteoblasts involves culturing hESCs or EBs with supplements (Sottile et al. 2003; Bielby et al. 2004; Cao et al. 2005). Adding these components also led to the differentiation of mesenchymal-like cells (Barberi et al. 2005). Plating intact EBs on human primary bone-derived cells, without addition of special factors, can also direct hESCs to form osteoblasts (Ahn et al. 2006). Osteogenesis can be facilitated in stem cells by spreading treated cells on PDLLA scaffold and engrafting in SCID mice (Bielby et al. 2004).

2.2.3 Skeletal muscle

Inducing the differentiation of mesenchymal-like cells derived from hESCs into skeletal muscle was achieved by culturing them with murine myoblasts. Apart from identification of molecular markers, the cells formed multinucleated myotubes (Barberi et al. 2005).

2.2.4 Adipocytes

Xiong et al. (2005) identified fat cells in differentiated EBs on the basis of the typical lipid droplets that appear in their cytoplasm, and confirmed the finding by demonstrating the presence of the relevant mRNA molecules. They also cultured the EBs in the presence of rosiglitazone, an agonist of an adipocyte related receptor (PPARγ), which increased the number of adipocyte-like cells. This increase was concomitant with higher leptin levels in the medium, and since this hormone is characteristic of adipocytes, its secretion points to a recapitulation of fat cell function by the differentiated stem cells (Xiong et al. 2005). It should be noted, however, that none of the markers used, including mRNA and leptin, was shown to co-localize with the cells possessing lipid droplets, and therefore further evidence is required to conclude definite adipocyte differentiation. Stronger evidence for adipocyte differentiation was obtained by culturing hESC-derived mesenchymal cells with exogenous factors (Barberi et al. 2005).

2.3 Intermediate Mesoderm

Very little is known about the differentiation of hESCs into intermediate mesoderm, which comprise the kidney and the urogenital system. Schuldiner et al. (2000) identified mRNA transcripts typical of the kidney in undifferentiated hESCs. Additional relevant transcripts appeared via EB formation, and a substantial induction of renal gene transcription was obtained by supplementing EB-derived cells with nerve growth factor (NGF). This molecule, along with hepatocyte growth factor (HGF), may have also promoted these cells' differentiation into the cells of the urogenital system (Schuldiner et al. 2000). No further evidence for differentiation along these paths has been obtained.

3. CONCLUSION

During gastrulation, the formation of mesoderm starts a cascade of events that leads to the development of various tissues through the intermediate differentiation into intermediate, dorsal (paraxial), and lateral mesoderm, which give rise to most of the body mass. The study of hESCs has allowed for the artificially directed differentiation of pluripotent cells into some of the progenies of these three mesodermal lineages.

REFERENCES

Ahn, S.E., Kim, S., Park, K.H., Moon, S.H., Lee, H.J., Kim, G.J., Lee, Y.J., Park, K.H., Cha, K.Y., and Chung, H.M. (2006) Primary bone-derived cells induce osteogenic differentiation without exogenous factors in human embryonic stem cells. Biochem. Biophys. Res. Commun., 340: 403–408.

Barberi, T., Willis, L.M., Socci, N.D., and Studer, L. (2005) Derivation of multipotent mesenchymal precursors from human embryonic stem cells. PLoS. Med., 2: e161.

Bielby, R.C., Boccaccini, A.R., Polak, J.M., and Buttery, L.D. (2004) In vitro differentiation and in vivo mineralization of osteogenic cells derived from human embryonic stem cells. Tissue Eng., 10: 1518–1525.

Bowles, K.M., Vallier, L., Smith, J.R., Alexander, M.R., and Pedersen, R.A. (2006) HOXB4 overexpression promotes hematopoietic development by human embryonic stem cells. Stem Cells, 24: 1359–1369.

Cao, T., Heng, B.C., Ye, C.P., Liu, H., Toh, W.S., Robson, P., Li, P., Hong, Y.H., and Stanton, L.W. (2005) Osteogenic differentiation within intact human embryoid bodies result in a marked increase in osteocalcin secretion after 12 days of in vitro culture, and formation of morphologically distinct nodule-like structures. Tissue Cell, 37: 325–334.

Carlson, B. (1988) Patten's Foundations of Embryology, 5th edn. McGraw-Hill, New York.

Chadwick, K., Wang, L., Li, L., Menendez, P., Murdoch, B., Rouleau, A., and Bhatia, M. (2003) Cytokines and BMP-4 promote hematopoietic differentiation of human embryonic stem cells. Blood, 102: 906–915.

Cerdan, C., Rouleau, A., and Bhatia, M. (2004) VEGF-A165 augments erythropoietic development from human embryonic stem cells. Blood, 103: 2504–2512.

Dvash, T., Mayshar, Y., Darr, H., McElhaney, M., Barker, D., Yanuka, O., Kotkow, K.J., Rubin, L.L., Benvenisty, N., and Eiges, R. (2004) Temporal gene expression during differentiation of human embryonic stem cells and embryoid bodies. Hum. Reprod., 19: 2875–2883.

Eiges, R., Schuldiner, M., Drukker, M., Yanuka, O., Itskovitz-Eldor, J., and Benvenisty, N. (2001) Establishment of human embryonic stem cell-transfected clones carrying a marker for undifferentiated cells. Curr. Biol., 11: 514–518.

Gaur, M., Kamata, T., Wang, S., Moran, B., Shattil, S.J., and Leavitt, A.D. (2006) Megakaryocytes derived from human embryonic stem cells: a genetically tractable system to study megakaryocytopoiesis and integrin function. J. Thromb. Haemost., 4: 436–442.

Gerecht-Nir, S., Cohen, S., Ziskind, A., and Itskovitz-Eldor, J. (2004a) Three-dimensional porous alginate scaffolds provide a conducive environment for generation of well-vascularized embryoid bodies from human embryonic stem cells. Biotechnol. Bioeng., 88: 313–320.

Gerecht-Nir, S., Dazard, J.E., Golan-Mashiach, M., Osenberg, S., Botvinnik, A., Amariglio, N., Domany, E., Rechavi, G., Givol, D., and Itskovitz-Eldor, J. (2005) Vascular gene expression and phenotypic correlation during differentiation of human embryonic stem cells. Dev. Dyn., 232: 487–497.

Gerecht-Nir, S., Osenberg, S., Nevo, O., Ziskind, A., Coleman, R., and Itskovitz-Eldor, J. (2004b) Vascular development in early human embryos and in teratomas derived from human embryonic stem cells. Biol. Reprod., 71: 2029–2036.

Gilbert, S. (2000) Developmental Biology, 6th edn. Sinauer Associates, Sunderland, MA.

Goldstein, R.S., Drukker, M., Reubinoff, B.E., and Benvenisty, N. (2002) Integration and differentiation of human embryonic stem cells transplanted to the chick embryo. Dev. Dyn., 225: 80–86.

He, J.Q., Ma, Y., Lee, Y., Thomson, J.A., and Kamp, T.J. (2003) Human embryonic stem cells develop into multiple types of cardiac myocytes: action potential characterization. Circ. Res., 93: 32–39.

Itskovitz-Eldor, J., Schuldiner, M., Karsenti, D., Eden, A., Yanuka, O., Amit, M., Soreq, H., and Benvenisty, N. (2000) Differentiation of human embryonic stem cells into embryoid bodies compromising the three embryonic germ layers. Mol. Med. 6: 88–95.

Karp, J.M., Ferreira, L.S., Khademhosseini, A., Kwon, A.H., Yeh, J., and Langer, R. (2005) Cultivation of human embryonic stem cells without the embryoid body step enhances osteogenesis in vitro. Stem Cells [Epub ahead of print].

Kaufman, D.S., Hanson, E.T., Lewis, R.L., Auerbach, R., and Thomson, J.A. (2001) Hematopoietic colony-forming cells derived from human embryonic stem cells. Proc. Natl. Acad. Sci. USA, 98: 10716–10721.

Kehat, I., Gepstein, A., Spira, A., Itskovitz-Eldor, J., and Gepstein, L. (2002) High-resolution electrophysiological assessment of human embryonic stem cell-derived cardiomyocytes: a novel in vitro model for the study of conduction. Circ. Res., 91: 659–661.

Kehat, I., Kenyagin-Karsenti, D., Snir, M., Segev, H., Amit, M., Gepstein, A., Livne, E., Binah, O., Itskovitz-Eldor, J., and Gepstein, L. (2001) Human embryonic stem cells can differentiate into myocytes with structural and functional properties of cardiomyocytes. J. Clin. Invest., 108: 407–414.

Kehat, I., Khimovich, L., Caspi, O., Gepstein, A., Shofti, R., Arbel, G., Huber, I., Satin, J., Itskovitz-Eldor, J., and Gepstein, L. (2004) Electromechanical integration of cardiomyocytes derived from human embryonic stem cells. Nat. Biotechnol., 22: 1282–1289.

Kim, S.J., Kim, B.S., Ryu, S.W., Yoo, J.H., Oh, J.H., Song, C.H., Kim, S.H., Choi, D.S., Seo, J.H., Choi, C.W., Shin, S.W., Kim, Y.H., and Kim, J.S. (2005) Hematopoietic differentiation of embryoid bodies derived from the human embryonic stem cell line SNUhES3 in co-culture with human bone marrow stromal cells. Yonsei. Med. J., 46: 693–699.

Laflamme, M.A., Gold, J., Xu, C., Hassanipour, M., Rosler, E., Police, S., Muskheli, V., and Murry, C.E. (2005) Formation of human myocardium in the rat heart from human embryonic stem cells. Am. J. Pathol., 167: 663–671.

Levenberg, S., Golub, J.S., Amit, M., Itskovitz-Eldor, J., and Langer, R. (2002) Endothelial cells derived from human embryonic stem cells. Proc. Natl. Acad. Sci. USA, 99: 4391–4396.

Levenberg, S., Huang, N.F., Lavik, E., Rogers, A.B., Itskovitz-Eldor, J., and Langer, R. (2003) Differentiation of human embryonic stem cells on three-dimensional polymer scaffolds. Proc. Natl. Acad. Sci. USA, 100: 12741–12746.

Lu, S.J., Li, F., Vida, L., and Honig, G.R. (2004) CD34 + CD38- hematopoietic precursors derived from human embryonic stem cells exhibit an embryonic gene expression pattern. Blood, 103: 4134–4141.

Mossman, A.K., Sourris, K., Ng, E., Stanley, E.G., and Elefanty, A.G. (2005) Mixl1 and oct4 proteins are transiently co-expressed in differentiating mouse and human embryonic stem cells. Stem Cells Dev., 14: 656–663.

Mummery, C., Ward-van Oostwaard, D., Doevendans, P., Spijker, R., van den Brink, S., Hassink, R., van der Heyden, M., Opthof, T., Pera, M., de la Riviere, A.B., Passier, R., and Tertoolen, L. (2003) Differentiation of human embryonic stem cells to cardiomyocytes: role of coculture with visceral endoderm-like cells. Circulation, 107: 2733–2740.

Narayan, A.D., Chase, J.L., Lewis, R.L., Tian, X., Kaufman, D.S., Thomson, J.A., and Zanjani, E.D. (2006) Human embryonic stem cell-derived hematopoietic cells are capable of engrafting primary as well as secondary fetal sheep recipients. Blood, 107: 2180–2183.

Passier, R., Oostwaard, D.W., Snapper, J., Kloots, J., Hassink, R.J., Kuijk, E., Roelen, B., de la Riviere, A.B., and Mummery, C. (2005) Increased cardiomyocyte differentiation from human embryonic stem cells in serum-free cultures. Stem Cells, 23: 772–780.

Qiu, C., Hanson, E., Olivier, E., Inada, M., Kaufman, D.S., Gupta, S., and Bouhassira, E.E. (2005) Differentiation of human embryonic stem cells into hematopoietic cells by coculture with human fetal liver cells recapitulates the globin switch that occurs early in development. Exp. Hematol., 33: 1450–1458.

Satin, J., Kehat, I., Caspi, O., Huber, I., Arbel, G., Itzhaki, I., Magyar, J., Schroder, E.A., Perlman, I., and Gepstein, L. (2004) Mechanism of spontaneous excitability in human embryonic stem cell derived cardiomyocytes. J. Physiol., 559: 479–496.

Schuldiner, M., Yanuka, O., Itskovitz-Eldor, J., Melton, D.A., and Benvenisty, N. (2000) Effects of eight growth factors on the differentiation of cells derived from human embryonic stem cells. Proc. Natl. Acad. Sci. USA, 97: 11307–11312.

Segev, H., Kenyagin-Karsenti, D., Fishman, B., Gerecht-Nir, S., Ziskind, A., Amit, M., Coleman, R., and Itskovitz-Eldor, J. (2005) Molecular analysis of cardiomyocytes derived from human embryonic stem cells. Dev. Growth Differ., 47: 295–306.

Snir, M., Kehat, I., Gepstein, A., Coleman, R., Itskovitz-Eldor, J., Livne, E., and Gepstein, L. (2003) Assessment of the ultrastructural and proliferative properties of human embryonic stem cell-derived cardiomyocytes. Am. J. Physiol. Heart Circ. Physiol., 285: H2355–H2363.

Sottile, V., Thomson, A., and McWhir, J. (2003) In vitro osteogenic differentiation of human ES cells. Cloning Stem Cells, 5: 149–155.

Thomson, J.A., Itskovitz-Eldor, J., Shapiro, S.S., Waknitz, M.A., Swiergiel, J.J., Marshall, V.S., and Jones, J.M. (1998) Embryonic stem cell lines derived from human blastocysts. Science, 282: 1145–1147.

Tian, X., Morris, J.K., Linehan, J.L., and Kaufman, D.S. (2004) Cytokine requirements differ for stroma and embryoid body-mediated hematopoiesis from human embryonic stem cells. Exp. Hematol., 32: 1000–1009.

Tian, X., Woll, P.S., Morris, J.K., Linehan, J.L., and Kaufman, D.S. (2006) Hematopoietic engraftment of human embryonic stem cell-derived cells is regulated by recipient innate immunity. Stem Cells, 24: 1370–1380.

Tzukerman, M., Rosenberg, T., Ravel, Y., Reiter, I., Coleman, R., and Skorecki, K. (2003) An experimental platform for studying growth and invasiveness of tumor cells within teratomas derived from human embryonic stem cells. Proc. Natl. Acad. Sci. USA, 100: 13507–13512.

Vodyanik, M.A., Bork, J.A., Thomson, J.A., and Slukvin, II. (2005) Human embryonic stem cell-derived CD34 + cells: efficient production in the coculture with OP9 stromal cells and analysis of lymphohematopoietic potential. Blood, 105: 617–626.

Wang, L., Li, L., Shojaei, F., Levac, K., Cerdan, C., Menendez, P., Martin, T., Rouleau, A., and Bhatia, M. (2004) Endothelial and hematopoietic cell fate of human embryonic stem cells originates from primitive endothelium with hemangioblastic properties. Immunity, 21: 31–41.

Wang, J., Zhao, H.P., Lin, G., Xie, C.Q., Nie, D.S., Wang, Q.R., and Lu, G.X. (2005a) In vitro hematopoietic differentiation of human embryonic stem cells induced by co-culture with human bone marrow stromal cells and low dose cytokines. Cell Biol. Int., 29: 654–661.

Wang, L., Menendez, P., Shojaei, F., Li, L., Mazurier, F., Dick, J.E., Cerdan, C., Levac, K., and Bhatia, M. (2005b) Generation of hematopoietic repopulating cells from human embryonic stem cells independent of ectopic HOXB4 expression. J. Exp. Med., 201: 1603–1614.

Woll, P.S., Martin, C.H., Miller, J.S., and Kaufman, D.S. (2005) Human embryonic stem cell-derived NK cells acquire functional receptors and cytolytic activity. J. Immunol., 175: 5095–5103.

Xiong, C., Xie, C.Q., Zhang, L., Zhang, J., Xu, K., Fu, M., Thompson, W.E., Yang, L.J., and Chen, Y.E. (2005) Derivation of adipocytes from human embryonic stem cells. Stem Cells Dev., 14: 671–675.

Xu, C., Inokuma, M.S., Denham, J., Golds, K., Kundu, P., Gold, J.D., and Carpenter, M.K. (2001) Feeder-free growth of undifferentiated human embryonic stem cells. Nat. Biotechnol., 19: 971–974.

Xu, C., Police, S., Rao, N., and Carpenter, M.K. (2002) Characterization and enrichment of cardiomyocytes derived from human embryonic stem cells. Circ. Res., 91: 501–508.

Xue, T., Cho, H.C., Akar, F.G., Tsang, S.Y., Jones, S.P., Marban, E., Tomaselli, G.F., and Li, R.A. (2005) Functional integration of electrically active cardiac derivatives from genetically engineered human embryonic stem cells with quiescent recipient ventricular cardiomyocytes: insights into the development of cell-based pacemakers. Circulation, 111: 11–20.

Zambidis, E.T., Peault, B., Park, T.S., Bunz, F., and Civin, C.I. (2005) Hematopoietic differentiation of human embryonic stem cells progresses through sequential hematoendothelial, primitive, and definitive stages resembling human yolk sac development. Blood, 106: 860–870.

Zhan, X., Dravid, G., Ye, Z., Hammond, H., Shamblott, M., Gearhart, J., and Cheng, L. (2004) Functional antigen-presenting leucocytes derived from human embryonic stem cells *in vitro*. Lancet, 364: 163–171.

CHAPTER 9

THREE-DIMENSIONAL CULTURE OF HUMAN EMBRYONIC STEM CELLS

SHARON GERECHT[1], JASON A. BURDICK[2], CHRISTOPHER CANNIZZARO[1], AND GORDANA VUNJAK-NOVAKOVIC[3]

[1] *Harvard-MIT Division of Health Sciences and Technology, Massachusetts Institute of Technology, Cambridge MA 02139*

[2] *Department of Bioengineering, University of Pennsylvania, Philadelphia PA 19104,*

[3] *Department of Biomedical Engineering, Columbia University, 1210 Amsterdam Avenue, MC 8904, New York, NY 10027*

1. INTRODUCTION

Human embryonic stem cells (hESCs) were initially derived in 1998 by Thomson and colleagues (Thomson et al. 1998). Due to their essentially unlimited capacity for self-renewal and differentiation and capability to give rise to any cell type in the body, these cells have been actively researched since their discovery. Human ESCs have enormous potential for two important areas: (a) regenerative medicine for therapeutics and (b) fundamental research of human development. The use of different hESC lines and variations of culture protocols and culture durations raise the fundamental question whether different preparations of undifferentiated hESCs are equivalent (see review by Hoffman and Carpenter 2005). Clearly, the interpretation of data, comparisons of results from different laboratories, and the use of hESC derivatives will all depend on our ability to culture hESCs in a controllable and reproducible fashion and to maintain and rigorously assess their characteristics. Ideally, the environments established *in vitro* for the derivation, propagation and differentiation of hESCs should resemble the environments that cells encounter *in vivo*.

In this chapter, we review the cultivation of hESCs in three-dimensional (3D) environments, which can provide *rigorous control over the cell microenvironment* within a setting that is designed to *mimic the native developmental milieu* (e.g., that of an early blastocyst, or that associated with development of specific cell/tissue types). The approach we discuss is biomimetic in nature,

J.R. Masters et al (eds.), Embryonic Stem Cells, 149–172.

as it tends to capture various aspects of the native environment, using two components:

- *Scaffold* that provides a structural and logistic template for cell attachment, growth and differentiation
- *Bioreactor* that controls the environmental conditions, maintains all parameters of interest at target levels, and subjects the cells to molecular and physical regulatory signals

Our focus is on 3D systems for culture of hESCs (not including murine ESCs or human germ cells), all of which were established in recent years. We discuss the 3D settings for the *growth of undifferentiated hESCs* and for the *directed differentiation of expanded hESCs into various cell lineages*, in the overall context of derivation of hESC-based cell sources for fundamental research and regenerative medicine. In all cases, the two components of such 3D systems—a biomaterial scaffold and a bioreactor—are described, and detailed protocols are provided for each step of the process. Lastly, our review of the criteria and methods used for characterization of hESCs and their derivatives is only briefly covered since this important aspect of hESC cultivation is covered in other chapters of this book.

2. STATE OF THE ART

Consistency of cell properties: The success rates for deriving hESC lines range from 5% to 100%, reflecting the differences and inconsistencies in procedures used in different laboratories. Human ESC isolation procedures vary as well (Hoffman and Carpenter 2005). However, despite these differences in the derivation process, all hESC lines derived to date exhibit similar expression patterns of standard stem cell markers. It is possible that the various conditions used are all permissive to some extent for cultivation of various hESC preparations. Additionally, it is possible that the differences between hESCs from different culture systems are not seen due to low fidelity of current methods used to characterize hESCs.

Methods for hESC characterization: Standard methods for evaluation of hESCs include the expression of molecular markers and the capacity of the cells to differentiate into various lineages. Recently, the capacity of hESCs to proliferate (self-renew) over extended periods at a constant rate and the euploid and epigenetic status of the cells are considered important additional criteria (Hoffman and Carpenter 2005). For differentiated cells derived from hESCs, the assessment methods are those routinely used for characterization of primary tissue cells, and they vary from one cell type to another. In addition, for all hESC derivatives it is critically important to assess and document the lack of tumorigenicity.

Passaging: Standard culture protocols for expansion of undifferentiated hESCs involve cultivation in monolayers followed by either mechanical disaggregation or enzymatic dissociation of the cells. Mechanical passaging generally results in variable cluster size and cell distribution. Enzymatic passaging involves the use of enzymes of animal origin, such as bacterial collagenase or porcine trypsin, which carries the risk of zoonosis and can result in abnormal cell karyotype (Brimble et al. 2004). It has been recommended to culture hESCs in clusters (to preserve the integrity of culture) and to rigorously monitor the characteristics of the cells (to ensure consistency of the outcomes) (Hoffman and Carpenter 2005). However, the maintenance of cell density remains a problem. Development of new culture methods that help overcome the limitations of the current techniques would greatly improve the consistency of hESC proliferation and help ensure equivalency of the cells derived in independent experiments.

Maintenance of cell karyotype: How and whether the hESCs can be used as a source of cells for engineered tissues and regenerative medicine, drug screening, studies of development, models of disease, and many other applications depends on the fundamental properties of hESCs and their derivatives, which are in turn dependent on the methods we use to isolate, propagate, differentiate, and characterize the cells. Notably, the "normalcy" of these cells can depend on culture conditions. Most studies report the maintenance of normal karyotype in long-term cultures (e.g., Rosler et al. 2004), whereas some studies suggest that the accumulation of cytogenetic abnormalities may be related to the manner in which the cells are passaged (Brimble et al. 2004) and that hESCs propagated *in vitro* for even a few months can develop an abnormal karyotype (Buzzard et al. 2004; Draper et al. 2004). Data reported by Mitalipova and colleagues (Mitalipova et al. 2005) showed that the maintenance of normal karyotype (after 100 passages) was indeed possible if the passaging was done manually, whereas bulk passaging that involves the use of enzymes which can perpetuate aberrations from normal karyotype and alter gene expression patterns in hESCs.

Culture conditions: Established approaches for the *in vitro expansion of undifferentiated hESCs* involve monolayer cultures, either on a mouse or human feeder layer, or use of medium conditioned by cultivation of feeder layers (Xu C. et al. 2001, 2005; Proetzel and Wiles 2002; Richards et al. 2002; Amit et al. 2004; Stojkovic et al. 2005). Additional methods have been developed that include the use of medium supplemented by basic fibroblastic growth factor (bFGF), in cultures that either have no serum (Amit et al. 2000), or no feeder layers (Xu et al. 2001). The supplementation of high concentrations of bFGF to culture medium containing serum replacement enabled the maintenance of hESCs expressing normal characteristics (karyotype, molecular markers, pluripotency, telomerase activity) (Wang et al. 2005; Xu, C. et al. 2005; Xu, R.H. et al. 2005). Established approaches for the *in vitro differentiation of hESCs* involve the generation of embryoid bodies (EBs) with cells forming all three layers: mesoderm, ectoderm, and endoderm. The specific lineages of differentiated cells are then obtained by sorting the cell populations from dissociated EBs. Alternative methods discussed in this chapter include directed differentiation of hESCs propagated in culture into specific cell lineages (Hoffman and Carpenter 2005).

Biomaterial substrates for hESC culture: Cultures of undifferentiated hESCs have been maintained on substrates that belong to two general classes: (a) feeder layers (mouse or human origin, alive or inactivated), and (b) biopolymers (Matrigel, laminin or fibronectin in the presence of conditioned medium). Although Matrigel represents an improvement over the use of feeder layers, its use is not without problems. Matrigel is of animal origin, contains a variety of defined and undefined components (laminin, collagen IV, entactin, heparan sulfate proteoglycan, and many different growth factors), and has a composition that varies from one batch to another. The use of a single matrix such as laminin (human from placenta, mouse or from tumors) or fibronectin (from human, bovine or mouse plasma, from human foreskin fibroblasts) has also been successful in the maintenance of hESCs (Xu et al. 2001; Amit et al. 2004). In sum, although the use of a single substrate for hESC growth is a considerable step forward over the use of feeder layers, the substrates we currently use contain undefined components, and have batch-to-batch variability.

A new generation of biomaterials that can mimic the regulatory characteristics of natural extracellular matrices (ECMs) is now being developed and used as a 3D environment for fundamental studies of cell function and tissue development, and for application in regenerative medicine (see review by Lutolf and Hubbell 2005). Clearly, even the best synthetic biomaterials we currently have lack the complexity of natural ECMs, and have only a limited capacity for presenting the cells with spatial and temporal profiles of multiple molecular and physical regulatory factors. However, progress is being made and the combined advances in polymer science, engineering, and cell biology are leading towards the development of materials that can help recapitulate signaling involved in stem cell growth and differentiation during normal morphogenesis. The methods for hESC propagation and differentiation in 3D culture described in this chapter include the use of some of these novel biomaterials, such as hyaluronic acid hydrogels that are chemically, structurally, and mechanically designed to capture some of the features of native ECMs (Anderson et al. 2004; Burdick et al. 2004; Khademhosseini et al. 2006).

3. CULTURE REQUIREMENTS

Human ESCs have been maintained under a variety of conditions and culture durations using a range of culture media, cell attachment substrates, cell lines, passage numbers, and regulatory factors (such as bone morphogenic proteins BMPs, fibroblast growth factors (FGFs), Wnts). In many instances, it is difficult to compare the results obtained in various experiments because of differences in experimental conditions, cell properties and culture durations. It is even more difficult to define which conditions are optimal, because the final selection of culture methods and their standardization requires more insight into the regulatory pathways and the molecular factors controlling these pathways. Finally, the observations from these studies are likely affected by the 2D setting of the cultures (which are distinctly different from the 3D setting of a developing blastocyst), the lack of control of additional developmentally relevant factors—in particular oxygen—and the lack of spatial and temporal profiling of factors which are intrinsic for normal development. Culture systems similar to the *in vivo* environment, with more precise control of multiple regulatory factors and the ability to subject the cells to gradients of factors, would greatly advance the optimization of culture conditions for desired cell outcomes (Gerecht-Nir et al. 2006; Radisic et al. 2006, in press).

During normal development, stem cells reside in a 3D environment of a developing blastocyst, where they are engaged in a cross-talk with the surrounding cells and ECM. Biologists are increasingly turning to 3D cell cultures, where they are observing the patterns of gene expression and other biological activities that more closely mirror what happens in living organisms (Jacks et al. 2002; Abbot 2003; Postovit et al. 2006). There is a growing awareness that the specific context of the in vivo stem cell "niche" needs to be reproduced *in vitro* in order to create a system that will have sufficient fidelity to tease apart the biochemical signaling between the cells and their environment.

Well-defined and controllable culture conditions are required to help establish much needed consistency of protocols used in multiple laboratories. The general requirements for hESC culture include:

- Chemical and structural design of the cell culture substrate
- The use of chemically defined media with no components of animal origin
- Establishment of spatially uniform initial cell distributions in a range of cell densities
- Close control of the culture parameters (pH, levels of nutrients, growth factors, metabolites, oxygen) in the cell microenvironment
- Ability to subject the cells to spatial and temporal profiles of regulatory molecules (e.g., oxygen concentration over the time in culture)
- Imaging compatibility (e.g., fluorescence) to monitor the progression of culture in real time without interruption

Additional specific requirements may be determined by the intended use of the hESCs. In some cases, it will be required to propagate the hESCs and maintain their undifferentiated properties and high proliferation rate. These cells will then be subjected to selective differentiation in a separate system, for example by using tissue engineering scaffolds and bioreactors. In other cases, maintenance of undifferentiating hESCs in culture will be followed by directed cell differentiation within the same system. Clearly, the design of the culture system will depend on the set of tasks that will need to be performed in each particular case. In all cases, however, the overall goal is to have control over the characteristics of hESCs and their derivatives and to rigorously test the cells at all stages of culture to ensure that there are no artifacts or aberrations that would affect the experimental observations and the ultimate use of the cells.

We describe here four different, complementary methods for the cultivation of hESCs in 3D environments, using biomaterial scaffolds and cell culture devices (bioreactors):

- *Method 1* involves the use of porous scaffolds made of synthetic polymers for cultivation of differentiated cells from EBs grown using conventional methods.
- *Method 2* involves the use of alginate scaffolds for the culture of undifferentiated hESCs and generation of EBs.
- *Method 3* involves the use of hyaluronic acid-based hydrogels for encapsulation and maintenance of undifferentiated hESCs.
- *Method 4* involves the use of hyaluronic acid-based hydrogels in conjunction with microarray bioreactors for directed differentiation of hESCs.

3.1 Method 1: Cultivation of Differentiated hESCs on Porous Scaffolds

Scope and objectives: hESC differentiation can be induced in monolayer culture or by removing the cells from their feeder layer and growing them in suspension, where they form EBs. Chemical cues provided directly by growth factors or indirectly by feeder cells induce ESC differentiation toward specific lineages within the EBs. However, cell growth and differentiation in EBs are rather spontaneous, and it has been difficult to control cell proliferation and differentiation into higher-order structures. Levenberg and colleagues examined the use of porous, biodegradable scaffolds made of synthetic polymers for the cultivation of early differentiating hESCs isolated from EBs (Levenberg et al. 2003, 2005).

In one study (Levenberg et al. 2003), 3D tissue constructs were obtained with characteristics of neural tissue, cartilage, and liver using various growth factors supplements. They report that tissue constructs implanted in severe combined immunodeficient (SCID) mice continued to express specific differentiation markers and vascularize.

In another study (Levenberg et al. 2005), neuronal differentiation of hESCs in 3D porous polymer scaffolds was induced using neurotrophic factors. In both cases, porous degradable polymer scaffolds created a supportive environment for the growth of differentiating hESCs and their organization into tissue-like structures.

3.1.1 Experimental design

A schematic presentation of the experimental design for Method 1 is shown in Figure 1. The scaffolds were seeded with cells derived from 4- and 9-day-old EBs. EBs were trypsinized, and either mixed with Matrigel and seeded on scaffolds, or seeded directly on scaffolds coated with fibronectin. Scaffold was a porous structure made from a blend of 50% poly(lactic-co-glycolic acid) (PLGA) and 50% poly(L-lactic acid), with a void volume of 90%, and interconnected pores ranging from 250 to 500 μm. The resulting constructs were grown

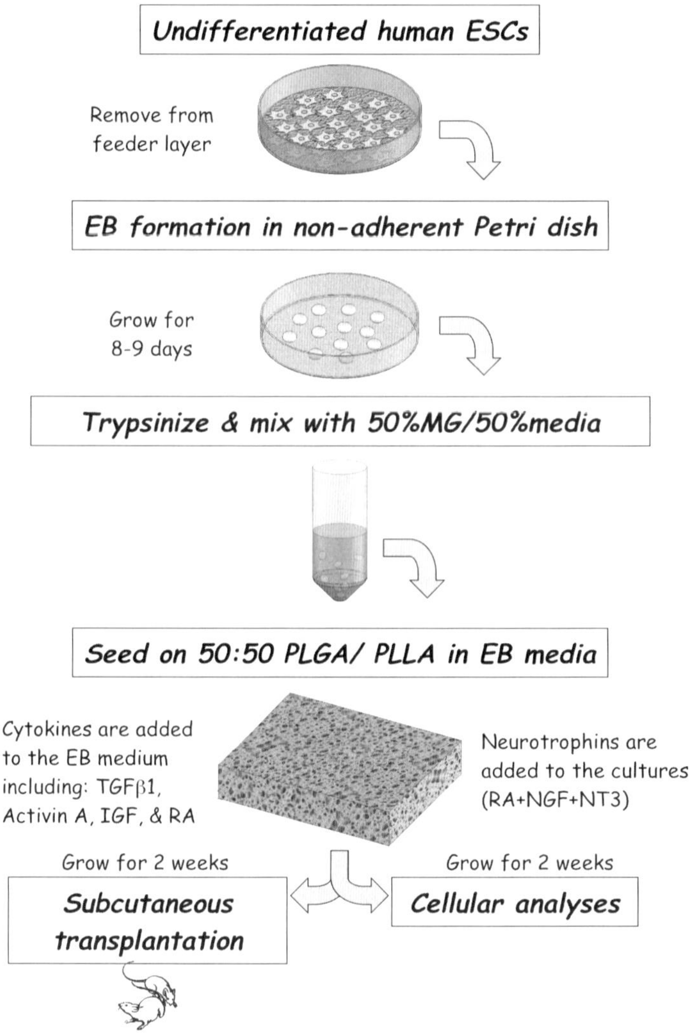

Figure 1. Experimental design for Method 1.

in culture medium supplemented with one or more cytokines for a period of two weeks. In one study, medium was supplemented with one or more of the following cytokines: retinoic acid (RA), activin-A, transforming growth factor β (TGF-β1), and insulin-like growth factor-I (IGF-I), and the final constructs were implanted into SCID mice for an additional 2 weeks. In another study, a combination of neurotrophic factors was added to the culture medium, constructs were grown for 2 weeks and analyzed for cell proliferation, differentiation, and formation of tissue-like structures.

3.1.2 Description of methods

Scaffold fabrication: Scaffolds consisting of a 50/50 blend of poly(lactic-co-glycolic acid) (Boehringer Ingelheim, Ingelheim, Germany, MW ~25 kDa) and poly(L-lactic acid) (PLA, Polysciences, Warrington, PA, MW ~300 kDa) were fabricated by a salt-leaching process as described previously (Levenberg et al. 2002) with pores in the range of 250–500 μm. Scaffolds were cut into rectangular pieces (~4 × 4 × 1 mm), sterilized overnight in 70% (vol/vol) ethanol and washed three times in phosphate buffered saline prior to cell seeding. The porous structure of the scaffolds was determined by sputter coating with gold and visualizing on a scanning electron microscope.

Cell culture: hESCs (H9 line) were grown on mouse embryonic fibroblasts (MEF; Cell Essential, Boston, MA) in knockout medium as previously described (Itskovitz-Eldor et al. 2000). To induce formation of EBs, hESC colonies were dissociated with 1 mg/mL collagenase Type IV and suspended in differentiation medium without lymphocyte inhibitory factor (LIF) and bFGF in Petri dishes (Itskovitz-Eldor et al. 2000).

Cell differentiation on Matrigel and on scaffolds: For seeding in Matrigel, 8- to 9-day-old EBs were trypsinized, and $0.8 \cdot 10^6$ cells were mixed in 25 μl of a 50% (vol/vol) medium and Matrigel (growth factor reduced, BD Biosciences, Bedford, MA). EB medium was supplemented with one of the following growth factors: TGF-β1 (2 ng/mL), activin-A (20 ng/mL), and IGF-I (10 ng/mL) (R & D Systems), and RA (300 ng/mL) (Sigma). The cell-Matrigel mixture solidified in a six-well Petri dish in a 37 °C incubator and was detached from the dish using a sterile blade. Four milliliters of EB medium containing a specific growth factor was added. *For seeding on scaffolds*, $0.8 \cdot 10^6$ cells (either undifferentiated hESCs or 8-day EBs) were seeded into each scaffold by using 25 μl of a mixture containing 50% (vol/vol) of Matrigel and the respective EB medium. After seeding the cells, scaffolds were cultured in six-well Petri dishes in their respective medium. For some experiments, scaffolds were soaked in 50 μg/mL fibronectin (Sigma) for 1 h and washed in PBS, and the cells were seeded without the use of Matrigel in 25 μl of EB medium.

Tissue processing and immunohistochemical staining: Tissue constructs were fixed for 6 h in 10% neutral buffered formalin, embedded in paraffin and sectioned to 5 μm. For histological evaluation, sections were stained with hematoxylin and eosin (H&E), trichrome, and safranin-O. For immunohistochemical evaluation, sections were stained with the following primary antibodies: anti-human α-feto-protein (AFP) (1:2,500), cytokeratin-7 (1:25), CD31(1:20), albumin (1:100), vimentin (1:50), S100 (1:100), Desmin (1:150), Myogenin (1:150), and Insulin (1:100) (all from Dako), anti-human β_{III}-tubulin (Sigma, 1:500), nestin (Transduction Laboratories, 1:1,000), CD34 (Labvision, Fremont, CA, 1:20), antihuman stage-specific embryonic antigen 4 (SSEA4, Hybridoma bank, University of Iowa, Ames, 1:4), and Tra 1–60 (a gift from Peter Andrews, University of Sheffield, Sheffield, U.K., 1:10). For proliferation studies, culture medium was incubated with 10 μl of BrdUrd (Sigma) for 3 h before tissues were harvested, fixed, and stained by mouse anti-BrdUrd antibodies (1:1,000). (For details, please see Levenberg et al. 2003).

RT-PCR analysis: RNA was isolated by an RNEasy Mini kit (Qiagen, Valencia, CA). RT-PCR was carried out by using a Qiagen OneStep RT-PCR kit with 10 units of RNase inhibitor (GIBCO) and 40 ng of RNA. The amplified products were separated on 1.2% agarose gels with ethidium bromide (E Gel, Invitrogen). (For details see Levenberg et al. 2003).

Transplantation into SCID mice: After 2 weeks of cultivation, tissue constructs were implanted subcutaneously in the dorsal region of 4-week-old SCID mice (CB.17.SCID, Taconic Farms). Scaffolds without cells were used as controls. The implants were retrieved after an additional 2 weeks and evaluated histologically.

3.1.3 Summary of results

Formation of tissue constructs by early differentiating hESCs on porous scaffolds: After 2 weeks of *in vitro* culture, primitive tissue structures were found throughout the scaffolds with tissue-specific markers observed depending on the growth factor used. Specifically, supplementation of IGF resulted in the formation of open tubular structures lined by a single layer of cytokeratin-positive cuboidal-to-columnar epithelial cells. Supplementation of RA induced the formation of small circular multilayered bodies and an increase in the fraction of cytokeratin-positive areas, approaching levels found in adult lung. Collagen production, demonstrated by trichrome stain, and cell-matrix organization were markedly influenced by growth factor supplementation to the culture medium. In addition, 3D capillary-like networks containing cells displaying endothelial surface markers were observed.

2D-3D growth and the effect of cell growth substrate: The 2D fibronectin-coated dish supported some cell differentiation but could not support the formation of 3D structures. Matrigel alone failed to support the hESC growth and 3D organization beyond the formation of capillary networks from vascular progenitor cells. With respect to the differentiation and organization of cells grown on a scaffold or within EBs, higher expression of differentiation-associated proteins such as cytokeratin, AFP, and nestin was found on the scaffolds. This finding correlates with a more complete organization of epithelial tubular structures and neural tube-like rosettes. The EB population had very heterogeneous structures and protein expression levels. Consequently, polymer scaffolds were more suitable than EBs from the perspective of directed cell differentiation and the homogeneity of cell populations. The small size of the EBs and high heterogeneity between individual EBs may limit their utility for generating large numbers of cells needed to engineer functional tissues for transplantation applications.

Neuronal differentiation: After 2 weeks of *in vitro* cultivation, the constructs were partially filled with differentiating tissue. Neural structures (i.e., rosettes) were found throughout the constructs, and the number and maturity of the tissue structures depended on the addition of RA, NGF, and NT-3. In the presence of neurotrophins, the rosette structures consisted of a more defined ring structure with elongated and oriented nuclei. In addition, neurotrophins induced the formation of more pronounced and larger lumens as compared to control cultures. A significant increase in the number of neural structures was observed in the presence of NGF and NT-3, for hESCs isolated from 4-day-old EBs and in the presence of NT-3 alone or in combination with RA for 9-day-old EBs.

Subcutaneous implantation: After 2 weeks, implants contained viable cells and blood vessels formed from both human and host cells, in some cases containing intraluminal red blood cells. Immunostaining with cytokeratin, β_{III}-tubulin, and AFP antibodies indicated that the implanted constructs continued to express these human proteins. In certain instances, the constructs continued to differentiate after implantation, in the direction mediated by the cytokine treatment during *in vitro* culture.

Vasculogenesis: Vascularization of tissue-engineered structures is essential in maintaining cell viability over clinically useful thicknesses (the penetration depth of oxygen in most vascularized tissues is only 100–200 μm, Radisic et al. 2006). It is thus important that capillary-like networks were observed throughout the cultured constructs, and especially those seeded with cells derived from 4-day-old EBs and treated with NGF. The presence of RA in the culture medium appeared to inhibit endothelial differentiation and formation of capillary networks. The inhibitory effect of RA on endothelial vessel formation was also shown with differentiating hESCs derived from 8-day-old EBs.

3.2 Method 2: Generation of EBs from Undifferentiated hESCs in Porous Alginate Scaffolds

Scope and objectives: The cultivation of EBs from undifferentiated hESCs is an *in vitro* analogue of the early stages of embryonic development *in vivo*. A representative and successful method for the *in vitro* formation of EBs involved the cultivation of undifferentiated hESCs encapsulated in alginate scaffolds, (Gerecht-Nir et al. 2004a). In contrast, a study that employed the seeding of undifferentiated hESCs into porous PLLA/PLGA scaffolds failed to generate EBs (Levenberg et al. 2003). It thus appears that the confined environment of the pore structure in alginate scaffolds was the factor that mediated the formation of a homogenous population of EBs starting from dissociated undifferentiated hESCs.

Alginate scaffolds are characterized by a macromolecular structure resembling the ECM and they enable efficient cell seeding and cultivation (Shapiro and Cohen 1997; Glicklis et al. 2000; Leor et al. 2000). The porosity of the alginate scaffolds can be controlled during fabrication, yielding a sponge-like material with more than 90% void volume and interconnected pores ranging from 50 to 200 μm (Zmora et al. 2002). The formation of EBs in alginate scaffolds was studied with respect to cell proliferation and differentiation in the scaffold-borne EBs, with an emphasis on the vasculogenesis process.

3.2.1 Experimental design

A schematic presentation of the experimental design for Method 2 is shown in Figure 2. Undifferentiated hESCs were removed from their feeder layer and inoculated into the scaffolds at three initial concentrations: high ($0.8–1 \times 10^6$ cells/scaffold), medium ($0.4 – 0.7 \times 10^6$ cells/scaffold) and low ($0.1–0.25 \times 10^6$ cells/scaffold). The scaffolds used in the study were fabricated from alginate, in the form of porous 5 mm diameter × 2 mm thick discs, with void volume of ~90%), and a network of interconnected round pores with diameters of 50–200 μm (Zmora et al. 2002). hESC-alginate constructs were cultured for a period of 30 days either statically or in a rotating bioreactor (Gerecht-Nir et al. 2004a).

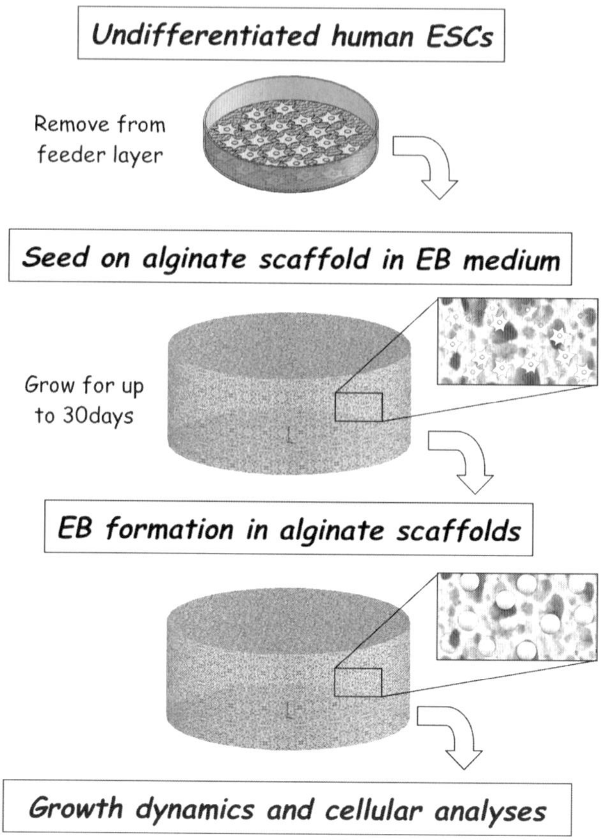

Figure 2. Experimental design for Method 2.

3.2.2 Description of methods

hESCs: Undifferentiated hESCs (H9.2 and H13 lines) were grown on an inactivated MEF layer, in growth medium consisting of 80% Knockout DMEM (KO-DMEM, Gibco Invitrogen Co, San Diego, CA), supplemented with 20% Knockout Serum Replacement (KSR), 4 ng/mL basic FGF, 1 mM L-glutamine, 0.1 mM β-mercaptoethanol, and 1% nonessential amino acid stock (Invitrogen Corporation, Carlsbad, CA). Cells were passaged every 4–6 days using 1 mg/mL Type IV collagenase (Invitrogen Corporation, Carlsbad, CA). For the control group with static EB formation, hESCs were removed from the feeder layer using either 1 mg/mL Type IV collagenase or 5mM EDTA (Promega, Madison, WI) in PBS and cultured in suspension in 50 mm nonadherent petri dishes (Corning) in medium consisting of 80% KO-DMEM, 20% defined fetal bovine serum (FBSd; HyClone), 1 mM L-glutamine, and 1% nonessential amino acid (all from Gibco-BRL). Dynamic formation of hEBs was carried out using a rotating bioreactor, as previously described (Gerecht-Nir et al. 2004a).

Scaffold preparation: Porous 3D scaffolds were prepared from pharmaceutical-grade alginate, Protanal LF 5/60 or LF120 (FMC Biopolymers, Drammen, Norway), which have a high glucuronic acid (G) content (65–75%) and solution viscosities (1% w/v, 25°C) of 50 and 200 cP, respectively. Scaffolds were prepared using a four-step process: (a) preparation of sodium alginate solutions (1 to 3% (w/v); (b) cross-linking of the alginate by adding the bivalent cross-linker calcium gluconate; (c) freezing the cross-linked alginate at –20°C; and (d) lyophilization to produce a sponge-like scaffold. The scaffolds were sterilized using ethylene oxide and stored at room temperature until use. The final scaffolds were in the form of discs (5 mm in diameter × 2 mm thick), had a void volume of ~90% porosity and pore sizes ranging from 50 to 200 µm (Shapiro and Cohen 1997; Zmora et al. 2002).

Cell seeding and cultivation: Dynamic cell seeding onto the scaffold was performed using a previously established method (Dar et al. 2002). Undifferentiated hESCs were collected, counted and concentrated according to the desired seeding cell number into 10–20 µl of hEB medium. The cell-suspension was then applied to the scaffolds, followed by centrifugation (1500 rpm for 3 min) and the addition of 200 µl of EB medium. After 12–24 h, the scaffolds were placed in 12-well plates (Nunc, Roskilde, Denmark) with 1 mL of fresh medium.

EB size, histology and immunohistochemistry: For size analysis, scaffolds were digested using PBS and the diameter of the scaffold-borne EBs was calculated as described before (Gerecht-Nir et al. 2004a). For histological analyses, scaffolds seeded with cells were fixed in 10% neutral-buffered formalin for 1 h at room temperature, dehydrated in graded ethanols (70–100%), embedded in paraffin, sectioned to 6–8 µm and stained with hematoxylin/eosin. Immunostaining was performed with a Dako LSAB+ staining kit with specific antihuman CD34, antihuman glial fibrillary acidic protein (GFAP), AFP (all from Dako, Denmark), and SSEA4 (kindly provided by Prof. P. Andrews, University of Sheffield, UK). Mouse IgG isotype-matching (R&D Systems Minneapolis MN, USA) or secondary antibody alone (from Dako LSAB+ staining kit), were used as a control. For quantification, at least 20 EBs per scaffold (n = 5) of three different experiments were scored for positive CD34+ voids. The degree of vascularization was calculated as the number of positive voids per EB.

Viability assay: The numbers of viable cells were determined by the XTT Kit (Sigma, St Louis MO, USA). The cell-seeded scaffolds were incubated for 4 hr with medium containing 20% (v/v) XTT solution. For analysis, 150 μl of the medium were sampled, placed in a 96-plate well and read by a microplate reader at 450 nm. The cell viability was determined according to the standard curve of known viable cell concentrations (Gerecht-Nir et al. 2004).

Scanning electron microscopy: Scaffolds were fixed for 1 hr in 3% glutaraldehyde in 0.1M sodium cacodylate, dehydrated in graduated alcohol (70–100%), and dried. The samples were coated with gold and examined using Philips XL30 (FEI company, Eindhoven, The Netherlands)

3.2.3 Summary of results

Scaffold properties: In their dry state, the scaffolds had compressive (Young's) moduli ranging from 385 ± 213 to 1,136 ± 264 kPa. The LF5/60 scaffolds degraded faster than LF120 scaffolds (Zmora et al. 2002). The hydrophilic nature of alginate enabled rapid hydration in culture medium, and resulted in efficient cell seeding with spatially uniform cell distributions throughout the scaffold volume (Gerecht-Nir et al. 2004b).

Bioreactor cultivation with and without scaffolds: When compared to the EBs formed without the scaffolds in the rotary bioreactor (Gerecht-Nir et al. 2004a), the scaffold-borne EBs were smaller in size (250 to 900 μm after 1 month of culture), spherical in shape and with a minimal tendency for agglomeration. Unlike the EBs formed in the bioreactors, the scaffold-borne hEBs were less uniform in size, probably reflecting the variability of scaffold pore size.

Effects of alginate material: The adherence of the cells and the number and size of the resultant hEBs depended on the initial cell seeding concentration and the type of alginate used to make the scaffolds. Seeding hESCs onto the LF5/60 scaffolds resulted in the adherence of about 65% of the initially added cells within 24 h, irrespective of the initial cell seeding concentration. The cells aggregated to form EBs within 48 h. Although the formation of EBs was not affected by the cell seeding concentration, the density of forming EBs increased concomitant with the increase in the initial cell seeding concentration, as occurs during EB formation in Petri dishes. With time, the LF5/60 scaffold-borne EBs grew in size, ruptured scaffolds due to their relatively poor mechanical strength and fast degradation, and were released into the medium from day 15 of culture.

In the LF120 alginate scaffolds, almost all of the cells adhered when seeding with low cell concentration suspensions, but no EBs were formed under these conditions. At medium and high cell concentrations, about 80% or 60% of the cells adhered to the scaffolds, respectively, and formed EBs within 48 h. Scanning electron micrographs of the hESC-seeded scaffolds after 1 month of cultivation revealed that the forming EBs occupied the entire pore volume, sometime extending outside the pores. Seeding the scaffolds with either high or medium cell concentrations yielded EBs with a similar size, which grew in size with time, eventually reaching a diameter ranging from 250 to 900 μm after a month of culture. Apparently, scaffold degradation with time and the increase in scaffold pore size enabled the growth of EBs beyond the initial pore size of 100 μm. At medium cell seeding concentrations, EBs formed mainly within the scaffold pores and were distributed evenly over the entire scaffold volume.

Cell viability: During EB formation within alginate scaffolds, there was a two-fold increase in the number of viable cells within the first week of culture, comparable to numbers reported for static culture (Gerecht-Nir et al. 2004b). Starting from the second week in culture, the increase in viable cell concentration in the EBs cultured in the scaffold system in a bioreactor was twice as high as that in the static culture, but lower than in the bioreactor culture of EBs without scaffolds. This may be due either to the better control over the aggregation and agglomeration of EBs in the scaffold-less bioreactor system, as compared to the scaffold-bioreactor system.

Cell morphology and differentiation: The overall morphology of EBs was similar in the scaffold-bioreactor system, scaffold-less bioreactor system and static dishes. Different cell types and tissue-like structures such as epithelial sheets and tubes, connective tissues and various voids could be observed in the scaffold-borne EBs which remained entrapped inside the scaffold pores, as well as in those that were released from the scaffold into the culture medium. Undifferentiated cells within the scaffold-borne EBs were examined by SSEA4, which is a known marker specific for primate cells of the inner cell mass stage (Thomson et al. 1998). After 1 week of differentiation, no SSEA4+ cells could be detected in any of the culture systems. Positive immuno-labeling of representative tissues of the three germ layers demonstrated that the scaffold-borne EBs maintained their capability of differentiating into representatives of the three germ layers: ectoderm, endoderm and mesoderm. It seems that the confining environment of the scaffolds helped control the morphology and size of EBs without altering the patterns of morphogenesis.

Vasculogenesis within the scaffold-borne EBs: Numerous voids were located within cells lining the scaffold walls or around scaffold pores. The majority of these structures were formed by CD34+ cells, and resulted in relatively complex structures compared to those formed in other systems (Gerecht-Nir et al. 2004). Twice as many voids with CD34+ cells were observed in scaffold-borne EBs compared to EBs formed in static Petri dishes. Thus, the alginate environment seems to enhance vessel formation as compared to the unconfined environments of the Petri dish and rotating bioreactor. The scaffold itself provides an initial template for the cells to adhere and interact with each other. The environment of the medium-filled pores allowed the cells to aggregate in a manner similar to that in suspension. It is also possible that alginate scaffolds induced signaling processes which favor vasculogenesis in the forming EBs. Such culture conditions are not available in the static Petri dishes or in the rotating bioreactors.

3.3 Method 3: Maintenance of Undifferentiated hESCs in Hyaluronic Acid (HA) Hydrogels

Scope and objectives: Monolayer cultures are the standard method for propagation of undifferentiated hESCs. While this method has enabled much progress in hESC research, there are two concerns that can limit the utility of this simple method. The first one is undefined composition, variability between batches, and the hazard of zoonosis associated with the use of components of animal origin. This concern has been eliminated, at least in part, by using systems with chemically defined components (please see the Introduction for details and references). The other concern is that a cell monolayer is distinctly different from the 3D architecture of a developing blastocyst, where hESCs are embedded in an ECM, which in turn regulates their growth and differentiation. Notably, the hyaluronic acid (HA) content is greatest in undifferentiated cells and during early embryogenesis, and then decreases at the onset of differentiation (Toole 2001). To address the need for controllable maintenance of undifferentiated hESC in a well-defined 3D environment, hESCs were encapsulated in a HA hydrogel scaffold (Gerecht-Nir et al. in revision). Hydrogels were selected because they may be composed of biologically recognized molecules, have a high water content to promote cell viability, and are structurally and mechanically similar to the native ECM of many tissues.

3.3.1 Experimental design

A schematic presentation of the experimental design for Method 3 is shown in Figure 3. Undifferentiated hESCs (lines H1, H9, and H13) were removed from their feeder layer and encapsulated in HA hydrogel by photopolymerization. Encapsulated hESCs were propagated in their undifferentiated state for over 40 days (30 population doublings). At timed intervals, cells could be released and recultured either on a feeder layer or in HA hydrogels, and evaluated.

3.3.2 Description of methods

hESCs: Three different lines of hESCs (WA9, WA13 and WA1, passages 19 – 40) were grown on inactivated MEFs in growth medium consisting of 80% Knockout DMEM, supplemented with 20% KSR, 4 ng/mL bFGF, 1 mM L-glutamine, 0.1 mM β-mercaptoethanol, 1% nonessential amino acid stock (Invitrogen Corporation, Carlsbad, CA). hESCs were passaged every 4 to 6 days using 1mg/mL Type IV collagenase (Invitrogen Corporation, Carlsbad, CA).

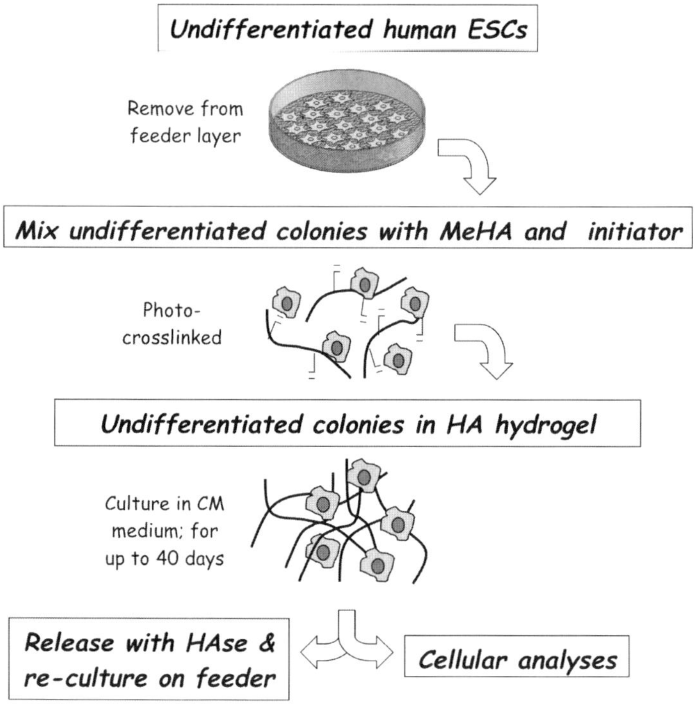

Figure 3. Experimental design for Method 3.

hESC encapsulation and release: Methacrylated HA was synthesized as previously described (Burdick et al. 2005) dissolved at a concentration of 2% in PBS containing 0.05% 2-methyl-1-[4-(hydroxyethoxy)phenyl]-2-methyl-1-propanone (Irgacure 2959, I2959) and hESCs were added (0.5–1 × 10^7 cells/mL precursor solution). The mixture was pipetted into a sterile mold (50 µL volume per well, to obtain discs measuring 5mm in diameter × 2mm thick), and photopolymerized (~10 mW/cm^2 UV light, BlakRay, for 10 min). Dextran-acrylate macromer was prepared as described previously (Ferreira et al. 2002). hESCs were encapsulated within the dextran using the same procedures as for HA hydrogels.

To release encapsulated hESCs, HA constructs were incubated for 24 h in hESC growth medium containing 1000 or 2000 U/mL hyaluronidase (Sigma, St. Louis, MO). For reculture, cells were collected, centrifuged, washed three times with PBS to remove any hydrogel residues, resuspended in growth medium, and cultured on MEF-coated dishes using standard methods (Carpenter et al. 2003; Schatten et al. 2005). For EB formation, hESCs were cultivated in nonadherent Petri dishes.

HA receptors and stem cell/differentiation markers: hESCs were removed from MEFs or released from hydrogels and filtered through a 40 µm mesh strainer (BD, San Jose, CA). Expression of alkaline phosphatase (AP) was considered as an indicator of hESCs in an undifferentiated state. Intrastain kit (Dako

California Inc. Carpinteria, CA) was used for the fixation and permeabilization of cell suspensions, according to the manufacturer's instructions. Dissociated hESCs were blocked with 5% FBS/PBS, incubated with antihuman CD44 clone A3D8 (Sigma, St. Louis, MO), or IgG antibody (R&D systems, Minneapolis, MN) for 30 min, and washed with PBS, followed by incubation with donkey anti-mouse FITC (Vector Labs Burlingame, CA) for 15min. Cells were stained with APC conjugated antihuman AP or PE conjugated antihuman SSEA4 (both from R&D systems, Minneapolis, MN) for stem cell markers or with FITC conjugated antihuman CD31 (BD, San Jose, CA) as marker of differentiation. hESCs were analyzed using FACSCalibur (BDIS) and Cell Quest software (BDIS).

Metabolic assay: Proliferating cells were identified by the XTT kit (Sigma, St. Louis MO). Undifferentiated hESCs cultured in the presence of macromer in concentrations of 10 and 50 μl/mL, on Matrigel, and within HA cultures were incubated for 4 h in medium containing 20% (v/v) XTT solution. For analysis, 150 μl of the medium was removed, placed in a 96-plate and read in a microplate reader at 450 nm. XTT was also used for visual analysis of viable cells within hydrogels in which HA constructs were incubated for 4 h in medium containing 20% (v/v) XTT solution and examined using inverted light microscopy (Nikon Diaphot system).

Immunohistochemistry: HA constructs were either embedded in histo-gel or directly fixed in 10% neutral-buffered formalin (Sigma, St. Louis, MO), dehydrated in graded alcohols (70 – 100%), embedded in paraffin, sectioned to 4 μm, and stained with hematoxylin/eosin. Immunostaining was performed using a Dako LSAB+ staining kit (Dako California Inc. Carpinteria, CA) with specific anti tumor rejection antibody (TRA)-1-60, anti TRA-1-81, and anti CD44 clone P3H9 (Chemicon Temecula, CA). Mouse IgG isotype-matching (R&D systems, Minneapolis, MN) or secondary antibody alone (from Dako LSAB+ staining kit) served as negative controls. For proliferation assessment, anti-Ki67 (BD Pharmingen, San Jose, CA) was used. For apoptotic assessment, TUNEL assay (Roche Applied Science, Indianapolis, IN) was performed according to the manufacturer's instructions and sections were stained for anti-Caspase-3 (Cell Signaling, Beverly, MA). For quantification, three gels were scored for positive cells.

Immunofluorescence and confocal microscopy: hESC colonies grown on MEFs and HA—hESC constructs were fixed *in situ* with accustain (Sigma, St. Louis, MO) for 20–25 min at room temperature, blocked with 5% FBS, and stained with one of the following primary antibodies: antihuman SSEA4, anti-TRA-1-60, anti-TRA-1-81, anti-Oct 3/4, anti-CD44 clone P3H9, anti-Tubulin III isoform (all from Chemicon Temecula, CA), anti-CD44 clone A3D8 (Sigma, St. Louis, MO), anti-CD168 (Novo Castra, Newcastle upon Tyne, UK), anti-CD31, anti-α-fetoprotein (Dako California Inc. Carpinteria, CA), anti-Hyal 1 and Hyal 2 (kindly provided by Inna Gitelman from Ben-Gurion University of the Negev, Israel). Cells were then rinsed three times with PBS (Invitrogen corporation, Carlsbad, CA) and incubated for 30 min with suitable FITC-conjugated (R&D systems, Minneapolis, MN) or Cy3-conjugated (Sigma, St. Louis, MO) secondary antibodies. DAPI (2 μg/mL; Sigma, St Louis, MO) or To-pro 3 (1:500; Molecular Probe, Invitrogen corporation, Carlsbad, CA) were added during the last rinse. IgG isotype-matching using mouse or goat (both from R&D systems, Minneapolis, MN) or secondary antibody alone served as controls. The immuno-labeled cells were examined using either fluorescence microscopy (Nikon TE300 inverted microscope) or confocal laser scanning microscopy (Zeiss LSM510 Laser scanning confocal).

HA binding and uptake: The binding assay of fluorescein-labeled hyaluronan was performed as previously described (Evanko and Wight 1999). hESCs were cultured on coverslips. After gentle washing, human fluorescein-labeled hyaluronan (100 μg/mL, Sigma, St Louis, MO) was added to the growth medium for 16 h at 4°C. Following three washes with ice-cold PBS, the cells were fixed in 100% ice-cold acetone for 10 min, air-dried, and then rehydrated 15 min in PBS. Processed cells were further stained with anti-CD44 or anti-CD168 and examined.

RT-PCR: Total RNA was extracted using TriZol (Gibco Invitrogen Co., San Diego, CA), according to manufacturer's instructions. Total RNA was quantified by a UV spectrophotometer and 1μg was used for each RT sample. One step RT-PCR kit (Qiagen Inc, Valencia, CA) was used according to manufacturer's instructions. RT reaction mix was used for negative controls. PCR conditions consisted of: 5 min at 94°C (hot start), 30–40 cycles (actual number noted below) of: 94°C for 30 sec, annealing temperature 60°C for 30 sec, 72°C for 30 sec. A final 7 min extension at 72°C was performed. Primers used include:

HYAL1 sense 5′GGGCACCTACCCCTACTACACG3′,
antisense 5′CATCTGTGACTTCCCTGTGCC3′;
HYAL2 sense 5′TGGCCCACGCCTCAAGGTGCC3′,
antisense 5′GGCCATGGAGGGCGGAAGCA3′;
HYAL3 sense 5′AGCACACTGTGAGGCCCGCTTT3′,
antisense 5′GGGGATGTCGGTGCCCAACAA3′;
PH20 5′CTTAGTCTCACAGAGGCCAC3′,
5′TACACACTCCTTGCTCCTGG3′. The amplified products were separated on 2% agarose gels containing ethidium bromide.

3.3.3 *Summary of results*

Hyaluronic acid in hESC cultures: It was observed that MEF that form feeder layers for hESC cultivation produce high levels of HA, and that abundant HA-binding sites were located intracellularly in undifferentiated hESCs. Furthermore, undifferentiated hESCs expressed high levels of CD44 and CD168. Undifferentiated cells were characterized by intracellular expression of CD44 and either membrane or intracellular expression of CD168.

Encapsulation of hESCs in HA hydrogels: Throughout the cultivation in HA hydrogels, hESCs remained viable. Importantly, cells were present in the form of undifferentiated hESC colonies expressing undifferentiated markers. At any time during culture, encapsulated cells could be released using hyaluronidase and either re-encapsulated for further propagation, or plated in monolayers on MEFs, or used to grow engineered tissue constructs.

Specificity of HA hydrogels: In contrast to the proliferation of undifferentiated hESC colonies in the HA system, dextran hydrogels induced hESC differentiation and the formation of EBs. Notably, HA hydrogels act as a unique microenvironment for the propagation of hESCs, likely due to the regulatory role of HA in the maintenance of hESCs in their undifferentiated state, *in vitro* and *in vivo*. The addition of human FL-HA to the culture of hESCs on MEFs resulted in the localization of HA receptors to the cell membranes, first at the edges of cell colonies and then at their centers. FL-HA was internalized through the membrane receptors and localized within the cells, indicating receptor-mediated internalization of HA by hESCs. Immunofluorescence of hESC colonies cultured on MEFs revealed that densely packed colonies expressed human hyaluronidase Hyal 1 and 2. RT-PCR analysis corroborated that hESCs express high levels of expression of Hyal 2, one of the isoforms of human hyaluronidase.

In sum, viable and actively proliferating hESCs can be maintained in their undifferentiated state when cultured in HA hydrogels, and released without the loss of cell viability. hESC survival and proliferation were likely associated with the presence of developmentally relevant signals and the ability of the cells to remodel HA hydrogel. Networks of HA maintain proliferating hESCs in their undifferentiated state (in contrast to other 3D environments studied, or cell monolayers on HA) and under chemically defined conditions (in contrast to soluble HA, MEFs, Matrigel, and human serum).

3.4 Method 4: Differentiation of hESCs in HA Hydrogels Cultured in Microbioreactors

Scope and objectives: The complexity of parameters that mediate hESC differentiation brought about the need for high throughput experiments that can form the basis for directed differentiation of hESCs under optimal and controlled *in vitro* conditions. To derive culture parameters, quantitative studies of the individual and interactive effects of soluble and physical factors are needed, involving in most cases cascades of multiple molecular and physical regulatory factors. The most advanced existing bioreactors available until now can provide *either* local control of oxygen and pH *or* subject the cells to biophysical stimuli, but not the two sets of factors concurrently. Advances in biomaterial and bioreactor design were combined to develop culture systems that have the necessary cues and signals to provide microenvironmental control *and* biophysical regulation of cultured hESCs. This approach also allowed studies of signaling pathways via the use of molecular inhibitory factors in conjuction with the contact guidance and biophysical regulatory signals.

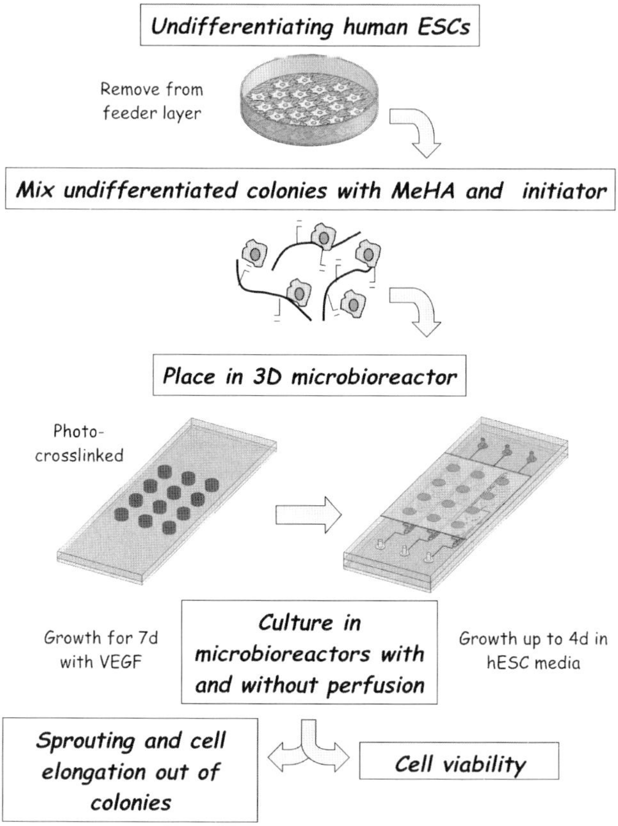

Figure 4. Experimental design for Method 4.

3.4.1 Experimental design

A schematic presentation of the experimental design for Method 4 is shown in Figure 4. Undifferentiated hESCs (lines H9 and H13) were removed from their feeder layer, encapsulated in HA hydrogel by photopolymerization and cultured in an array-type microbioreactor. The bioreactor was designed in two layers of polydimethylsiloxane (PDMS) incorporating an array of wells. The first layer is attached directly to a glass slide via plasma treatment of both surfaces.

To start the culture, the wells are filled with the HA hydrogel precursor solution (methacrylated HA macromer and photoinitiator) mixed with hESCs, and the hydrogel is then cross-linked *in situ* by photopolymerization. A second layer of PDMS, containing microfluidic channels of 100 μm in width, is placed above and each well is closed with a thin layer of PDMS and glass cover slip. The channels and the thin layer of PDMS were designed to reduce bubbles generation and avoid channel obstruction. The system of microfluidic channels delivers medium independently to the individual wells, and the outlet medium is recovered from each well via a separate set of channels.

The basic design of the system includes an array of 4 × 4 wells (2 mm in diameter × 3 mm high) connected with 100 μm diameter channels that allow flow rates of culture medium as low as 0.1 mL/min. Human ESCs were cultured for up to 4 days in growth media compositions. A system that was studied in detail was the vascular differentiation of hESCs encapsulated in HA hydrogel. The bioreactor array allowed systematic variation of culture parameters with minimal consumption of hESCs and expensive growth factors, provided precise control of the cellular microenvironment, and enabled visual insight without interruption (e.g., monitoring the formation of hESC colonies of the formation of capillary networks).

3.4.2 Description of methods

hESCs: Undifferentiated hESCs (line H9 and H13 p19–40) were grown on inactivated MEFs in growth medium consisting of 80% KO-DMEM, supplemented with 20% KSR, 4 ng/mL bFGF, 1 mM L-glutamine, 0.1 mM β-mercaptoethanol, 1% nonessential amino acid stock (Invitrogen Corporation, Carlsbad, CA). Cells were passaged using 1 mg/mL Type IV collagenase (Invitrogen Corporation, Carlsbad, CA).

Microencapsulation of hESCs: HA (50 kDa, Lifecore) was dissolved in deionized water and adjusted to a pH of 8.0 with 5 N NaOH. Methacrylic anhydride (Aldrich) was slowly added and the reaction mixture was incubated overnight at room temperature. The product was dialyzed for purification, lyophilized, and stored as a powder at 0°C. The methacrylated HA was dissolved in PBS containing 0.05% 2-methyl-1-[4-(hydroxyethoxy)phenyl]-2-methyl-1-propanone (Irgacure 2959, I2959) and hESCs were added (0.5–1 × 10^7 cells/mL precursor solution). The mixture was pipetted into a sterile microbioreactor (20–30 μl), and photopolymerized (~10 mW/cm^2 UV light, BlakRay, 10 min). Cell-gel constructs were cultivated either in hESC growth medium or in endothelial cell medium (PromoCell, Germany) supplemented with (100ng/mL) vascular endothelial growth factor (VEGF) (R&D systems, Minneapolis, MN).

Viability assay: The cell viability was studied by a fluorescence assay (Molecular Probes) for adherent and nonadherent cells, that detects live and dead cells simultaneously using calcein AM and ethidium homodimer-1 (EthD-1) dye. The calcein is retained within live cells and converted enzymatically in green fluorescent dye (ex/em ~495 nm/~515 nm), whereas EthD-1 enters cells with damaged membranes and binds to nucleic acids, thereby producing a bright red fluorescence in dead cells (ex/em ~495 nm/~635 nm). The HA-hESCs constructs were washed with PBS to remove serum esterase activity generally present in serum-supplemented growth media, because esterase can increase extracellular fluorescence by hydrolyzing calcein AM. The HA was covered by 100 μL of the combined fluorescent dyes according to manufacturer instructions and incubated for 90 min at room temperature. The labeled cells were analyzed using fluorescence microscopy (Nikon TE300 inverted microscope).

Colonies morphology: HA—hESCs constructs were fixed *in situ* with accustain (Sigma, St Louis, MO) for 20–25 min at room temperature. For morphology assessment, colonies were examined using inverted light microscopy. Cells were stained with antihuman smooth muscle actin or CD34 (both from Dako California Inc. Carpinteria, CA). Constructs were then rinsed three times with PBS (Invitrogen corporation, Carlsbad, CA) and incubated for 30 min with suitable Cy3-conjugated (Sigma, St Louis, MO) secondary antibody. DAPI (2μg/mL; Sigma, St Louis, MO) or To-pro 3 (1:500; Molecular Probe, Invitrogen corporation, Carlsbad, CA) was added to the final wash. IgG isotype-matching (R&D systems, Minneapolis, MN) or secondary antibody alone served as control. The immuno-labeled cells were examined using either fluorescence microscopy or confocal laser scanning microscopy.

3.4.3 Summary of results

Cell encapsulation: Colony organization within the microwells could be detected after 24 h of hESC encapsulation in HA hydrogels. The bioreactor design enabled monitoring of the colony organization of hESCs in various culture conditions and medium perfusion rates. Medium perfusion was essential for the maintenance of cell viability. In static (non-perfused) controls, cell viability decreases substantially. Notably, dead cells surrounded even the viable cell colonies detected at the borders of the hydrogel. Perfusion can wash out free radicals while delivering fresh nutrients and oxygen to the cells, thus resulting in enhanced cellular viability and function. This level of environmental control was not possible using other, previously established bioreactor designs for hESC cultivation.

Vascular differentiation: To examine the use of the microbioreactor system for control over environmental cues playing a role during early stages of angiogenesis, cell elongation and sprouting within HA hydrogel were evaluated. hESCs were microencapsulated and cultured for 1 week in endothelial cell media containing 100 ng/mL of VEGF. Cell sprouting, elongation, and branching of hESC colonies were markedly enhanced in the perfusion microbioreactor compared to the static cultures. Staining for vascular markers suggested that most of the sprouting cells are α smooth muscle actin positive, and that some of these cells were positive for CD34.

REFERENCES

Abbot, A. (2003) Biology's new dimension. Nature, 424: 870–872.

Amit, M., Carpenter, M.K., Inokuma, M.S., Chiu, C.P., Harris, C.P., Waknitz, M.A., Itskovitz-Eldor, J., and Thomson, J.A. (2000) Clonally derived human embryonic stem cell lines maintain pluripotency and proliferative potential for prolonged periods of culture. Dev. Biol., 227: 271–278.

Amit, M., Shariki, C., Margulets, V., and Itskovitz-Eldor, J. (2004) Feeder layer- and serum-free culture of human embryonic stem cells. Biol. Reprod., 70: 837–845.

Anderson, D.G., Burdick, J.A., and Langer, R. (2004) Materials science. Smart biomaterials. Science, 305: 1923–1924.

Brimble, S.N., Zeng, X., Weiler, D.A., Luo, Y., Liu, Y., Lyons, I.G., Freed, W.J., Robins, A.J., Rao, M.S., and Schulz, T.C. (2004) Karyotypic stability, genotyping, differentiation, feeder-free maintenance, and gene expression sampling in three human embryonic stem cell lines derived prior to August 9, 2001. Stem Cells Dev., 13: 585–597.

Burdick, J.A., Chung, C., Jia, X., Randolph, M.A., and Langer, R. (2005) Controlled degradation and mechanical behavior of photopolymerized hyaluronic acid networks. Biomacromolecules, 6: 386–391.

Burdick, J.A., Khademhosseini, A., and Langer, R. (2004) Fabrication of gradient hydrogels using a microfluidics/photopolymerization process. Langmuir, 20: 5153–5156.

Buzzard, J.J., Gough, N.M., Crook, J.M., and Coleman, A. (2004) Karyotype of human ES cells during extended culture. Nat. Biotechnol., 22: 381–382.

Carpenter, M.K., Chunhui, Xu., Daight, C.A., Antosiewiczm J.E., and Thomsonm J.A. (2003) Protocols for the maintenance of human embryonic stem cells. In: Human Embryonic Stem Cells, Chiu, A. and Rao, M.S. (eds.), Humana Press Totowa, NJ.

Dar, A., Shachar, M., Leor, J., and Cohen, S. (2002) Optimization of cardiac cell seeding and distribution in 3D porous alginate scaffolds. Biotechnol. Bioeng., 80: 305–312.

Draper, J.S., Smith, K., Gokhale, P., Moore, H.D., Maltby, E., Johnson, J., Meisner, L., Zwaka, T.P., Thomson, J.A., and Andrews, P.W. (2004) Recurrent gain of chromosomes 17q and 12 in cultured human embryonic stem cells. Nat. Biotechnol., 22: 53–54.

Evanko, S.P. and Wight, T.N. (1999) Intracellular localization of hyaluronan in proliferating cells. J. Histochem. Cytochem., 47: 1331–1342.

Ferreira, L., Gil, M.H., and Dordick, J.S. (2002) Enzymatic synthesis of dextran-containing hydrogels. Biomaterials, 23: 3957–3967.

Gerecht-Nir, S., Cohen, S., and Itskovitz-Eldor, J. (2004a) Three-dimensional porous alginate scaffolds provide a conducive environment for generation of well-vascularized embryoid bodies from human embryonic stem cells. Biotechnol. Bioeng., 86: 493–502.

Gerecht-Nir, S., Cohen, S., Ziskind, A., and Itskovitz-Eldor, J. (2004b) Bioreactor cultivation enhances the efficiency of human embryoid body (hEB) formation and differentiation. Biotechnol. Bioeng., 88: 313–320.

Gerecht-Nir, S., Radisic, M., Park, H., Boublik, J., Cannizzaro, C., Langer, R., and Vunjak-Novakovic, G. (2006) Biophysical regulation of cardiogenesis. Int. J. Dev. Biol., 50: 233–243.

Gerecht-Nir, S., Burdick, J.A., Ferreira, L.S., Townsend, S.A., Langer, R., and Vunjak-Novakovic, G. Propagation of undifferentiated human embryonic stem cells in hyaluronic acid hydrogels. PNAS (in review).

Glicklis, R., Shapiro, L., Aqbaria, R., Merchuk, J.C., and Cohen, S. (2000) Hepatocyte behavior within three-dimensional porous alginate scaffolds. Biotechnol. Bioeng., 67: 344–353.

Hoffman, L.M. and Carpenter, M.K. (2005) Characterization and culture of human embryonic stem cells. Nat. Biotechnol., 23: 699–708.

Itskovitz-Eldor, J., Schuldiner, M., Karsenti, D., Eden, A., Yanuka, O., Amit, M., Soreq, H., and Benvenisty, N. (2000) Differentiation of human embryonic stem cells into embryoid bodies compromising the three embryonic germ layers. Mol. Med., 6: 88–95.

Jacks, T. and Weinberg, R.A. (2002) Taking the study of cancer cell survival to a new dimension. Cell, 111: 923–925.

Khademhosseini, A., Eng, G., Yeh, J., Fukuda, J., Blumling, J. 3rd., Langer, R., and Burdick, J.A. (2006) Micromolding of photocrosslinkable hyaluronic acid for cell encapsulation and entrapment. Biomed. Mater. Res. A., Jun 20; [Epub ahead of print].

Leor, J., Aboulafia-Etzion, S., Dar, A., Shapiro, L., Barbash, I., Battler, A., Granot, Y., and Cohen, S. (2000) Bioengineered cardiac grafts: a new approach to repair the infarcted myocardium. Circulation, 102: 56–61.

Levenberg, S., Golub, J.S., Amit, M., Itskovitz-Eldor, J., and Langer, R. (2002) Endothelial cells derived from human embryonic stem cells. Proc. Natl. Acad. Sci. U.S.A, 99: 4391–4396.

Levenberg, S., Huang, N.F., Lavik, E., Rogers, A.B., Itskovitz-Eldor, J., and Langer, R. (2003) Differentiation of human embryonic stem cells on three-dimensional polymer scaffolds. Proc. Natl. Acad. Sci. U.S.A, 100: 12741–12746.

Levenberg, S., Burdick, J.A., Kraehenbuehl T., and Langer R. (2005) Neurotrophin-induced differentiation of human embryonic stem cells on three-dimensional polymeric scaffolds. Tissue Eng., 11: 506–512.
Lutolf, M.P. and Hubbell, J.A. (2005) Synthetic biomaterials as instructive extracellular microenvironments for morphogenesis in tissue engineering. Nat. Biotechnol., 23: 47–55.
Mitalipova, M.M., Rao, R.R., Hoyer, D.M., Johnson, J.A., Meisner, L.F., Jones, K.L., Dalton, S., and Stice, S.L. (2005) Preserving the genetic integrity of human embryonic stem cells. Nat. Biotechnol., 23: 9–20.
Postovit, L.M., Seftor, E.A., Seftor, R.E., and Hendrix, M.J. (2006) A three-dimensional model to study the epigenetic effects induced by the microenvironment of human embryonic stem cells. Stem Cells 24: 501–505.
Proetzel, G. and Wiles, M.V. (2002) The use of a chemically defined media for the analyses of early development in ES cells and mouse embryos. Methods Mol. Biol., 185: 17–26.
Radisic, M., Malda, J., Epping, E., Geng, W., Langer, R., and Vunjak-Novakovic, G. (2006) Oxygen gradients correlate with cell density and cell viability in engineered cardiac tissue. Biotechnol. Bioeng., 93: 332–343.
Radisic, M., Park, H., Gerecht-Nir, S., Cannizzaro, C., Langer, R., and Vunjak-Novakovic, G. Biomimetic approach to cardiac tissue engineering. Philosophical Transactions of the Royal Society of London (in press).
Richards, M., Fong, C.Y., Chan, W.K., Wong, P.C., and Bongso, A. (2002) Human feeders support prolonged undifferentiated growth of human inner cell masses and embryonic stem cells. Nat. Biotechnol., 20: 933–936.
Rosler, E.S., Fisk, G.J., Ares, X., Irving, J., Miura, T., Rao, M.S., and Carpenter, M.K. (2004) Long-term culture of human embryonic stem cells in feeder-free conditions. Dev. Dyn., 229: 259–274.
Schatten, G., Smith, J., Navara, C., Park, J.H., and Pedersen, R. (2005) Culture of human embryonic stem cells. Nat. Methods, 2: 455–463.
Shapiro, L. and Cohen, S. (1997) Novel alginate sponges for cell culture and transplantation. Biomaterials, 18: 583–590.
Stojkovic, P., Lako, M., Przyborski, S., Stewart, R., Armstrong, L., Evans, J., Zhang, X., and Stojkovic M. (2005) Human-serum matrix supports undifferentiated growth of human embryonic stem cells. Stem Cells, 23: 895–902.
Thomson, J.A., Itskovitz-Eldor, J., Shapiro, S.S., Waknitz, M.A., Swiergiel, J.J., Marshall, V.S., and Jones, J.M. (1998) Embryonic stem cell lines derived from human blastocysts. Science, 282: 1145–1147.
Toole, B.P. (2001) Hyaluronan in morphogenesis. Semin. Cell Dev. Biol., 12: 79–87.
Wang, L., Li, L., Menendez, P., Cerdan, C., and Bhatia, M. (2005) Human embryonic stem cells maintained in the absence of mouse embryonic fibroblasts or conditioned media are capable of hematopoietic development. Blood, 105: 4598–4603.
Xu, C., Inokuma, M.S., Denham, J., Golds, K., Kundu, P., Gold, J.D., and Carpenter, M.K. (2001) Feeder-free growth of undifferentiated human embryonic stem cells. Nat. Biotechnol., 19: 971–974.
Xu, C., Rosler, E., Jiang, J., Lebkowski, J.S., Gold, J.D., O'Sullivan, C., Delavan-Boorsma, K., Mok, M., Bronstein, A., and Carpenter, M.K. (2005) Basic fibroblast growth factor supports undifferentiated human embryonic stem cell growth without conditioned medium. Stem Cells, 23: 315–323.
Xu, R.H., Peck, R.M., Li, D.S., Feng, X., Ludwig, T., and Thomson, J.A. (2005) Basic FGF and suppression of BMP signaling sustain undifferentiated proliferation of human ES cells. Nat. Methods, 2: 185–190.
Zmora, S., Glicklis, R., and Cohen, S. (2002) Tailoring the pore architecture in 3-D alginate scaffolds by controlling the freezing regime during fabrication. Biomaterials, 23: 4087–4094.

CHAPTER 10

EXTRAEMBRYONIC CELL DIFFERENTIATION

LYLE ARMSTRONG[1,2] AND MAJLINDA LAKO[1,2]

[1]*Centre for Stem Cell Biology and Developmental Genetics, University of Newcastle, Newcastle upon Tyne, UK*

[2]*Institute of Human Genetics, University of Newcastle, Newcastle upon Tyne, UK*

1. INTRODUCTION

Embryonic stem cell (ESC) lines, derived from the inner cell mass (ICM) of mammalian blastocysts are characterised by the phenomenon of pluripotency, the ability to differentiate into any of the cell types found in the adult. Early studies suggested that the fate decision required to produce the cells of either the trophectoderm or the ICM removes the ability of the ICM to differentiate into trophectoderm (Pedersen et al. 1986). Subsequent studies in human ESC have shown that differentiation of trophectodermal cells spontaneously is indeed possible thereby expanding the repertoire of human embryonic stem cells (hESC) pluripotency (Xu et al. 2002). The trophectoderm gives rise to many of the subsequent cell lineages that produce the placental tissues and components of the yolk sac and are thus essential to the progression of embryo development. However, there are a few notable extraembryonic components arising from the ICM. This chapter describes the formation of these cell types in addition to those of the trophectoderm.

2. ORIGINS OF EXTRAEMBRYONIC STRUCTURES

2.1 Pre-Implantation Development

It is helpful to briefly review the origins of embryonic and extraembryonic structures in the developing embryo. The progression of developmental events is summarised in Figures 1 and 2, but the changes in cell potency leading up to the first obvious differentiation, formation of the trophectoderm, apparently take place 24–36 h prior to the event. The cells or blastomeres of the early

J.R. Masters et al (eds.), Embryonic Stem Cells, 173–188.

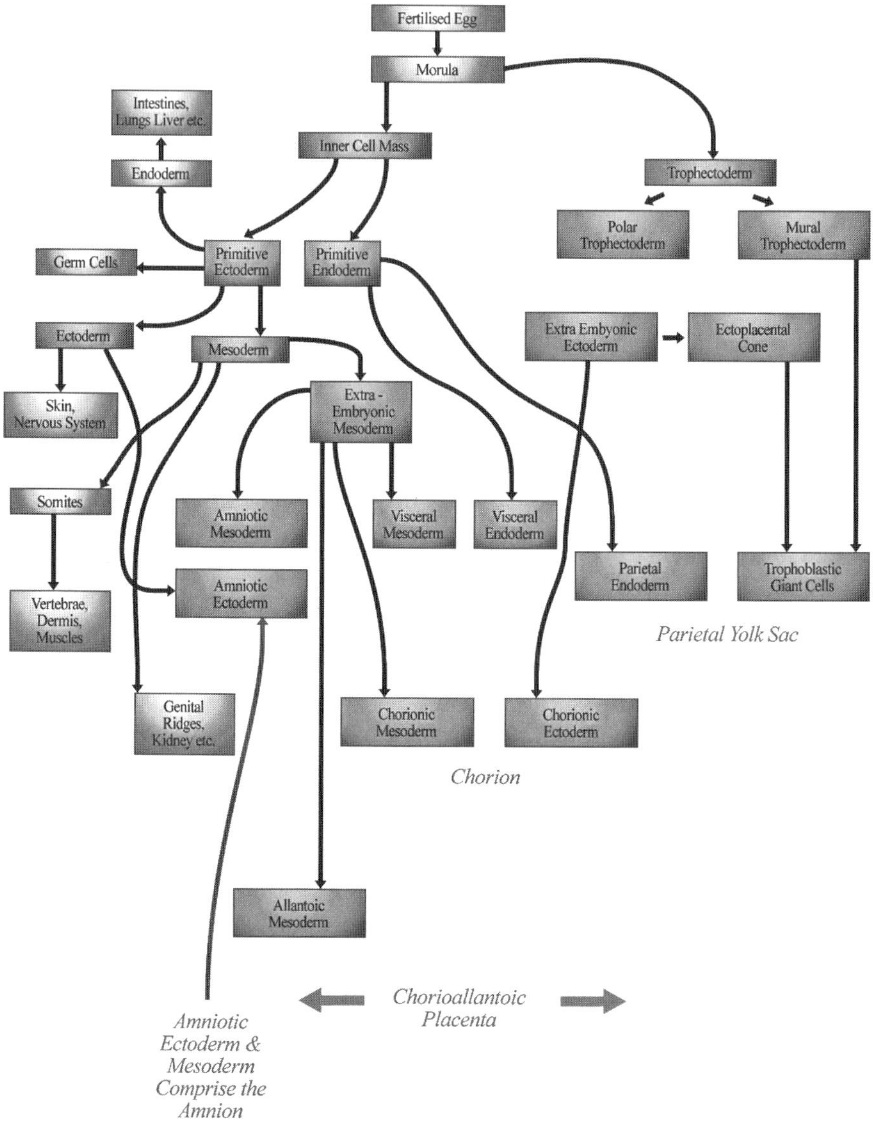

Figure 1. Tissues arising in the pre-implantation and early post-implantation embryo. The diagram represent the types of tissue which differentiate from the initial zygote and demonstrates which of these contribute towards extraembryonic structures.

cleavage stage embryos (two cells and four cells) are most probably equally totipotent since they can be cultured in isolation to give rise to individual mice. By the eight cell stage, the blastomeres have lost this capacity, although they can still contribute to a wide range of tissues when recombined with other blastomeres

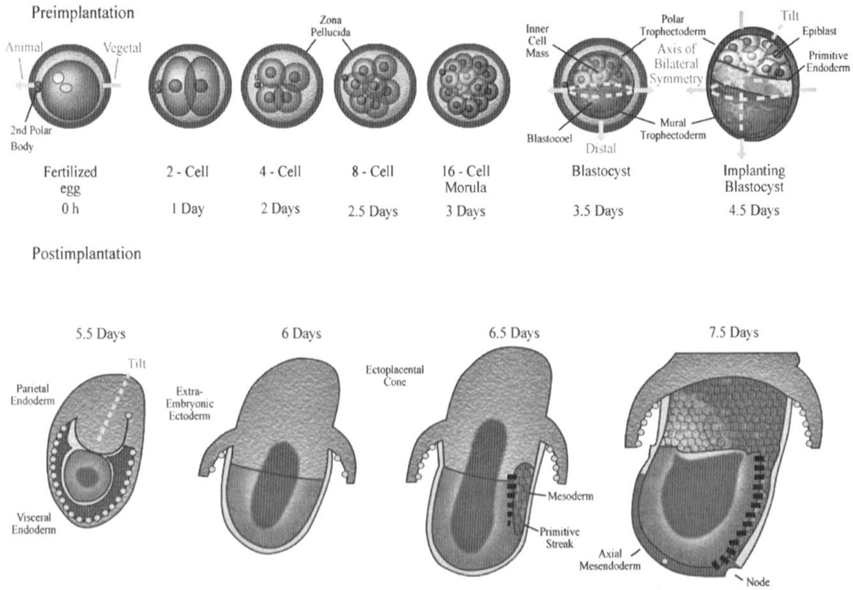

Figure 2. Developmental stages of the pre-implantation and early post-implantation mammalian embryo. This represents the structures of the early embryo and correlates these with the tissue types shown in Figure 1. The data used to construct this image are derived from mouse but are largely applicable to other mammalian embryos.

in the technique of morula aggregation. As development proceeds past the 16 cell stage, there is a further restriction in the potency of the cells, which eventually results in the formation of trophectoderm and ICM. The first evidence of this process is morula compaction, resulting from an increase in the calcium dependent adhesiveness of the cells causing them to increase their degree of contact (Khang et al. 2005). Development of apical and basal membrane and cytoplasmic domains, a process referred to a polarisation, is dependent on this increase in cell-to-cell contact and ensures that blastomeres which find themselves on the outside of the compacting morula are more committed to form trophectoderm, while those inside form the ICM. By the blastocyst stage, this process is irreversible.

The process of polarisation induces changes in the membrane structure such that they begin to resemble the cells of many epithelial tissues (Larue et al. 1994). Scanning electron microscopy shows the presence of numerous microvilli on their outside poles while the inner surfaces are smooth and moreover, there are considerable differences in the expression of transmembrane receptors. For example, the EGF receptor is localised to the basolateral surface of the trophectoderm (Dardik et al. 1992). Despite this knowledge, the final chain of molecular events leading to the partition of the ICM and trophectoderm is unknown. Two theories have been proposed to account for the partition, the first of which suggests that different membrane and cytoplasmic molecules such as glycoprotein receptors are expressed by outside and inside cells after compaction and that this is responsible for establishing differences in the developmental potentials of the inner and outer cells (Antczak and Van Blerkom 1997). Another hypothesis is that a network of junctions between the inner and outer cells needs to be established prior to differentiation so that they will be subjected to different microenvironments to which they respond appropriately by differentiating into either ICM or trophectoderm (Gardner 1983; Johnson et al. 1986; Pratt 1989).

2.2 Post-Implantation Development

The blastocyst hatches from the zona pellucida ~4–5 days post-coitum in mouse and 8 days in humans. Implantation in the wall of the uterus will occur soon thereafter. The blastocyst will normally attach via the mural trophectoderm so that the cells destined to become the tissues of the developing embryo protrude into the lumen of the uterus (Figure 2). The trophectoderm undergoes considerable post-implantation changes. For example, the cells of the mural trophectoderm cease proliferation, develop polytene chromosomes and grow much larger (Varmuza et al. 1988). These cells are now referred to as trophoblast giant cells and will later contribute to the formation of the parietal yolk sac in combination with cells of the parietal endoderm. The polar trophectoderm continues to proliferate and can now make one of two fate decisions. It may differentiate towards either the extraembryonic ectoderm of the egg cylinder stage or encapsulate the embryo and replace the giant cells derived from the mural trophectoderm eventually forming the ectoplacental cone. The extraembryonic ectoderm forms a finger-like projection which pushes down into the blastocoel cavity and the leading edge of this projection comprises the derivatives of the ICM. However, as other segments of the embryo begin to develop, particularly the extraembryonic mesoderm, the extraembryonic ectoderm recedes until it is restricted to the chorion.

The extraembryonic ectoderm and ectoplacental cone have an interesting additional property in that they may give rise to trophoblast stem cell (TSC) lines *in vitro* (Quinn et al. 2006). This process is analogous to the derivation of ESC lines from the ICM, but TSC lines are restricted to differentiation into extraembryonic ectoderm, ectoplacental cone, and trophoblast giant cells only and seem to require different culture conditions and signalling pathways to maintain proliferation. TSC lines may also be derived from blastocysts by culturing in the presence of FGF4, Heparin, and primary embryonic fibroblast conditioned medium (Tanaka et al. 1998). TSC lines are not pluripotent and do not express many of the genes associated with pluripotency such as Oct4 or Nanog (Nichols et al. 1998) but they do express some other genes in common with ESC, such as FoxD3 which is essential for the successful derivation of TSC lines (Tompers et al. 2005). TSC lines are as much a product of the tissue culture environment as ESCs and *in vivo* switching of trophectodermal to ICM or epiblast fate has never been observed. In the laboratory, however, it is possible to derive trophoblast cells from ESCs and switching the culture conditions to those which favour TSC gives rise to cell lines which are morphologically very similar to TSC (Rossant 2001).

The ICM continues its own programme of development during this period. Cells on the free surface facing into the blastocoelic cavity differentiate into the primitive endoderm, which will progress to form the parietal and visceral endoderms, which in turn will contribute to the parietal and visceral yolk sac, respectively. The cells behind the primitive endoderm are referred to as the epiblast or primitive ectoderm and it is these which will eventually produce all of the cell types of the developing foetus and they represent the last stage at which the phenomenon of pluripotency may be said to exist until the emergence of the germ line cells. In the period between implantation and gastrulation, the epiblast cells divide rapidly and undergo differentiation into the three definitive germ layers whilst losing many of the molecular markers associated with pluripotency such as Oct4, Nanog, and alkaline phosphatase expression and the ability to contribute to embryonic development following injection of isolated epiblast cells into mouse blastocysts (Bradley et al. 1984). The differentiation of epiblast cells towards the mesoderm lineage has one final contribution to make towards extraembryonic tissues in that it extends both above and below the primitive streak region and covers an area which is beyond the boundary formed by the endometrium and is thus formally considered to be extraembryonic. This extraembryonic mesoderm forms the cavity of the visceral yolk sac but will also contribute to the amniotic mesoderm which together with amniotic ectoderm cells derived from the ectoderm germ layer will form the amnion.

Chorionic mesoderm also forms from the initial mesodermal cells and contributes to the formation of the chorion in concert with cells of the chorionic ectoderm which arises from the polar trophectoderm (see Figure 1). Finally, the growth of the allantoic mesoderm is of particular importance to the embryo since this is the site in which the primordial germ cells will be specified and begin their migration via the developing hindgut endoderm to lodge in the developing genital ridge (Lawson et al.1999; Anderson et al. 2000). There is little information on the development of the cell types needed to form this tissue from ESC cultures.

3. MOLECULAR EVENTS LEADING TO DIFFERENTIATION OF TROPHECTODERM

3.1 Expression of Key Genes in the Pre-Implantation Embryo

A key gene which undergoes downregulation in the course of trophectoderm differentiation is the POU transcription factor Oct4 (encoded by *Pou5f1*). This gene has been extensively characterised as a regulator of ESC pluripotency and is expressed in the ICM of mouse and human embryos and ESCs (Adjaye et al.

2005). An important application of ESCs is understanding embryonic development, a fact which is often overshadowed by their potential usefulness as a source of differentiated cells for regenerative medicine. Elegant gene-targeting studies in mouse ESC have demonstrated that reduced levels of Oct4 expression will induce differentiation into trophectoderm, whilst overexpression will direct the murine ESC to become mesoderm and primitive endoderm (Niwa et al. 2000). Reducing the level of Oct4 mRNA using short interfering RNAs in both human and mouse ESC also induces trophectoderm differentiation in addition to primitive endoderm differentiation (Velkey and O'Shea 2003; Matin et al. 2004). The mechanism by which OCT4 downregulation is initiated or how loss of this protein in human ESC results in differentiation is still far from clear but it has been suggested that bone morphogenetic protein 4 (BMP4), a member of the transforming growth factor-β superfamily, can induce the differentiation of human ESC to trophoblast (Xu et al. 2002). Microarray hybridisation of cDNAs from culture of H1 human ESC grown in the presence of 100 ng/mL BMP4 showed the upregulation of many genes associated with the trophoblast lineage, such as *TFAP2*, *MSX2*, and *GATA2* and *GATA3*. Moreover, the trophoblast cells derived in this way were capable of synthesising placental gene products such the α- and β- subunits of chorionic gondatotropin, lutenising hormone, and placental growth factor, indicating function. In addition, genes associated with ESC pluripotency (*OCT4* and *TERT*—telomerase reverse transcriptase subunit) were significantly downregulated. The mechanism by which BMP4 can initiate signal cascades that result in alterations to the human ESC gene transcription profile that causes them to differentiate is not known. However, transcripts of several BMP receptors are present in morula and blastocyst stage mouse embryos and transcripts of the BMPs exist in the maternal tissues surrounding the embryo (Peng 2003). BMP receptors are also present on human ESC.

Embryos of Oct4 mutant mice die around the time of implantation, and only trophectoderm cells can be obtained from these (Nichols et al. 1998). This had led to the speculation that trophectoderm is the default state of the embryo in the murine system and that this must be overridden by the presence of Oct4. Several other genes have been identified which promote trophectoderm differentiation and one of the most interesting of these is *Caudal related transcription factor 2* (*Cdx2*) (Strumpf et al. 2005), expression of which is observed from the late morula stage. Knockout of *Cdx2* results in an inability to produce trophectoderm and leads to pre-implantation lethality (Beck et al. 2003). Moreover, inducible overexpression of *Cdx2* in mouse ESC led to trophectoderm differentiation, although Cdx2 alone is not sufficient as spontaneous differentiation of a mutant ESC line in which both alleles of the *Cdx2* gene had been removed by gene targeting was capable of forming trophectoderm that was indistinguishable from the wild type. It is probable that *Cdx2* and *Oct4* respond to the molecular cues that are set up during morula compaction. Immunocytochemical staining of pre-implantation embryos reveals that Cdx2 levels are much higher in the outer cells of the morula. Since both Cdx2 and Oct4 can be autoregulated (Niwa et al. 2005), if either of them respond to molecular signals that will result in an imbalance between their expression levels, then a reciprocal inhibition system may result in their mutually exclusive expression in trophectoderm and ICM.

3.2 Experimental Procedures to Derive Trophectoderm from Human and Mouse ESC

3.2.1 BMP4

The procedure used to derive trophectoderm from human ESC lines was devised by Thomson's group at the WiCell Institute, Madison WI and may be summarised as follows. Matrigel coated plastic culture plates were prepared (Xu et al. 2001) and the human ESC lines H1, H7, and H9 were plated onto these as colonies and maintained in hESC culture medium conditioned with mitotically inactive mouse embryonic fibroblasts and supplemented with 4 ng/mL human bFGF. Single cells from ESC colonies obtained by treatment with trypsin/EDTA solution were plated at low density and BMP4 (R&D systems, Minneapolis, MN, 100 ng/ml) was added. Within 2 weeks, some single cells will form syncytial cells which, after treatment with the Golgi complex blocking agent, Brefeldin A (Sigma, StLouis, MO, 1.25 μg/mL), may be fixed by exposure to 2% paraformaldehyde. Evidence for differentiation towards trophoectodermal lineages can be obtained by staining the fixed cells with mouse anti-human chorionic gonadotropin β followed by fluorescein labelled rabbit anti-mouse IgG antibody (Pierce, Rockford IL) at 1:200. The nuclei can be counterstained with Hoechst 33342 (Sigma) and visualised by epifluorescence microscopy.

3.2.2 siRNA knockdown of Oct4 in ESC

The following procedure from Velkey and O'Shea (Velkey and O'Shea 2003) relies upon RNA interference methodology to decrease the levels of Oct4 transcript present in mouse ESC, thereby forcing them to follow a trophectodermal differentiation pathway. RNAi was enhanced by the development of vectors containing RNA polymerase type III promoters such as the U6 small nuclear RNA promoter (U6) (Miyagishi and Taira 2002) or H1 promoter (Brummelkamp et al. 2002) driving expression of a single RNA transcript that folds into a hairpin siRNA. This permits constitutive expression of siRNAs which can maintain permanent knockdown of gene expression.

A specific vector (pCU-Octi) was constructed such that a hairpin siRNA template corresponding to nucleotides 670–688 of the mouse Oct4 sequence would be expressed under the control of the U6/H1 promoter. The fluorescent protein DsRed2 (Clontech) is also expressed under the control of a CMV promoter so that transfected cells may be easily visualised and/or enriched by fluorescence activated cell sorting. The construct was transfected into mouse D3 ESC grown on 0.1% gelatin-coated plastic ware in DMEM (Invitrogen, Carlsbad CA) containing

10% fetal bovine serum (FBS) which was batch tested for ESC compatibility, L-glutamine (Invitrogen, 0.224 g/mL), HEPES (Invitrogen, 1.33 g/mL), 2-mercaptoethanol (Sigma, StLouis, MO, 10^{-4} M) and human recombinant leukemia inhibitory factor (LIF) (Oncogene research products, San Diego, CA, 1,000 units/mL). The cells were seeded onto 6-well plates at 7.5×10^5 cells per well and after 24 h transfected with the pCU-Octi vector using Lipofectamine Plus reagent (Invitrogen) in serum free DMEM. After 3 h, the medium was replaced by normal ESC culture medium as detailed above. Subsequently, 36 h later the cells were dissociated with 0.25% trypsin/1 mM EDTA then resuspended in phosphate buffered saline (PBS) and separated by fluorescent-activated cell sorter (FACS). The instrument used was the Coulter Elite ESP using a 514 nm argon excitation laser with a 575 nm bandpass filter. The cells sorted on the basis of DsRed 2 fluorescence were plated either in 0.1% gelatin-coated 35 mm dishes or on coverslips at a density of 150 cells/mm^2 then cultured for a further 5.5 days in ESC medium plus 100 units/mL of penicillin and 100 μg/mL of streptomycin. After the culture period, cells were fixed by exposure to 2% paraformaldehyde/PBS and examined by immunohistochemical staining with antibodies directed against Oct4 and cytokeratin endoA. Cells on coverslips were also fixed using 2% glutaraldehyde/0.1 M Sorensen's phosphate buffer and used for scanning electron microscopic studies.

siRNA mediated knockdown of Oct4 resulted in the formation of cells that were morphologically similar to trophoblast giant cells with thinly spread cytoplasm and pronounced nuclear bulges. Interestingly, these cells appeared to "surround" undifferentiated ESC in a manner reminiscent of the blastocyst.

Similar studies confirmed the utility of siRNA for reducing the expression level of *OCT4* and differentiation of ESCs towards a trophectodermal lineage (Matin et al. 2004). Double stranded 21 mer siRNA were obtained (Qiagen, Valencia CA) and transfected into either hESC (Wisconsin H7 and H14) or embryonal carcinoma cells (NTera2 and 2102Ep cell lines) using the following method:

Cells were harvested with 0.25% trypsin, 1 mM EDTA in PBS without Ca^{2+} and Mg^{2+} (for EC cells) or 0.05% trypsin, 1 mM EDTA in PBS without Ca^{2+} and Mg^{2+} (for ESC) and plated in 6-well plates at 2×10^4 per cm^2. The next day, when the cultures were 30–50% confluent, siRNA was introduced into the cells using the Oligofectamine transfection reagent (Invitrogen). In brief, 10 μL siRNA (20 μM solution) was incubated with 4 μL Oligofectamine in 190 μL Optimem (Invitrogen) for 20 min; the mixture was then added to the cells in a final volume of 1.2 mL. The transfected cells were cultured and were fed daily with fresh medium until they were analysed by flow cytometry, which indicated reduction of the hESC surface marker proteins SSEA3 and TRA-1-60 5 days after treatment with *OCT4* siRNA. In this timescale, the expression of *CDX2* and hCG was strongly upregulated, which indicates the formation of trophectodermal cells.

3.2.3 Overexpression of Cdx2/Eomesodermin in murine ESC

Once again, mouse ESC were cultured in the absence of feeder cells in Glasgow minimal essential medium (GMEM) supplemented with 10% fetal calf serum (FCS), 1 mM sodium pyruvate, 10^{-4} M 2-mercaptoethanol, 1× non-essential

amino acids and 1,000 U/mL of LIF on gelatin-coated dishes. Overexpression of Cdx2 and Eomesodermin is achieved using an episomal tranfection system (Niwa et al. 2005). Cdx2 and Eomesodermin were amplified by reverse transcriptase-polymerase chain reaction (RT-PCR) using total RNA from trophectoderm stem cells with the following primer sets:
Cdx2 S: AAACATGTACGTGAGCTACCTTCC
Cdz2 AS: AAAGTACTGGGTGACAGTGGAGTTT
Eomesodermin S: AAAGCATGCAGTTGGGAGAGCAGCTCC
Eomesodermin AS: AATGCTCTAGGCACTTGTGTAAAAAGCA

The PCR amplicons were subcloned into the pCAG-IP vector (Niwa et al. 2002) and 2 μg of this plasmid was transfected into 30,000 MGZ5 ESC using Lipofectamine 2000 (invitrogen). The cells were replated into 60 mm dishes and 24 h after transfection were placed under puromycin selection (1 μg/mL) and the effects of transgene overexpression on the morphology of ESC was scored after 6 days. Most surviving cells differentiated towards trophectoderm in a manner similar to the differentiation induced by downregulation of Oct4 and the cells obtained were characterised by enlarged or multiple nuclei and expression of the trophectoderm surface marker Cadherin 3 (Brulet et al. 1980).

A hormone inducible vector for overexpression of Cdx2 was produced by amplifying the entire open reading frame of the gene using the following primer set:
Cdx2S2: CCTCGAGCCAACATGTACGTGAGCTACCTT
Cdx2AS2: TCAACTAGTCTGGGTGACTGAGGAGTT
The amplified DNA fragment was digested with the restriction enzymes *XhoI* and *SpeI*. The ligand binding domain of mutant mouse estrogen receptor was amplified with the following primer set;
mESRS: TTCATGACTAGTCGAAATGAAATGGGTGCT
mESRAS: AGCGGCCGCTCAGATCGTGTTGGGGAAGCC
This fragment was digested with *SpeI* and *NotI* and both this and the Cdx2 fragment were subcloned into pCAG-IP which had been previously digested with *XhoI/NotI* resulting in the creation of pCAG-CDX2ER-IP. Nearly 40 μg of this vector was linearised with *SalI* and electroporated into ZHB Tc4 ESC at 800 V/3 μF in a 0.4 cm cuvette using the Gene Pulser (BioRad). Surviving cells were plated under puromycin (1 μg/mL) selection for 8 days until colonies of resistant cells were obtained. Many of these clones were able to undergo differentiation to trophectoderm by addition of 4-hydroxytamoxifen (Tx, Sigma, 1 μg/mL) to the culture medium.

3.2.4 Derivation of trophectodermal stem cells

Derivation of TSC is carried out in a manner somewhat similar to ESC, except the ICM or outgrowths from it in culture need to be removed and discarded. In mouse embryos they may be isolated at the blastocyst stage or from single blastomeres. Typically, blastocyst or the isolated extraembryonic ectoderm (late blastocyst) is plated onto mitotically inactivated primary embryonic fibroblasts after the method of Tanaka et al. (1998) and cultured in RPMI 1640 medium supplemented with 20% FBS, 50 μg/mL penicillin/streptomycin, 1 mM sodium pyruvate, 100 mM 2-mercaptoethanol, 2 mM L-glutamine, 25 ng/mL FGF4, and 1 μg/mL heparin. Outgrowths from the attached blastocysts may be disaggregated with 0.25% trypsin/EDTA after ~4 days and plated onto new feeder cells. From these cultures, several lines of TSC should become established.

Alternatively, single blastomeres may be removed from eight-cell morula stage pre-implantation embryos (mouse) by cutting a hole in the zona pellucida with a piezo-activated drilling pipette. These cells can be aggregated individually with existing ESC lines labelled with green fluorescent protein (GFP) and grown under ESC culture conditions until non-GFP positive outgrowths appear from the ES colonies (Chung et al. 2006). This normally requires 24–48 h culture in the presence of 2000 IU of murine LIF and 50 μM MEK1 inhibitor. Once the non-GFP positive outgrowths have achieved a certain size (typically more than 20 cells) they are removed manually and plated on their own feeder cells. Outgrowths which resemble the morphology of trophectoderm or extraembryonic endoderm may then be cultured in the above ESC medium supplemented further with 50 ng/mL FGF4 and should proceed to give TSC lines.

4. DIFFERENTIATION OF EMBRYONIC STEM CELLS TO OTHER EXTRAEMBRYONIC CELL TYPES

4.1 Primitive Endoderm

4.1.1 Differentiation of primitive endoderm

After segregation of the trophoblast, the next differentiation event to occur in the pre-implantation embryo is the partition of the ICM into the cells of the epiblast and the extraembryonic endoderm. ESCs have frequently been used to model this event *in vitro* especially since we expect them to be good representations of the true ICM cells. Upon aggregation *in vitro*, ESC undergo spontaneous differentiation into extraembryonic endoderm like cells (Coucouvanis and Martin 1995, 1999) which express specific markers such as *GATA4*, *GATA6*, *Laminin*, and *Collagen IV* (Bielinska et al. 1999) while *Oct4* undergoes downregulation. The GATA transcription factors are highly conserved among species and are central to the processes of embryonic development and the maintenance of the differentiated state of adult cells. GATA4 and GATA6 are among the few genes upregulated in the primitive endoderm and several studies have shown that they have overlapping roles depending on the technique used to induce ESC differentiation. If mouse ESC are allowed to differentiate spontaneously, they tend to aggregate into embryoid bodies within 48 h of LIF removal and it seems likely that upregulation of GATA4 is one response to cellular aggregation. GATA4 will then induce GATA6 which then collaborates with GATA4 to induce differentiation. GATA4 and GATA6 also interact since higher levels of GATA4 are thought to repress GATA6. This regulatory loop may serve to balance the relative expressions of these two factors at precise levels. Further evidence for the involvement of GATA4 and GATA6 comes from studies of ectopic overexpression of these genes in ESCs, which is sufficient to induce differentiation towards extraembryonic endoderm (Fujikura et al. 2002), although the full range of downstream target genes is not yet clear. Finally, primitive endoderm expresses both Indian hedgehog and bone morphogenetic protein 2 (BMP2) (Maye et al. 2000).

4.1.2 Visceral and parietal endoderm

These next differentiation stages from primitive endoderm may rely upon extracellular signals such as BMP2 to induce differentiation to visceral endoderm. There is some evidence to suggest that visceral endoderm is the signal requiring pathway and that parietal endoderm is simply the default pathway that occurs to primitive endoderm in the absence of external signals. This mechanism probably applies to differentiation in both the embryo and an embryoid body model system since, in the embryo, parietal endoderm forms as the primitive endoderm cells move away from the epiblast and migrate along the trophectoderm, thus removing them from the potential source of BMP2 in the maternal tissues of the uterus. Both parietal and visceral endoderms require the continued expression of GATA4 and GATA6. A known downstream target of GATA6 is HNF4 which seems to be restricted to the developing visceral endoderm (Duncan et al. 1997) in mouse embryos. Embryoid bodies derived from HNF4 knockout ESC form the morphological equivalent of the endoderm and express many endoderm markers such as GATA4, Apo-E, and vHNF-1 but they fail to express later markers of the visceral endoderm such as AFP, TTR, and ApoAI. These genes seem to be downstream targets of HNF4. There is also evidence to suggest that the Hedgehog family member Indian Hedgehog plays a role in promoting the differentiation of visceral endoderm.

Parietal endoderm on the other hand is probably specified by the action of one more *SOX* genes, particularly *SOX7* and *SOX17* (Niimi et al. 2004). SOX7 is involved in regulation of GATA6 expression (Futaki et al. 2004), but SOX17 is a downstream target of GATA6 as are other markers of the parietal endoderm such as HNF1b, Laminin-1, FoxA2, and type IV collagen.

The homoeobox transcription factor Nanog has been proposed as a major regulator of pluripotency in mouse and human ESCs (Chambers et al. 2003; Mitsui et al. 2003). Depletion of Nanog from murine ESC results in loss of pluripotency, reduction in cell growth, and differentiation into the extraembryonic endoderm lineage (Hatano et al. 2005). Thus, it was suggested that Nanog might act as a transcriptional repressor of GATA4 and GATA6. However, the presence of two unusually strong activation domains in the C-terminus of the Nanog protein (Pan and Pei 2005) suggests that it may be more likely to act as both transcriptional activator and repressor. Also, the differentiation pathway taken by the cells is dependent upon the absolute level of Nanog protein. Complete absence results in primitive endoderm formation whereas a twofold downregulation induces mouse ESC to form the three primitive germ layers of mesoderm, endoderm, and ectoderm, implying that specific amounts of Nanog are required to define cell fates, in a manner similar to that observed for Oct4. In human ESC growing as monolayers, knockdown of *NANOG* and *OCT4* using siRNA seems to produce extraembryonic cell types only, with no evidence of formation of the primitive germ layers (Hyslop et al. 2005). Two days after transfection of *NANOG* siRNA, the cells begin to adopt an enlarged, flattened morphology and, after 4 days, virtually all the cells in the culture are of this type. Examination of the transfected cells by flow cytometry for markers such as SSEA-4 and TRA-1-60, which are typical of undifferentiated human ESC, indicated that considerable differentiation had taken place. Real time RT-PCR indicated the expression of several genes of the extraembryonic endoderm lineage such as *GATA4* and *GATA6*, while there was no significant increase in markers of other differentiation pathways such as *BRACHYURY* (mesoderm), *FGF5* (ectoderm), or *PAX6* (neuroectoderm). Some induction of the early trophectodermal markers *CDX2* and *GATA2* was observed and, by day 4, later genes such as hCG alpha and hCG beta could be detected. The presence of extraembryonic endodermal cells was confirmed by the emergence of genes specific to parietal and visceral endoderm such as *AFP* and *LAMININ B1*, although these did not appear when the monolayers of human ESC were allowed to differentiate spontaneously. Perhaps this reflects differences between this culture system and the embryoid body method.

4.1.3 Experimental procedures to derive primitive endoderm, visceral and parietal endoderm cells from ESC

4.1.3.1 Spontaneous differentiation in embryoid bodies: In the case of mouse ESCs grown either on mitotically inactivated feeder cells or on gelatin in the presence of LIF, formation of embryoid bodies is induced simply by removal from these culture conditions. This may be achieved in either of two ways according to operator preference:

1. Culture of ESC in "hanging drops." ESCs grown to confluence on tissue culture surfaces treated with 0.1% gelatin in PBS are harvested by 0.25% trypsin EDTA. Then they are resuspended at 3×10^4 cells/mL in GMEM (Gibco BRL) with 7.5% NaHCO3, non-essential amino acids, 100 mM L-glutamine and 50 mM pyruvate, 0.1 mM 2-mercaptoethanol and FCS (10%) with LIF (Chemicon, 1 μL/mL). About 10–20 μL drops of this suspension are "spotted" onto the inner surface of the lids of 10 cm square bacterial culture plates containing 5 mL sterile water and then the lids are placed over the water-containing plate bases and incubated at 37°C in 5% CO_2. After 48 h, the embryoid body suspension is collected by knocking the lids to dislodge the drops and collected by aspiration. Embryoid bodies are sedimented at low speed (300 rpm/5 min) and resuspended in fresh medium in 10 cm bacterial plates. These cells may be grown in culture for up to 20 days by performing medium changes every 2 days.
2. Confluent cultures of ESCs may be harvested by trypsinisation as above and plated at an appropriate density (2×10^5 cells/mL) in GMEM (Gibco BRL)

with 7.5% NaHCO3, non-essential amino acids, 100 mM L-glutamine and 50 mM pyruvate, 0.1 mM 2-mercaptoethanol, and FCS (10%) and allowed to aggregate to form embryoid bodies. At various time points, embryoid bodies may be isolated and disrupted to examine the profile of differentiated cells. Disruption to a single-cell suspension without losing viability is best performed using Accutase (Chemicon).

The formation of embryoid bodies from human ESC is slightly more difficult in that they do not form stable, compact aggregations of cells with the same ease as mouse ES cells. Typically, human ESC are cultured on mitotically inactive mouse embryonic fibroblasts until just before the point where passaging would normally be required. The colonies are harvested by treatment with 1.0 mg/mL collagenase in Knockout-DMEM (Invitrogen) at 37°C in 5% CO_2 (4 min). The medium is replaced by normal human ESC culture medium containing 80% Knockout-DMEM (Invitrogen, Paisley, UK), 100 μM β-mercaptoethanol (Sigma, Dorset UK), 1 mM L-glutamine (Invitrogen), 100 mM non-essential amino acids (Invitrogen), 20% serum replacement (SR, Invitrogen), 1% penicillin-streptomycin (Sigma), and 8 ng/mL FGF2 (Invitrogen). And colonies are collected by mechanical dissaggregation using a 25-gauge hypodermic needle. The suspended colonies are sedimented (300 rpm, 3 min) and resuspended at high density in ESC differentiation medium containing 80% Knockout-DMEM (Invitrogen, Paisley, UK), 100 μM β-mercaptoethanol (Sigma, Dorset UK), 1 mM L-glutamine (Invitrogen), 100 mM non-essential amino acids (Invitrogen), 20% FBS (Hyclone), 1% penicillin-streptomycin (Sigma) in coated suspension dishes (Costar) and incubated at 37°C in 5% CO_2. After 24 h, embryoid bodies should have formed, although there will still be cells and cell debris in the medium. Collection of the embryoid bodies followed by gravity sedimentation should permit these extraneous cells to be removed.

Formation of human embryoid bodies may be facilitated by culture in bioreactor systems. ESC colonies harvested by collagenase treatment are re-suspended in the above differentiation medium and then left to aggregate in 50 mL total volume bioreactor (Synthecon, Houston, TX) at a rotation speed of 13 rpm. The whole bioreactor assembly is placed in an incubator at 37°C in 5% CO_2 and after 1 week will produce embryoid bodies of uniform size and shape which express markers of all germ layers as well as trophectoderm and primitive endoderm.

4.1.3.2 Knockdown of NANOG expression using siRNA: Human ESC lines H1 (WiCell) and hES-NCL1 (University of Newcastle, UK) were plated onto matrigel in the presence of mouse embryonic fibroblast conditioned medium 24 h before transfection. Target mRNA sequences for siRNA mediated knockdown were as follows: NANOG, AACCAGACCUGGAACAAUUCA (Accession no. NM_024865, 808–828, and AY455283) and mutated NANOG, AAC**G**AGACC**A**UGAAC**G**AUUCA. These siRNAs were obtained from Ambion (Austin, TX, http://www.ambion.com) and were transfected into human ESC at a concentration of 100 nM using Lipofectamine 2000 in accordance with manufacturer's instructions. Briefly, the siRNA–Lipofectamine 2000 complex was prepared in OptiMEM reduced serum medium by mixing a 1:2 ratio of siRNA to Lipofectamine and cells were incubated with these complexes for 24 h after which the transfection was repeated again. After day 2, the cells begin to show enlarged, flattened morphology and after 4 days express many of the markers typical of extraembryonic endoderm and trophectoderm.

5. SUMMARY AND FUTURE DIRECTIONS

There have been few studies which identify extraembryonic mesoderm or the further development of visceral mesoderm or allantoic mesoderm from human ESCs. It is probable that these cell types require the presence and precise positioning of many other cell types in the developing embryo and perhaps differentiation of embryonic stem cells either as monolayers or as embryoid bodies cannot recapitulate this process. This does not detract from the potential usefulness of embryonic stem cell cultures in modelling the early events needed for the differentiation and function of the extraembryonic tissues and their contribution to the formation of the placenta and support of the developing organism.

REFERENCES

Adjaye, J., Huntriss, J., Herwig, R., BenKahla, A., Brink, T.C., Wierling, C., Hultschig, C., Groth, D., Yaspo, M.L., Picton, H.M., Gosden, R.G., and Lehrach, H. (2005) Primary differentiation in the human blastocyst: comparative molecular portraits of inner cell mass and trophectoderm cells. Stem Cells, 23(10): 1514–1525.

Anderson, R., Copeland, T.K., Scholer, H., Heasman, J., and Wylie, C. (2000) The onset of germ cell migration in the mouse embryo. Mech. Dev., 91(1–2): 61–68.

Antczak, M. and Van Blerkom, J. (1997) Oocyte influences on early development: the regulatory proteins leptin and STAT3 are polarized in mouse and human oocytes and differentially distributed within the cells of the preimplantation stage embryo. Mol. Hum. Reprod., 3(12): 1067–1086.

Beck, F., Chawengsaksophak, K., Luckett, J., Giblett, S., Tucci, J., Brown, J., Poulsom, R., Jeffery, R., and Wright, N.A. (2003) A study of regional gut endoderm potency by analysis of Cdx2 null mutant chimaeric mice. Dev. Biol., 255: 399–406.

Bielinska, M., Narita, N., and Wilson, D.B. (1999) Distinct roles for visceral endoderm during embryonic mouse development. Int. J. Dev. Biol., 43(3): 183–205.

Bradley, A., Evans, M., Kaufman, M.H., and Robertson, E. (1984) Formation of germ-line chimaeras from embryo derived teratocarcinoma cell lines. Nature, 309: 255–256.

Brulet, P., Babinet, C., Kemler, R., and Jacob, C. (1980) Monoclonal antibodies against trophectoderm specific markers during mouse blastocyst formation. Proc. Natl. Acad. Sci. USA, 77(7): 4113–4117.

Brummelkamp, T.R., Bernards, R., and Agami, R. (2002) A system for stable expression of short interfering RNAs in mammalian cells. Science, 296(5567): 550–553.

Chambers, I., Colby, D., Robertson, M., et al. (2003) Functional cloning of Nanog, a pluripotency sustaining factor in embryonic stem cells. Cell, 30: 643–655.

Chung, Y., Klimanskaya, I., Becker, S., Marh, J., Lu, S.J., Johnson, J., Meisner, L., and Lanza, R. (2006) Embryonic and extraembryonic stem cell lines derived from single mouse blastomeres. Nature, 439(7073): 216–219.

Coucouvanis, E. and Martin, G.R. (1995) Signals for death and survival: a two-step mechanism for cavitation in the vertebrate embryo. Cell, 83(2): 279–287.

Coucouvanis, E. and Martin, G.R. (1999) BMP signaling plays a role in visceral endoderm differentiation and cavitation in the early mouse embryo. Development, 126(3): 535–546.

Dardik, A., Smith, R.M., and Schultz, R.M. (1992) Colocalization of transforming growth factor-alpha and a functional epidermal growth factor receptor (EGFR) to the inner cell mass and preferential localization of the EGFR on the basolateral surface of the trophectoderm in the mouse blastocyst. Dev. Biol., 154(2): 396–409.

Duncan, S.A., Nagy, A., and Chan, W. (1997) Murine gastrulation requires HNF-4 regulated gene expression in the visceral endoderm: tetraploid rescue of Hnf-4(–/–) embryos. Development, 124(2): 279–287.

Fujikura, J., Yamato, E., Yonemura, S., Hosoda, K., Masui, S., Nakao, K., Miyazaki Ji, J., and Niwa, H. (2002) Differentiation of embryonic stem cells is induced by GATA factors. Genes Dev., 16(7): 784–789.

Futaki, S., Hayashi, Y., Emoto, T., Weber, C.N., and Sekiguchi, K. (2004) Sox7 plays crucial roles in parietal endoderm differentiation in F9 embryonal carcinoma cells through regulating Gata-4 and Gata-6 expression. Mol. Cell Biol., 24(23): 10492–10503.

Gardner, R.L. (1983) Origin and differentiation of extraembryonic tissues in the mouse. Int. Rev. Exp. Pathol., 24: 63–133.

Hatano, S.Y., Tada, M., Kimura, H., et al. (2005) Pluripotential competence of cells associated with Nanog activity. Mech. Dev., 122: 67–79.

Hyslop, L., Stojkovic, M., Armstrong, L., Walter, T., Stojkovic, P., Przyborski, S., Herbert, M., Murdoch, A., Strachan, T., and Lako, M. (2005) Downregulation of NANOG induces differentiation of human embryonic stem cells to extraembryonic lineages. Stem Cells, 23(8): 1035–1043.

Johnson, M.H., Chisholm, J.S., Fleming, T.P., and Houliston, E. (1986) A role for cytoplasmic determinants in the development of the early mouse embryo? J. Embryol. Exp. Morphol. (Suppl.) 97: 97–121.

Khang, I., Sonn, S., Park, J.H., Rhee, K., Park, D., and Kim. K. (2005) Expression of epithin in mouse preimplantation development: its functional role in compaction. Dev. Biol., 281(1): 134–144.

Larue, L., Ohsugi, M., Hirchenhain, J., and Kemler, R. (1994) E-cadherin null mutant embryos fail to form a trophectoderm epithelium. Proc. Natl. Acad. Sci. USA, 91(17): 8263–8267.

Lawson, K.A., Dunn, N.R., Roelen, B.A., Zeinstra, L.M., Davis, A.M., Wright, C.V., Korving, J.P., and Hogan, B.L. (1999) Bmp4 is required for the generation of primordial germ cells in the mouse embryo. Genes Dev., 13(4): 424–436.

Matin, M.M., Walsh, J.R., Gokhale, P.J., Draper, J.S., Bahrami, A.R., Morton, I., Moore, H.D., and Andrews, P.W. (2004) Specific knockdown of Oct4 and beta2-microglobulin expression by RNA interference in human embryonic stem cells and embryonic carcinoma cells. Stem Cells, 22(5): 659–668.

Maye, P., Becker, S., Kasameyer, E., Byrd, N., and Grabel, L. (2000) Indian hedgehog signaling in extraembryonic endoderm and ectoderm differentiation in ES embryoid bodies. Mech. Dev., 94(1–2): 117–132.

Mitsui, K., Tokuzawa, Y., Itoh, H., et al. (2003) The homeoprotein Nanog is required for maintenance and pluripotency in mouse epiblast and ES cells. Cell, 113: 631–642.

Miyagishi, M. and Taira, K. (2002) U6 promoter-driven siRNAs with four uridine 3′ overhangs efficiently suppress targeted gene expression in mammalian cells. Nat. Biotechnol., 20(5): 497–500.

Nichols, J., Zevnik, B., Anastassiadis, K., Niwa, H., Klewe-Nebenius, D., Chambers, I., Scholer, H., and Smith, A. (1998) Formation of pluripotent stem cells in the mammalian embryo depends on the POU transcription factor Oct4. Cell, 95(3): 379–391.

Niimi, T., Hayashi, Y., Futaki, S., and Sekiguchi, K. (2004) SOX7 and SOX17 regulate the parietal endoderm-specific enhancer activity of mouse laminin alpha1 gene. J. Biol. Chem., 279(36): 38055–38061.

Niwa, H., Masui, S., Chambers, I., Smith, A.G., and Miyazaki, J.I. (2002) Phenotypic complementation establishes requirements for specific POU domain and generic transactivation function of Oct3/4 in embryonic stem cells. Mol. Cell Biol., 22(5): 1526–1536.

Niwa, H., Miyazaki, J., and Smith, A.G. (2000) Quantitative expression of Oct-3/4 defines differentiation, dedifferentiation or self-renewal of ES cells. Nat. Genet., 24(4): 372–376.

Niwa, H., Toyooka, Y., Shimosato, D., Strumpf, D., Takahashi, K., Yagi, R., and Rossant, J. (2005) Interaction between Oct3/4 and Cdx2 determines trophectoderm differentiation. Cell, 123: 917–929.

Pan, G. and Pei, D. (2005) The stem cell pluripotency factor Nanog activates transcription with two unusually potent subdomains at its C-terminus. J. Biol. Chem., 280: 1401–1407.

Pedersen, R.A., Wu, K., and Balakier, H. (1986) Origin of the inner cell mass in mouse embryos: cell lineage analysis by microinjection. Dev. Biol., 117(2): 581–595.

Peng, C. (2003) The TGF-beta superfamily and its roles in the human ovary and placenta. J. Obstet. Gynaecol. Can., 25(10): 834–844.

Pratt, H. (1989) Marking time and space: chronology and topography in the early mouse embryo. Int. Rev. Cytol., 117: 99–130.

Quinn, J., Kunath, T., and Rossant, J. (2006) Mouse trophoblast stem cells. Methods Mol. Med., 121: 125–148.

Rossant, J. (2001) Stem cells from the mammalian blastocyst. Stem Cells, 19: 477–482.

Strumpf, D., Mao, C.A., Yamanaka, Y., et al. (2005) Cdx2 is required for correct cell fate specification and differentiation of trophectoderm in the mouse blastocyst. Development, 132: 2093–2102.

Tanaka, S., Kunath, T., Hadjantonakis, A.K., Nagy, A., and Rossant, J. (1998) Promotion of trophoblast stem cell proliferation by FGF4. Science, 282(5396): 2072–2075.

Tompers, D.M., Foreman, R.K., Wang, Q., Kumanova, M., and Labosky, P.A. (2005) Foxd3 is required in the trophoblast progenitor cell lineage of the mouse embryo. Dev. Biol., 285(1): 126–137.

Varmuza, S., Prideaux, V., Kothary, R., and Rossant, J. (1988) Polytene chromosomes in mouse trophoblast giant cells. Development, 102: 127–134.

Velkey, J.M. and O'Shea, K.S. (2003) Oct4 RNA interference induces trophectoderm differentiation in mouse embryonic stem cells. Genesis, 37: 18–24.

Xu, C., Inokuma, M.S., Denham, J., Golds, K., Kundu, P., Gold, J.D., and Carpenter, M.K. (2001) Feeder-free growth of undifferentiated human embryonic stem cells. Nat. Biotechnol., 19(10): 971–974.

Xu, R.H., Chen, X., Li, D.S., Li, R., Addicks, G.C., Glennon, C., Zwaka, T.P., and Thomson, J.A. (2002) BMP4 initiates human embryonic stem cell differentiation to trophoblast. Nat. Biotechnol., 20(12): 1261–1264.

CHAPTER 11

PANCREATIC CELL DIFFERENTIATION

BETTINA FISHMAN[1], HANNA SEGEV[2],
AND JOSEPH ITSKOVITZ-ELDOR[1,2]
[1]*The Bruce Rappaport Faculty of Medicine, Technion-Israel Institute of Technology*
[2]*The Department of Obstetrics and Gynecology, Rambam Medical Center, Haifa, Israel*

1. BACKGROUND AND SIGNIFICANCE

Diabetes mellitus is a major health problem affecting more than 5% of the global population and is the most common metabolic disorder (Mandrup-Poulsen 1998). Diabetes mellitus takes two forms: Type I (insulin-dependent) is caused by an autoimmune destruction of the insulin-producing β-cells. Type II (noninsulin-dependent), results from a combination of reduced insulin sensitivity and impaired function of the insulin-secreting β-cells. Present treatments for diabetes fail to offer a cure and do not prevent secondary complications associated with diabetes, such as diabetic retinopathy, nephropathy, and neuropathy (Mandrup-Poulsen 1998). Early treatment of patients by restoration of their β-cell function through pancreas or islet transplantation can both free the patients from their dependency on insulin and prevent related complications (Juang et al. 1996; Meyer et al. 1998; Weir and Bonner-Weir 1998). A potential cure for this disease is transplantation therapy whereby islets are transplanted into the patient. However, there are limited numbers of donor organs that restricts the use of this procedure. Another potential treatment is the use of endocrine stem cells to produce insulin-producing cells for transplantation therapy. Embryonic stem (ES) cells are a potential source of endocrine stem cells.

Human embryonic stem (hES) cells are self-renewing pluripotent cells obtained from the inner cell mass of human blastocysts (Thomson et al. 1998; Reubinoff et al. 2000). hES cell lines and clones can retain normal karyotypes even after long-term culture. The unique features of ES cells are their ability to be cultured indefinitely in an undifferentiated state and their capacity to differentiate into cells representative of all three body lineages: ectoderm, mesoderm, and endoderm (Thomson and Marshall 1998; Thomson et al. 1998; Itskovitz-Eldor et al. 2000; Reubinoff et al. 2000).

J.R. Masters et al (eds.), Embryonic Stem Cells, 189–209.

2. INSULIN EXPRESSION IN HUMAN EMBRYONIC STEM CELLS

Assady et al. (2001) and Schuldiner et al. (2001) demonstrated spontaneous differentiation of hES cells into insulin-producing cells. H9 cells were grown in high-density adherent cell culture or in suspension as embryoid bodies, and were able to express low levels of insulin after 30 days in culture. We have presented a method for forming insulin-producing cells derived from hES cells (Segev et al. 2004), the protocol for which is described below in detail.

In order to differentiate ES cells into insulin-producing cells, several strategies of *in vitro* differentiation have been proposed (Figure 1). Those strategies consist of two main approaches: genetic manipulation, induction of differentiation by various growth factors and growth conditions, or a combination of those two strategies. Genetic manipulation involves the insertion of different reporters such as green fluorescent protein or antibiotic resistance genes under the control of pancreas-specific promoters and using these reporter constructs to identify and select cells that undergo differentiation to insulin-producing cells when cells are allowed to spontaneously differentiate *in vitro*. Environmental change consists of induction of differentiation through multiple stepwise differentiation stages beginning with generation of EBs and changing growth conditions at each stage by addition of growth factors and nutritional. Nutritional changes in the glucose concentration or in the oxygen levels and the use of different cellular matrices.

Understanding the process of normal β-cell differentiation *in vivo* is crucial in order to mimic it *in vitro*. The pancreas develops from the endoderm, which is one of the three germ layers (ectoderm, mesoderm, and endoderm) from which the early epiblast is formed. Thus, several works have suggested differentiation protocols of ES cells into definitive endoderm.

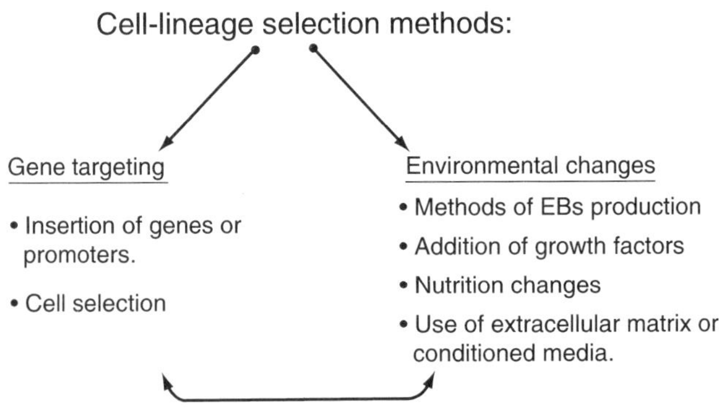

Figure 1. Strategies for in vitro differentiation.

3. DIFFERENTIATION OF EMBRYONIC STEM TO DEFINITIVE ENDODERM

The definitive endoderm gives rise to the epithelial lining of the respiratory and digestive tracts and to the thyroid, thymus, lungs, liver, and pancreas. It is formed during gastrulation, in which pluripotent epiblast cells are allocated to the three principal germ layers. Overexpression of Nodal promotes differentiation of mouse ES cells into mesoderm and endoderm at the expense of neuroectoderm formation (Pfendler et al. 2005). However hES cells cultured with Nodal showed prolonged expression of pluripotency marker genes and less induction of neuroectoderm markers (Vallier et al. 2004). Activin is another TGFβ family member which binds to the same receptors as Nodal (with the exception of the coreceptor cripto), triggering similar intracellular signaling events, and was therefore used to mimic Nodal activity *in vitro* (D'Amour et al. 2005). Differentiation of hES cells in the presence of activin A and low-serum concentrations for 4–5 days produced cultures highly enriched for definitive endoderm (D'Amour et al. 2005).

Lowering the serum concentration in the presence of activin A for 5 days resulted in an elevated expression of genes such as *Sox17*, Gooscoid (*Gsc*), *Foxa2*, and *Mixl1*. As these genes are also expressed in primitive/parietal/visceral endoderm, the expression of *Sox7*, which is not present in definitive endoderm, was examined. The population was further enriched to near homogeneity using the cell-surface receptor CXCR4.

In a similar approach, Yasunaga et al. (2005) used mES cells bearing the *GFP* and *CD25* marker genes in the *Gsc* and *Sox17* loci, respectively. This cell line allowed them to monitor the generation of Gsc^{+} $Sox17^{+}$ definitive endoderm and $Gsc^{-}Sox17^{+}$ visceral endoderm and to define culture conditions that differentially induced definitive and visceral endoderm. Seven surface markers, including *CXCR4*, were differentially expressed in the two populations. Gsc expression can be induced by activin A in serum-free conditions (Tada et al. 2005). The suggested pathway to definitive and visceral endoderm is illustrated in Figure 2.

Kubo et al. (2004) targeted GFP to the *brachyury* locus. In this experiment they demonstrated that endoderm develops from a $brachyury^{+}$ population that also displays a mesoderm potential – the mesoendoderm. Endoderm was induced in EBs either by limited exposure to serum or by culturing in the presence of activin A under serum-free conditions.

Ku et al. (2004) have found that EBs cultured in the presence of stage-specific concentrations of monothioglycerol and 15% fetal calf serum (FCS), followed by serum-free conditions, give rise to a population that expresses insulin I, insulin II, pancreatic duodenal homeobox 1 (Pdx1), and Sox17. Addition of activin βB, nicotinamide, and exendin-4 toward the end of the differentiation to later-stage culture increased insulin-positive cells to 2.73% of the total population as compared to 1% in the control culture.

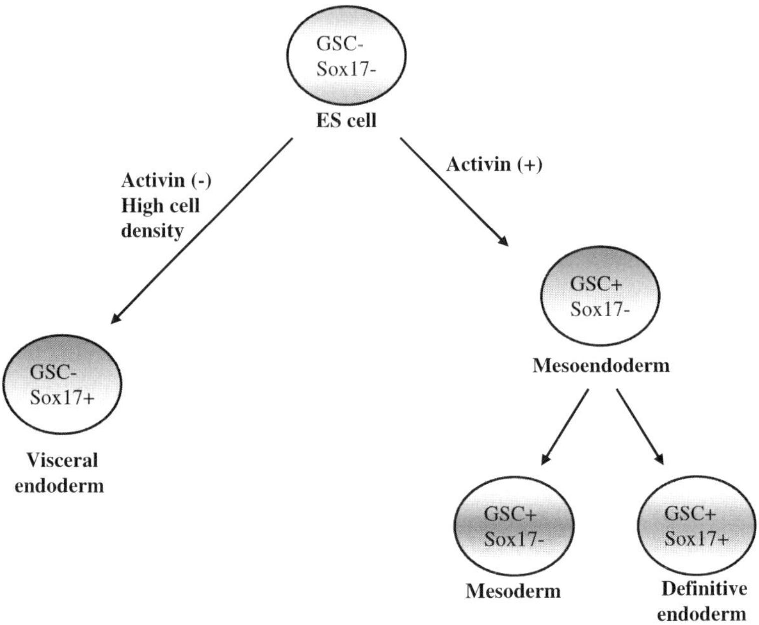

Figure 2. Identification of cell surface markers in ES cell differentiation. A differentiation pathway of ES cells into definitive and visceral endoderm was suggested by Yasunaga et al. (2005) by using two serum-free conditions. ES cells grown in serum-free medium with activin supplement differentiated into definitive endoderm and mesoderm cells through mesoendoderm, whereas cells grown at high density without activin differentiated into visceral endoderm. Five cell populations were sorted by FACS. (1) ES cells expressing E-cadherin (ECD) but negative for Gsc and Sox17: $Gsc^{-}Spx17^{-}$ ECD^{+}; (2) mesoendoderm cells which are Gsc^{+} $Sox17^{-}ECD^{+}$; (3) definitive endoderm cells which are Gsc^{+} $Sox17^{+}$ ECD+; (4) mesoderm cells which are Gsc+ $Sox17^{-}ECD^{-}$; and (5) visceral endoderm cells which are $Gsc^{-}Sox17^{+}$ ECD^{+}.

Because of the similarities between β-cell differentiation and neuroepithelial development (Edlund 2001), a transient expression of nestin was proposed to occur in human insulin-producing β-cell precursors similar to that seen in neuroepithelial differentiation (Zulewski et al. 2001; Abraham et al. 2002). Thus different protocols suggested differentiating hES cells into insulin-expressing cells by selecting nestin-positive cells (Lumelsky et al. 2001; Hori et al. 2002; Blyszczuk et al. 2003). However, recent studies using nestin-positive cells concluded that nestin is not a specific marker of β-cell precursors, although it may contribute to microvasculature (Humphrey et al. 2003; Treutelaar et al. 2003). Since other reports (Lammert et al. 2001) have suggested that signals from endothelial cells are critical to the growth of pancreatic endocrine cells during embryogenesis, it is possible that nestin-positive cells contribute to the developing vasculature of the pancreatic mesenchyme. Thus, the proliferation of nestin-positive cells and β-cells may be connected.

It has been suggested that during embryogenesis, cells expressing Neurogenin3 (Ngn3) are islet progenitors (Gu et al. 2002), and these $Ngn3^+$ cells give rise to the endocrine cells of the pancreas. Other reports (Chiang and Melton 2003) do not rule out the possibility that cells expressing glucagon, insulin, and Ngn3 eventually become adult β-cells.

4. DIFFERENTIATION OF MOUSE EMBRYONIC STEM CELLS USING ENVIRONMENTAL CHANGES

Lumelsky et al. (2001) published a protocol for differentiating mouse ES cells into insulin-secreting cells. The basis of their work was the hypothesis that similar mechanisms control the development of both the pancreas and the central nervous system (CNS). Based on these similarities, they suggested that strategies that induce production of neural cells from ES cells could potentially be adapted for endocrine pancreatic cells.

Thus they developed a multistep differentiation approach modifying the culture conditions used for the generation of nestin-positive cells. This protocol consisted of several steps (Figure 3). Four-day-old EBs were plated in a medium containing insulin, transferrin, selenium, and fibronectin (ITSF) that enriches for nestin-positive cells. Next, the cells were transferred to a medium containing N2, B27, and basic fibroblast growth factor (bFGF). bFGF and keratinocyte growth factor (KGF) were previously found to enhance the formation of islet-like clusters from ES cells (Schuldiner et al. 2000; Lumelsky et al. 2001; Soria et al. 2001; Ogneva and Martinova 2002). At the end of this stage, bFGF was withdrawn from the medium and nicotinamide was added. Nicotinamide is a poly-synthetase (ADP-ribose) inhibitor known to induce differentiation and increase β-cell mass in cultured human fetal pancreatic cells (Otonkoski et al. 1993).

Using this protocol, Lumelsky et al. (2001) were able to differentiate mouse ES cells into islet-like clusters. The cells created by this method were able to produce and secrete insulin, but only in small amounts per cell compared to the normal islets of Langerhans.

Hori at al. (2002) modified this protocol by substituting B27, which was added in the Lumelsky protocol at the stage that induces the differentiation of insulin-secreting cells, for PI3K inhibitors such as LY294002 (Figure 4). They hypothesized that this modification might lead to the formation of cells with greater similarity to pancreatic islets, induce a predominant insulin + cell component, a minor neuronal component, and reduce cellular proliferation.

This protocol was based on previous work which showed that *in vitro* treatment of human fetal pancreas with nicotinamide and LY29400 increases the total endocrine cell number and insulin content while reducing DNA synthesis (Ptasznik et al. 1997). In addition, treatment of neuroendocrine cell lines with wortmanin, another PI3K inhibitor, prevented neurite outgrowth (Kimura et al. 1994). The cells produced by this protocol expressed insulin, PDX1, GLUT2, and glucokinase. Transplanting those cells into STZ-induced diabetic mice resulted in reduction of

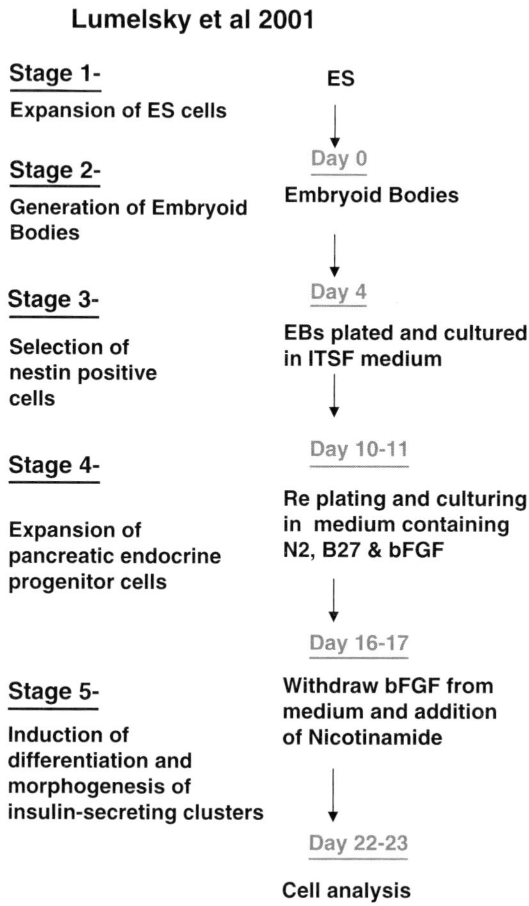

Figure 3. A schematic representation of the differentiation protocol suggested by Lumelsky (2001) for generating insulin-secreting islet-like clusters from undifferentiated mESs.

blood glucose, and increased survival in comparison to sham transplanted mice. Graft removal 3 weeks after engraftment resulted in increased mortality.

Hansson et al. (2004) repeated and further investigated the reports of Lumelsky (2001) and Hori (2002). The cells were cultured according to the protocol described by Lumelsky, as well as using a PI3 kinase inhibitor as described by Hori et al. The cells released insulin when glucose was added to the medium, but C-peptide release was not detected. Hansson claimed that the lack of C-peptide secretion indicated that the release of insulin was not the result of *de novo* insulin biosynthesis by the cells but a result of insulin that had been taken up from the medium. In addition, many insulin + cells contained small, condensed nuclei, suggesting apoptosis, or necrosis. More cells with these characteristics were seen following treatment with PI3K inhibitor, which is known to cause apoptosis.

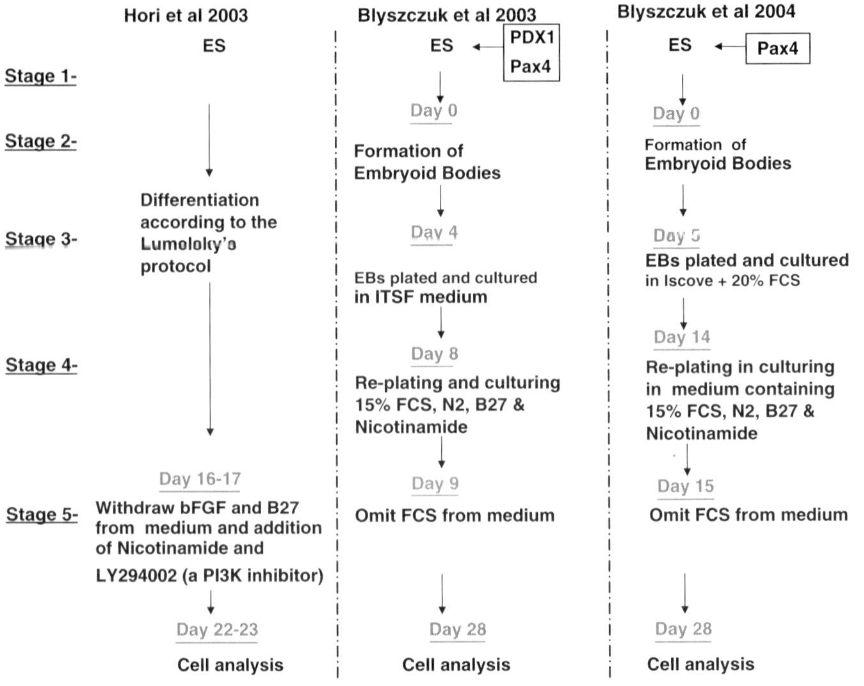

Figure 4. An outline of differentiation protocols for mES cells as suggested by Hori et al. (2002) and Blyszczuk (2003, 2004). Hori (2002) followed the differentiation protocol suggested by Lumelsky et al. (2001) with some modifications: the B27 supplement was withdrawn from the last stage and a PI3 kinase inhibitor, LY294002, was added. Blyszczuk et al. (2003, 2004) in their protocol used mESs transfected with Pdx1 or Pax4 and modified the protocol suggested by Lumelsky et al. (2001).

Another modification to the original protocol was proposed by Bai et al. (2005). Since glucagon-like peptide-1 (GLP-1) was shown in previous work to induce the differentiation of β cells from ductal progenitor cells, Bai et al. added 100 nM GLP-1 or 10 nM exendin-4 to Stage 5 of the differentiation protocol. The cells secreted low levels of insulin in response to glucose, along with C-peptide.

Using a different modification, our group was able to show the formation of insulin-secreting cells from human ES cells (Segev et al. 2004). The modification included two main changes: (a) reducing the glucose concentration in the last steps (medium III); and (b) introducing an aggregation step at the end of the protocol (Figure 5). Low glucose combined with nicotinamide has previously been suggested to increase the insulin content in β-cells differentiated from mouse ES cells (Soria et al. 2000, 2001). In addition, the aggregation contributes to the enrichment of insulin-producing cells and insulin secretion. Decreasing the glucose concentration in the growth medium from 3,151 to 901 mg/L during our protocol resulted in an increase in insulin secretion in response to glucose,

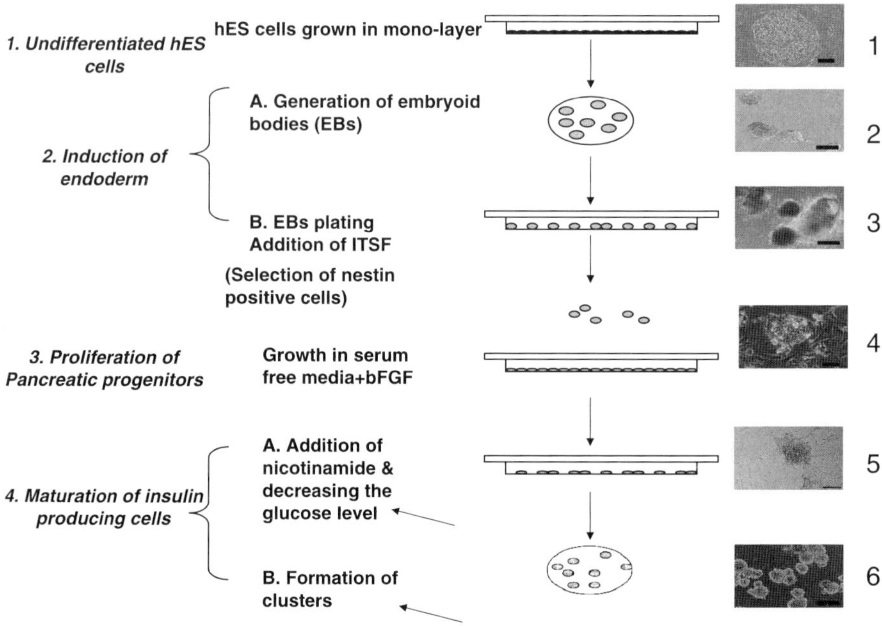

Figure 5. General outline of the differentiation protocol suggested by Segev et al. (2004). The protocol consists of several stages. Stage 1: Growth of undifferentiated hES cells (bar = 10 μM). Stage 2: Formation of EBs (bar = 30 μM). Stage 3: Plating EBs in *medium I*: (DMEM/F12 1:1, Insulin–Transferrin–Selenium–fibronectin and 1 mM glutamine) for 1 week (bar = 30 μM). Stage 4: Dissociation of the cells and plating them in *medium II*: (DMEM/F12 1:1 with N2 and B27 media, 1 mM glutamine and 10 ng/mL bFGF) for 1 week (bar = 5 μM). Stage 5: Change to medium III (removal of bFGF, addition of 10 mM of nicotinamide, and reduction of the glucose concentration from 3,151 to 901 mg/L) (bar = 10 μM). Stage 6: Dissociation of the cells and growing them in suspension in Petri dishes with *medium III* (bar = 10 μM).

from 2.13 ± 1.32 to 8.64 ± 3.42 μu/mL/10^5 cells/h. A more dramatic increase in insulin secretion to 225.8 ± 78.5 μu/mL/10^5 cells/h was obtained by the formation of clusters. Transcripts for insulin were shown by RT-PCR and *in situ* hybridization, along with transcripts for proinsulin processing enzymes, PC1/3 and PC2, indicating that Stage 6 cells acquired the ability to synthesize and process proinsulin to mature insulin. Transcripts for the two components of the K_{ATP}^+ channel, Sur1 and Kir6.2, and for Glut2 and Glucokinase, which participate in signal-secretion coupling in pancreatic β-cells, were also detected. In addition, transcription factors Pdx1, Nkx6.1, Isl1, Pax4, Pax6, Ngn3, and islet amyloid polypeptide (IAPP) were also present in Stage 6 clusters. Both insulin and C-peptide were also shown by immunofluorescence in Stage 6 clusters.

The use of a cluster phase has been previously demonstrated by Zhao et al. (2002) and others (Bonner-Weir et al. 2000; Itkin-Ansari et al. 2000) as a useful method for long-term maintenance of human islets *in vitro*. Using repeated cycles of aggregation and plating of cells obtained from postmortem human islets, Zhao et al. (2002) succeeded in maintaining the cells for 4 months without losing their potential for expressing insulin. This work introduced the aggregation step, which not only increased the percentage of the insulin-expressing cells, but also improved their survival from 1 week as mono-layer to a month or more as clusters.

A different differentiation strategy was proposed by Shi et al. (2005). Their protocol consisted of three major steps based on the combined induction of activin A, all-trans retinoic acid, and other maturation factors (Figure 6). Step 1 is the formation of embryonic bodies. After 24–48 h, EBs were collected and replated into 10% FBS/DMEM without LIF on 1% matrigel-coated plates. Almost 2 h later, the EBs were cultured in 10% FBS/DMEM with 100 ng/mL activin A for 24 h. Then medium was switched to 10% FBS/DMEM for 6–8 h. Next, the differentiated EBs were cultured in 10% FBS/DMEM with 10 μM retinoic acid for another 24 h. Step 2: To expand insulin-producing precursors,

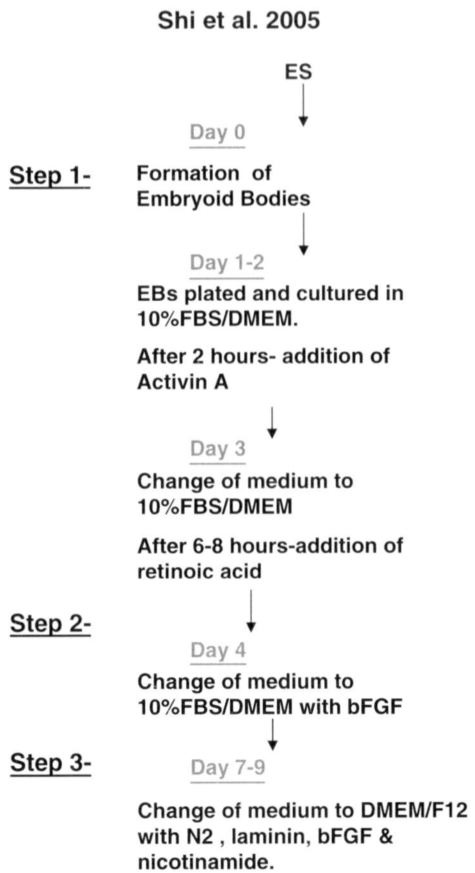

Figure 6. A differentiation protocol suggested by Shi et al. (2005). Mouse ES cells were allowed to differentiate into insulin-positive cells with the addition of activin A and retinoic acid.

the differentiated EB cells were cultured in 10% FBS/DMEM with 10 ng/mL bFGF for 3–5 days. Step 3: To mature the insulin-producing cells, the expanded cells in step 2 were switched to DMEM/F12 supplemented with N2, 1 mg/mL laminin, 10 ng/mL bFGF, and 10 mM nicotinamide, and cultured for 3–5 days. Following 2 weeks of differentiation, the mES cells differentiated into insulin-producing cells which secreted insulin in response to the glucose concentration. Using a GFP reporter gene linked to an insulin promoter system excluded the possibility of insulin uptake from the medium. In addition, transplantation of these insulin-positive cells into diabetic mice normalized blood glucose levels and improved their survival rates.

The role of retinoic acid was also demonstrated by Micallef et al. (2005). In this work, they used a mES cell line in which GFP was targeted to the Pdx1 gene. By monitoring GFP expression during the course of the differentiation of the ES cells, they were able to demonstrate that retinoic acid can regulate the commitment of ES cells to form $Pdx1^+$ cells. Retinoic acid was most effective when added to cultures at day 4 of ES differentiation, a period corresponding to the end of gastrulation in the embryo.

5. METHODS FOR CELL LINEAGE SELECTION

Strategies for *in vitro* differentiation usually result in an enrichment of several cell populations expressing markers of the desired cell type together with other undesired cell types. Even when cultures are enriched for certain cell types, the final cultures are always a heterogeneous mixture of cell types. The following methods have been suggested for selection of a desired cell population:

1. Purification of lineage-specific cells based on marker gene expression, detected by introduction of a transgene marker conferring drug resistance and/or cell sorting capacity (Klug et al. 1996; Muller et al. 2000; Soria et al. 2000; Soria 2001).
2. Engineered expression (or repression) of certain fate master genes.
3. Cell sorting separation (immunopurification) on the basis of a specific cell marker.

6. CELL TRAPPING SYSTEM

One approach was to use a cell trapping system in mES cells (Soria et al. 2000) (Figure 7). The cells were transfected with a plasmid bearing a neomycin selectable gene under the control of the insulin promoter. The plasmid also contained a gene conferring hygromycin resistance under a constitutively active promoter. The transfected cells were first cultured in hygromycin to select for stably transfected cells, then cultured in the absence of LIF to encourage the formation of EBs and finally in the antibiotic G418 (neomycin resistance) to select cells expressing factors that could activate the insulin promoter. For final

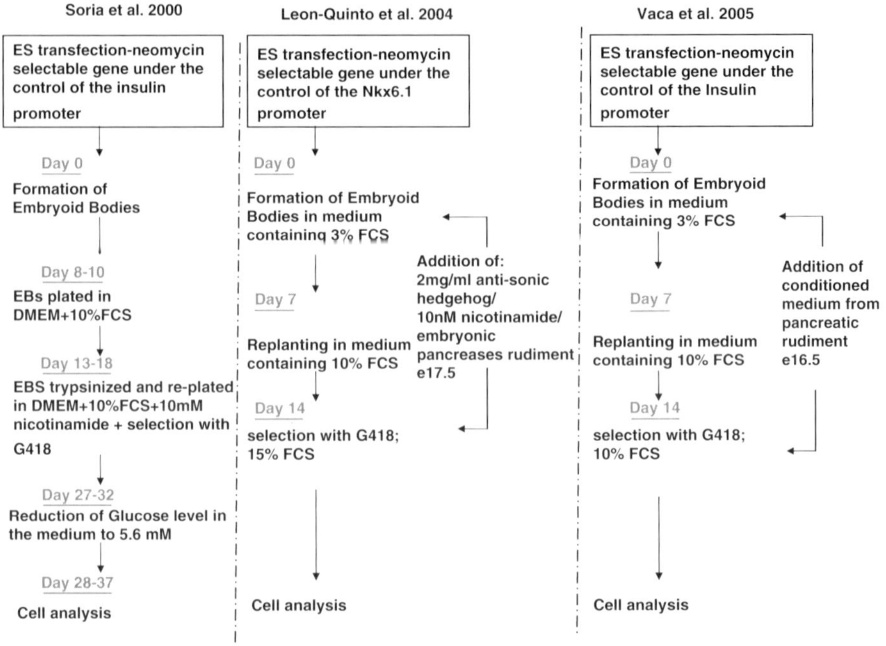

Figure 7. Examples of differentiation protocols that combined genetic manipulation and growth media changes. Soria et al. (2000; Leon-Quinto et al. 2004; Vaca et al. 2005) targeted mES with the insulin promoter and combined antibiotic cell selection with a maturation protocol. The maturation protocol combined an addition of nicotinamide and reduction of the glucose level at the last stage. mES cells targeted with insulin promoter were also used by Vaca (2005), while Leon-Quinto et al. (2004) used mES targeted with Nkx6.1 promoter. They both explored the use of soluble factors from embryonic pancreatic rudiments on the differentiation into insulin-producing cells.

differentiation and maturation, the resulting clones were trypsinized and plated in a Petri dish and grown for 2 weeks in DMEM supplemented with the antibiotic G418 and 10 mM nicotinamide. For the final maturation step, the glucose in the medium was reduced to 5.6 mM. One of the resultant clones contained 16.5 ng/μg protein of total insulin and secreted insulin at 46 pg/μg protein/30 min in 5 mM glucose, and at 318 pg/μg protein/30 min in 16.7 mM glucose. The cells (10^6 in total) were able to normalize blood glucose levels and restore body weight when implanted to mice with streptozotocin-induced diabetes. The selection with the antibiotic was followed by an improved maturation strategy. This included an exposure to low glucose and addition of 10 nM nicotinamide.

Moritoh et al. (2003) used a similar construct with mouse ES cells grown in feeder-free culture (Figure 8). Those cells were grown without a feeder layer in order to promote the expression of Pdx1 and therefore induce differentiation into insulin-producing cells. Undifferentiated cells (Stage 1) were dissociated and grown in suspension in Petri dishes (Stage 2). The Stage 2 EBs were replated on

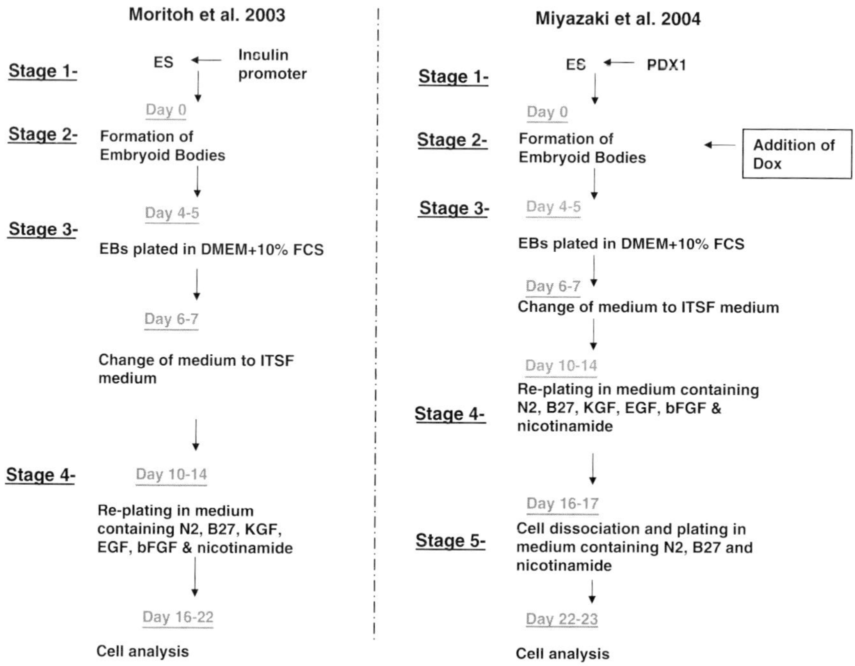

Figure 8. Differentiation protocols for mES cells into insulin-positive cells. Moritoh et al. (2003) modified the protocol suggested by Lumelsky et al. (2001). Moritoh targeted mESCs with the insulin promoter linked to a reporter gene. Miyazaki (2004) used regulated expression of the transcription factor Pdx1. The mES cells they established had exogenous Pdx1 expression which was regulated by Tet-off system by adding Dox at the EBs stage.

gelatin-coated plates in DMEM with 10% FCS. After 2 days the medium was changed to ITSFn medium, and the cells were incubated for 4–7 days. Growth in this medium resulted in enhanced cell death, and the surviving cells (Stage 3) were dissociated and replated on gelatinized plates at a concentration of $0.5–2 \times 10^5$ cells/cm^2 in DMEM/F12 with the addition of N2, hKGF, EGF, and bFGF in the presence of B27 and nicotinamide, and cultured for 6–8 days (Stage 4 cell clusters). At Stage 4 the number of cells expressing β-gal increased in both adherent colonies and floating spheres. These insulin-expressing cells coincided exactly with the β-gal positive cells. However, the insulin-positive cells were also stained for glucagon, indicative of their developmental immaturity.

Fluorescence activated cell sorting (FACS) or magnetic cell sorter (MACS) can be used by substituting the antibiotic resistance gene with either a GFP marker (as described by Muller et al. (2000) for cardiomyocyte separation) or CD4, respectively (David et al. 2005).

This cell lineage selection strategy may adopt multiple variants, such as using the promoter region of the Pdx1, Ngn3, Nkx6.1 genes (Leon-Quinto et al. 2004), or the pancreatic polypeptide (PP) promoter (Berna et al. 2001).

The Nkx6.1 promoter was also used to direct the differentiation of mouse ES cells into insulin-producing cells (Leon-Quinto et al. 2004) (Figure 7). In this work mouse ES cells were transfected with a plasmid containing the Nkx6.1 promoter upstream of the neomycin-resistance gene. EBs were first cultured in 3% FCS for 7 days followed by a week in 10% FCS, then 15% FCS, and selection with G418. To further induce differentiation they combined the reduction of the serum concentration (from 15% to 3%) with the addition of selected factors. The factors used were 2 μg/mL anti-sonic hedgehog (Shh) and 10 mM nicotinamide. *In vivo*, Shh is inhibited in the developing pancreas of embryonic mice, permitting the expression of Pdx1 and the subsequent cascade of pancreatic genes. In addition, the cells were cocultured with pancreas from embryos on day 17.5 (e17.5), in which the soluble factors secreted by the forming islets induced differentiation. The pancreatic rudiments were separated from the mES by nylon filters. Using this approach they were able to obtain cell cultures in which up to 20% of the cells coexpressed insulin and Pdx1. After neomycin selection, nearly 100% of the cells were positive for β-cell-specific genes and proteins (insulin, pdx1, nkx6.1, etc.). Cell survival was higher with nicotinamide, anti-Shh, or pancreatic rudiments than in the control. The cells demonstrated glucose-dependent insulin release. Transplanting these cells into diabetic mice resulted in glucose normalization.

Fetal pancreatic soluble factors and reduced serum concentration were also used by Vaca et al. (2005) to induce differentiation of mES into pancreatic-like islet cells (Figure 7). In addition, the insulin promoter linked to an antibiotic resistance gene was used to target the cells. Coculture of these cells with medium conditioned by pancreatic rudiments resulted in the appearance of transcripts and proteins found normally in β-cells. The cells stained positive for both insulin and C-peptide. Half of the cells obtained coexpressed two proteins essential for the stimulus secretion coupling process, such as Glut2 and insulin. The differentiated cells showed regulated insulin release and increased insulin and C-peptide content (2.7 ± 0.1 and 1.5 ± 0.3 ng/μg protein, respectively). These cells also demonstrated functional K channel activity after exposing them to ATP. In addition, diabetic mice into which these cells were transplanted, maintained normal glucose levels. None of the mice transplanted with the differentiated cells developed teratomas.

Identification of a precursor of the pancreatic β-cell or the islet cells together with a clearer understanding of the signals that drive β-cell differentiation could be very useful to generate improved selection strategies.

7. ENGINEERED EXPRESSION (OR REPRESSION) OF CERTAIN FATE-DETERMINANT MASTER GENES, SUCH AS PA × 4 OR PDX1

Expression of master genes during differentiation can induce differentiation to a specific cell lineage, such as MyoD for skeletal muscle or Pax6 in the ectoderm induced ectopic eye (Altmann et al. 1997; Tapscott 2005).

Transcription factors such as Pdx1, Ngn3, and Pax4 might act as master genes to promote the appearance of islet cell precursors, islet cells, and more specifically β-cells. Expression of Pdx1 in liver cells from human or mice (Ferber et al. 2000; Zalzman et al. 2005) was shown to promote trans-differentiation of liver cells into insulin-expressing cells that were able to cure diabetes in streptozotocin-treated mice. Nevertheless, the sole action of a transcription factor such as Pdx1 may not be sufficient and might require other changes such as improved growth conditions and addition of growth factors. Pdx1 may be sufficient for initiating, but not for completing endocrine differentiation. Pdx1-expressing cells initiate a program of pancreatic development but do not proceed to the final stage of differentiation. Combination of expression of several transcription factors was tested in chicken embryos (Grapin-Botton et al. 2001). Neither Pax6 plus Pdx1 nor Isl1 plus Pdx1 elicited insulin or glucagon expression. In contrast, coexpression of Pdx1 and Ngn3 produced further differentiation into glucagon or somatostatin-producing cells. Additional endocrine cell markers Pax6, Isl-1, NeuroD, and Nkx2.2 are ectopically induced by Ngn3. However, although Ngn3 is required for differentiation of all pancreatic lineages (Gradwohl et al. 2000), when expressed alone, combined with Pdx1, or even under the control of the Pdx1 promoter, it does not induce cells to become insulin-producing in the mouse (Apelqvist et al. 1999), nor in chicken (Grapin-Botton et al. 2001).

Blyszczuk et al. (2003) have shown that constitutive expression of Pax4 and to a lesser extent Pdx1 affects the differentiation of ES cells and significantly promotes the development of insulin-producing cells (Figure 4). Constitutive expression of Pax4 combined with selection of nestin$^+$ cells and histotypic culture conditions give rise to spheroids containing insulin-positive granules typical of embryonal and adult β-cells. In brief, wild-type, Pdx$^+$ and Pax4$^+$ ES cells were used to form EBs, which were selected as previously suggested by Lumelsky (2001). Approximately 28 days later the cell clusters were trypsinized and plated in Petri dishes and incubated overnight. Then the spheres were transferred into 100 mL Spinner flasks and cultured in the cell-spin system. The constitutive overexpression of Pax4 revealed a significant upregulation of genes involved in β-cell development and function resulting in an increased number of insulin-positive cells and in the amount of the insulin production. The results suggested that Pax4 might play a significant role in directing undifferentiated ES into endocrine insulin-producing cells. In parallel to the selective differentiation via nestin$^+$ cells, insulin levels was further enhanced when cells were further differentiated in a histotypic culture system as 3D spheroids. Transplantation of the wt and Pax4$^+$ insulin-producing cells was sufficient to preserve normal blood glucose levels in diabetic mice but some of these animals developed teratomas, therefore implying that further lineage selection is needed.

Miyazaki et al. (2004) tried to improve the effect of Pdx1 by regulating its expression during differentiation using a Tet-off system (Figure 8). The differentiation strategy was similar to that previously described (Moritoh et al. 2003)

(Figure 8). Removing Dox induced the expression of Pdx1. In control experiments, Dox was present in the differentiation stages or in the EBs stage but was absent in the subsequent stages. In the final stage of *in vitro* differentiation, cells treated with Dox (when Pdx1 is active) did not proliferate well. On the other hand, Dox- cells could be cultured for more than 2 months. Thus exogenous Pdx1 expression appeared to affect the growth of the differentiated cells.

Two nonallelic insulin genes are expressed in rodents. The insulin 2 gene is expressed in developing brain and yolk sac as well as in the pancreatic β-cells, whereas insulin 1 gene expression is restricted to the pancreatic β-cells. The insulin 2 gene was detected in ES cells that differentiated without exogenous Pdx1 expression as described previously (Moritoh et al. 2003), but Pdx1 expression throughout the differentiation stages clearly enhanced insulin 2 expression. Moreover, a number of pancreas-specific genes were strongly induced by the exogenous expression of Pdx1 during *in vitro* differentiation. In contrast, the exogenous expression of Pdx1 after EB formation did not enhance the expression of the insulin 2 gene or other genes associated with the development of the endocrine pancreas except for somatostatin and Kir6.2. Thus the expression of Pdx1 during EB formation is important for the induction of differentiation to the pancreatic lineage. On the other hand, genes that are specific for endocrine pancreas *in vivo* such as insulin 1, Glut2, and endogenous Pdx1 expression were not observed even under continuous Pdx1 expression. It might be speculated that the continuous expression of exogenous Pdx1 can enhance pancreatic progenitors during EB formation. Yet it may suppress the expression of some endocrine-specific genes in the final stage. In normal development, Pdx1 is temporally expressed in the pancreatic buds, and later its expression become restricted to the pancreatic β-cells.

8. CELL SORTING SEPARATION (IMMUNOPURIFICATION) ON THE BASIS OF SPECIFIC CELL MARKERS

The development of new technologies in the field of microarray and proteomics enables researchers to identify specific cell markers that in various combinations can be used to sort cells according to their fate, even without transfecting the cells with a specific marker. For example, Yasunaga et al. (2005) identified seven surface molecules that are expressed differentially in definitive or visceral endoderm. One of these markers is CXCR4 for which a monoclonal antibody is available and thus allowed them to monitor and distinguish cell types in the process of differentiation.

9. METHODS FOR ANALYZING INSULIN-PRODUCING CELLS

Different methods have been suggested to analyze the ability of differentiated cells to produce and secrete insulin. The classical methods include the measurement of insulin secretion by ELISA or RIA, insulin detection at the RNA level using RT-PCR, and immunostaining of the cells in order to detect insulin protein levels.

In 2003, Rajagopal et al. (2003) claimed that immunohistochemical detection of insulin in cells resulted from an uptake of insulin from the culture media and thus challenged prior works. Similar results were later obtained by Sipione et al. (2004) and by Hansson et al. (2004). In this paper Rajagopal proposed the use of several methods in order to prove true *de novo* insulin production. Those methods included: electron microscope analysis, RNA measurement by Northern analysis or *in situ* hybridization; protein-level analysis by C-peptide staining, functional ability by measuring metabolic labeling and demonstration of biphasic insulin secretion and transplantation assays.

C-peptide staining and secretion: C-peptide labeling of cells is an indication of pro-insulin synthesis. Several researchers have demonstrated costaining for C-peptide and insulin in the same cells (Hori et al. 2002; Blyszczuk et al. 2003, 2004; Segev et al. 2004) or C-peptide staining alone (Miyazaki et al. 2004) but others have found that different cell populations were stained for each antibody (Sipione et al. 2004).

C-peptide secretion is therefore a better indication of pro-insulin synthesis than insulin secretion. Hansson et al. (2004) have failed to observe *in vitro* C-peptide secretion in differentiated cells but others such as Paek et al. (2005) observed C-peptide secretion, but in less than 1% of secreted insulin. They therefore suggested that the mechanism of insulin secretion by these differentiating cells is a combination of sequestration and *de novo* synthesis.

Rajagopal et al. (2003) and others (Sipione et al. 2004) have shown the need to combine an assay for apoptosis of the differentiating cells in addition to insulin or C-peptide staining of the cells, as shown previously (Segev et al. 2004).

RNA analysis: Most protocols rely on RT-PCR to detect markers associated with endodermal or pancreatic development, and it is often assumed that these markers indicate cells of embryonic origin. However, the extraembryonic endoderm that is part of the yolk sac of the developing conceptus shares many characteristics with those of embryonic endoderm, indicating expression of the early transcription factor network. RT-PCR is a very sensitive method, and thus even small amounts of transcript can be detected. Therefore, insulin detected only by RT-PCR cannot be a proof for pancreatic β-cells. Detection of other pancreatic cell markers should also be performed. Such markers include the transcription factors: *Pdx1*, *Nkx6.1*, *Pax4*, and *Ngn3*. In addition other β-cell specific markers such as *Glut2* and *Glucokinase*, which participate in signal secretion coupling in pancreatic cells along with transcripts for pro-insulin and processing enzymes pro-hormone convertase 1/3 (*PC1/3*) and *PC2*, indicating the ability to synthesize and process proinsulin to mature insulin. Transcripts for the two components of the K^{+}_{ATP} channel, *Kir6.2* and *SUR1* are also important.

RNA chip analysis can be useful in identifying the true nature of the differentiating cells and to identify all the important transcripts.

Two nonallelic insulin genes are expressed in rodents. The insulin 2 gene is expressed in developing brain and yolk sac as well as in the pancreatic β-cells, whereas insulin 1 gene expression is restricted to the pancreatic β-cells. It is therefore essential to identify transcripts of insulin 1 in rodent cells.

In situ hybridization is an important tool to evaluate the number of cells in a population expressing insulin transcripts, as demonstrated by Segev et al. (2004). In order to compare and quantify the amount of insulin transcript in the differentiating cells, methods such as RNA blot or real-time PCR analysis are essential.

Staining with zinc-chelating dithizone: Dithizone selectively stains pancreatic β-cells crimson red (Shiroi et al. 2002), as they contain a large amount of zinc. Thus, it is often used in the process of selecting human pancreatic islets from cadaveric donors (Shiroi et al. 2002). Another zinc sensitive probe is Newport Green (Lukowiak et al. 2001). This probe can also be used for the identification and purification of human β-cells using confocal microscopy and cell sorting.

Electron microscopy: Electron microscopy analysis can be used to observe secretory granules with crystalline formation in the differentiating cells (Kahan et al. 2003). By immunoelectron microscopy, some researchers were able to detect the presence of insulin-specific immono-gold particles distributed mainly over the cores of secretory granules (Blyszczuk et al. 2003; Paek et al. 2005).

Immunostaining: In addition to insulin and C-peptide staining, staining of other β-cell or pancreatic progenitors markers play an important role in analyzing differentiating cells. Those markers include *Pdx1*, *Glut2*, *IAPP*, *FoxA2*, *Isl1* and better still, double staining of these markers with insulin, C-peptide, glucagon, or somatostatin (Kahan et al. 2003; Brolen et al. 2005).

Electrophysiological analysis: Pancreatic β-cells constitute a well communicating multicellular network that permits the coordination and synchronization of signal transmission within the islet of Langerhans necessary for proper insulin release. Blyszczuk et al. (2004) showed that in differentiated ES cells, the characteristics of the voltage-activated sodium and potassium channels and the calcium-dependent secretory activity showed similarity to embryonic β-cells. The presence of cells responsive to K_{ATP} channel agonists and glucose induced secretory activity in the $Pax4^{+}$ ES derived cells, represented a developmentally advanced status in comparison to wild type cells. K channel activity regulated by ATP has also been demonstrated by Vaca et al. (2005). The use of fluorescence recovery after photobleaching has been considered (Quesada et al. 2003). This technique has been validated as a reliable and noninvasive approach to monitor functional gap junctions in real time.

Transplantation assays: An important assay in order to prove *de novo* insulin production in differentiated cells is to transplant these cells in a diabetic animal (most common is diabetic mice). Diabetes can be induced by application of the β-cell toxin, streptozotocin. The direct contribution of the transplanted cells to the rescue can be demonstrated by the return of normoglycemia. This test can prove the concept of insulin production by the cells in response to glucose levels *in vivo*. Immunosuppressed mice are used in order to avoid transplant rejection. Several groups have demonstrated normoglycemia following transplantation of insulin-producing cells (Soria et al. 2000; Hori et al. 2002; Blyszczuk et al. 2003; Shi et al. 2005; Vaca et al. 2005), while others failed (Lukowiak et al. 2001; Hansson et al. 2004; Sipione et al. 2004). C-peptide secretion following glucose challenge and histology of the transplant are further needed. In some cases the final maturation of the differentiated cells occurs following transplantation. The most common place for this kind of transplantation is under the kidney capsule, yet space is limited, thus limiting the number of cells transplantable to this site. Because of this volume restriction, other sites such as the spleen have been suggested, even though the transplanted cells cannot be quantitatively recovered from these organs (reviewed by Colman 2004). A combination of incomplete β-cell destruction and nonideal cell transplant cells can alter the interpretation of the experiments since endogenous regeneration cannot be readily ruled out. Another point which should be considered when transplanting ES derived cells is the potential for teratoma production in the transplanted animals. Teratomas may occur when some of the transplanted cells are still in an undifferentiated state (Fujikawa et al. 2005). It is therefore important to ensure that a pure population of differentiated cells is transplanted without any undifferentiated cell contaminants.

Even though several differentiation protocols have been published in the past few years, the goal of obtaining functional β-cell like cells for transplantation still lies ahead of us.

REFERENCES

Abraham, E.J., Leech, C.A., Lin, J.C., Zulewski, H., and Habener, J.F. (2002) Insulinotropic hormone glucagon-like peptide-1 differentiation of human pancreatic islet-derived progenitor cells into insulin-producing cells. Endocrinology, 143: 3152–3161.

Altmann, C.R., Chow, R.L., Lang, R.A., and Hemmati-Brivanlou, A. (1997) Lens induction by Pax-6 in *Xenopus laevis*. Dev. Biol., 185: 119–123.

Apelqvist, A., Li, H., Sommer, L., et al. (1999) Notch signalling controls pancreatic cell differentiation. Nature, 400: 877–881.

Assady, S., Maor, G., Amit, M., et al. (2001) Insulin production by human embryonic stem cells. Diabetes, 50: 1691–1697.

Bai, L., Meredith, G., and Tuch, B.E. (2005) Glucagon-like peptide-1 enhances production of insulin in insulin-producing cells derived from mouse embryonic stem cells. J. Endocrinol., 186: 343–352.

Berna, G., Leon-Quinto, T., Ensenat-Waser, R., et al. (2001) Stem cells and diabetes. Biomed. Pharmacother., 55: 206–212.

Blyszczuk, P., Asbrand, C., Rozzo, A., et al. (2004) Embryonic stem cells differentiate into insulin-producing cells without selection of nestin-expressing cells. Int. J. Dev. Biol., 48: 1095–1104.

Blyszczuk, P., Czyz, J., Kania, G., et al. (2003) Expression of Pax4 in embryonic stem cells promotes differentiation of nestin-positive progenitor and insulin-producing cells. Proc. Natl. Acad. Sci. USA, 100: 998–1003. Epub 2003 Jan 13.

Bonner-Weir, S., Taneja, M., Weir, G.C., et al. (2000) In vitro cultivation of human islets from expanded ductal tissue. Proc. Natl. Acad. Sci. USA, 97: 7999–8004.

Brolen, G.K., Heins, N., Edsbagge, J., and Semb, H. (2005) Signals from the embryonic mouse pancreas induce differentiation of human embryonic stem cells into insulin-producing beta-cell-like cells. Diabetes, 54: 2867–2874.

Chiang, M.K. and Melton, D.A. (2003) Single-cell transcript analysis of pancreas development. Dev. Cell, 4: 383–393.

Colman, A. (2004) Making new beta cells from stem cells. Semin. Cell Dev. Biol., 15: 337–345.

D'Amour, K.A., Agulnick, A.D., Eliazer, S., et al. (2005) Efficient differentiation of human embryonic stem cells to definitive endoderm. Nat. Biotechnol., 23: 1534–1541. Epub 2005 Oct 28.

David, R., Groebner, M., and Franz, W.M. (2005) Magnetic cell sorting purification of differentiated embryonic stem cells stably expressing truncated human CD4 as surface marker. Stem Cells, 23: 477–482.

Edlund, H. (2001) Developmental biology of the pancreas. Diabetes, 50: S5–S9.

Ferber, S., Halkin, A., Cohen, H., et al. (2000) Pancreatic and duodenal homeobox gene 1 induces expression of insulin genes in liver and ameliorates streptozotocin-induced hyperglycemia. Nat. Med., 6: 568–572.

Fujikawa, T., Oh, S.H., Pi, L., et al. (2005) Teratoma formation leads to failure of treatment for type I diabetes using embryonic stem cell-derived insulin-producing cells. Am. J. Pathol., 166: 1781–1791.

Gradwohl, G., Dierich, A., LeMeur, M., and Guillemot, F. (2000) Neurogenin3 is required for the development of the four endocrine cell lineages of the pancreas. Proc. Natl. Acad. Sci. USA, 97: 1607–1611.

Grapin-Botton, A., Majithia, A.R., and Melton, D.A. (2001) Key events of pancreas formation are triggered in gut endoderm by ectopic expression of pancreatic regulatory genes. Genes Dev., 15: 444–454.

Gu, G., Dubauskaite, J., and Melton, D.A. (2002) Direct evidence for the pancreatic lineage: NGN3+ cells are islet progenitors and are distinct from duct progenitors. Development, 129: 2447–2457.

Hansson, M., Tonning, A., Frandsen, U., et al. (2004) Artifactual insulin release from differentiated embryonic stem cells. Diabetes, 53: 2603–2609.

Hori, Y., Rulifson, I.C., Tsai, B.C., et al. (2002) Growth inhibitors promote differentiation of insulin-producing tissue from embryonic stem cells. Proc. Natl. Acad. Sci. USA, 99: 16105–16110. Epub 2002 Nov 19.

Humphrey, R.K., Bucay, N., Beattie, G.M., et al. (2003) Characterization and isolation of promoter-defined nestin-positive cells from the human fetal pancreas. Diabetes, 52: 2519–2525.

Itkin-Ansari, P., Demeterco, C., Bossie, S., et al. (2000) PDX-1 and cell-cell contact act in synergy to promote delta-cell development in a human pancreatic endocrine precursor cell line. Mol. Endocrinol., 14: 814–822.

Itskovitz-Eldor, J., Schuldiner, M., Karsenti, D., et al. (2000) Differentiation of human embryonic stem cells into embryoid bodies compromising the three embryonic germ layers. Mol. Med., 6: 88–95.

Juang, J.H., Bonner-Weir, S., Ogawa, Y., Vacanti, J.P., and Weir, G.C. (1996) Outcome of subcutaneous islet transplantation improved by polymer device. Transplantation, 61: 1557–1561.

Kahan, B.W., Jacobson, L.M., Hullett, D.A., et al. (2003) Pancreatic precursors and differentiated islet cell types from murine embryonic stem cells: an in vitro model to study islet differentiation. Diabetes, 52: 2016–2024.

Kimura, K., Hattori, S., Kabuyama, Y., et al. (1994) Neurite outgrowth of PC12 cells is suppressed by wortmannin, a specific inhibitor of phosphatidylinositol 3-kinase. J. Biol. Chem., 269: 18961–18967.

Klug, M.G., Soonpaa, M.H., Koh, G.Y., and Field, L.J. (1996) Genetically selected cardiomyocytes from differentiating embronic stem cells form stable intracardiac grafts. J. Clin. Invest., 98: 216–224.

Ku, H.T., Zhang, N., Kubo, A., et al. (2004) Committing embryonic stem cells to early endocrine pancreas in vitro. Stem Cells, 22: 1205–1217.

Kubo, A., Shinozaki, K., Shannon, J.M., et al. (2004) Development of definitive endoderm from embryonic stem cells in culture. Development, 131: 1651–1662. Epub 2004 Mar 3.

Lammert, E., Cleaver, O., and Melton, D. (2001) Induction of pancreatic differentiation by signals from blood vessels. Science, 294: 564–567. Epub 2001 Sep 27.

Leon-Quinto, T., Jones, J., Skoudy, A., Burcin, M., and Soria, B. (2004) In vitro directed differentiation of mouse embryonic stem cells into insulin-producing cells. Diabetologia, 47: 1442–1451. Epub 2004 Jul 29.

Lukowiak, B., Vandewalle, B., Riachy, R., et al. (2001) Identification and purification of functional human beta-cells by a new specific zinc-fluorescent probe. J. Histochem. Cytochem., 49: 519–528.

Lumelsky, N., Blondel, O., Laeng, P., et al. (2001) Differentiation of embryonic stem cells to insulin-secreting structures similar to pancreatic islets. Science, 292: 1389–1394. Epub 2001 Apr 26.

Mandrup-Poulsen, T. (1998) Diabetes. BMJ, 316: 1221–1225.

Meyer, C., Hering, B.J., Grossmann, R., et al. (1998) Improved glucose counterregulation and autonomic symptoms after intraportal islet transplants alone in patients with long-standing type I diabetes mellitus. Transplantation, 66: 233–240.

Micallef, S.J., Janes, M.E., Knezevic, K., et al. (2005) Retinoic acid induces Pdx1-positive endoderm in differentiating mouse embryonic stem cells. Diabetes, 54: 301–305. Epub 2004 Dec 7.

Miyazaki, S., Yamato, E., and Miyazaki, J. (2004) Regulated expression of pdx-1 promotes in vitro differentiation of insulin-producing cells from embryonic stem cells. Diabetes, 53: 1030–1037.

Moritoh, Y., Yamato, E., Yasui, Y., Miyazaki, S., and Miyazaki, J. (2003) Analysis of insulin-producing cells during in vitro differentiation from feeder-free embryonic stem cells. Diabetes, 52: 1163–1168.

Muller, M., Fleischmann, B.K., Selbert, S., et al. (2000) Selection of ventricular-like cardiomyocytes from ES cells in vitro. FASEB. J., 14: 2540–2548.

Ogneva, V. and Martinova, Y. (2002) The effect of in vitro fibroblast growth factors on cell proliferation in pancreas from normal and streptozotocin-treated rats. Diabetes Res. Clin. Pract., 57: 11–16.

Otonkoski, T., Beattie, G.M., Mally, M.I., Ricordi, C., and Hayek, A. (1993) Nicotinamide is a potent inducer of endocrine differentiation in cultured human fetal pancreatic cells. J. Clin. Invest., 92: 1459–1466.

Paek, H.J., Morgan, J.R., and Lysaght, M.J. (2005) Sequestration and synthesis: the source of insulin in cell clusters differentiated from murine embryonic stem cells. Stem Cells, 23: 862–867. Epub 2005 May 11.

Pfendler, K.C., Catuar, C.S., Meneses, J.J., and Pedersen, R.A. (2005) Overexpression of Nodal promotes differentiation of mouse embryonic stem cells into mesoderm and endoderm at the expense of neuroectoderm formation. Stem Cells Dev., 14: 162–172.

Ptasznik, A., Beattie, G.M., Mally, M.I., et al. (1997) Phosphatidylinositol 3-kinase is a negative regulator of cellular differentiation. J. Cell Biol., 137: 1127–1136.

Quesada, I., Fuentes, E., Andreu, E., et al. (2003) On-line analysis of gap junctions reveals more efficient electrical than dye coupling between islet cells. Am. J. Physiol. Endocrinol. Metab., 284: E980–E987. Epub 2003 Jan 7.

Rajagopal, J., Anderson, W.J., Kume, S., Martinez, O.I., and Melton, D.A. (2003) Insulin staining of ES cell progeny from insulin uptake. Science, 299: 363.

Reubinoff, B.E., Pera, M.F., Fong, C.Y., Trounson, A., and Bongso, A. (2000) Embryonic stem cell lines from human blastocysts: somatic differentiation in vitro. Nat. Biotechnol., 18: 399–404.

Schuldiner, M., Yanuka, O., Itskovitz-Eldor, J., Melton, D.A., and Benvenisty, N. (2000) Effects of eight growth factors on the differentiation of cells derived from human embryonic stem cells. Proc. Natl. Acad. Sci. USA, 97: 11307–11312.

Segev, H., Fishman, B., Ziskind, A., Shulman, M., and Itskovitz-Eldor, J. (2004) Differentiation of human embryonic stem cells into insulin-producing clusters. Stem Cells, 22: 265–274.

Shi, Y., Hou, L., Tang, F., et al. (2005) Inducing embryonic stem cells to differentiate into pancreatic beta cells by a novel three-step approach with activin A and all-trans retinoic acid. Stem Cells, 23: 656–662.

Shiroi, A., Yoshikawa, M., and Yokota, H., et al. (2002) Identification of insulin-producing cells derived from embryonic stem cells by zinc-chelating dithizone. Stem Cells, 20: 284–292.

Sipione, S., Eshpeter, A., Lyon, J.G., Korbutt, G.S., and Bleackley, R.C. (2004) Insulin expressing cells from differentiated embryonic stem cells are not beta cells. Diabetologia, 47: 499–508. Epub 2004 Feb 14.

Soria, B. (2001) In-vitro differentiation of pancreatic beta-cells. Differentiation, 68: 205–219.

Soria, B., Roche, E., Berna, G., et al. (2000) Insulin-secreting cells derived from embryonic stem cells normalize glycemia in streptozotocin-induced diabetic mice engineering pancreatic islets. Diabetes, 49: 157–162.

Soria, B., Skoudy, A., and Martin, F. (2001) From stem cells to beta cells: new strategies in cell therapy of diabetes mellitus. Diabetologia, 44: 407–415.

Tada, S., Era, T., Furusawa, C., et al. (2005) Characterization of mesendoderm: a diverging point of the definitive endoderm and mesoderm in embryonic stem cell differentiation culture. Development, 132: 4363–4374. Epub 2005 Sep 1.

Tapscott, S.J. (2005) The circuitry of a master switch: myod and the regulation of skeletal muscle gene transcription. Development, 132: 2685–2695.

Thomson, J.A. and Marshall, V.S. (1998) Primate embryonic stem cells. Curr. Top. Dev. Biol., 38: 133–165.

Thomson, J.A., Itskovitz-Eldor, J., Shapiro, S.S., et al. (1998) Embryonic stem cell lines derived from human blastocysts. Science, 282: 1145–1147.

Treutelaar, M.K., Skidmore, J.M., Dias-Leme, C.L., et al. (2003) Nestin-lineage cells contribute to the microvasculature but not endocrine cells of the islet. Diabetes, 52: 2503–2512.

Vaca, P., Martin, F., Vegara-Meseguer, J., et al. (2005) Induction of differentiation of embryonic stem cells into insulin secreting cells by fetal soluble factors. Stem Cells, 18: 18.

Vallier, L., Reynolds, D., and Pedersen, R.A. (2004) Nodal inhibits differentiation of human embryonic stem cells along the neuroectodermal default pathway. Dev. Biol., 275: 403–421.

Weir, G.C. and Bonner-Weir, S. (1998) Islet transplantation as a treatment for diabetes. J. Am. Optom. Assoc., 69: 727–732.

Yasunaga, M., Tada, S., Torikai-Nishikawa, S., et al. (2005) Induction and monitoring of definitive and visceral endoderm differentiation of mouse ES cells. Nat. Biotechnol., 23: 1542–1550. Epub 2005 Nov 27.

Zalzman, M., Anker-Kitai, L., and Efrat, S. (2005) Differentiation of human liver-derived, insulin-producing cells toward the beta-cell phenotype. Diabetes, 54: 2568–2575.

Zhao, M., Christie, M.R., Heaton, N., et al. (2002) Amelioration of streptozotocin-induced diabetes in mice using human islet cells derived from long-term culture in vitro. Transplantation, 73: 1454–1460.

Zulewski, H., Abraham, E.J., Gerlach, M.J., et al. (2001) Multipotential nestin-positive stem cells isolated from adult pancreatic islets differentiate ex vivo into pancreatic endocrine, exocrine, and hepatic phenotypes. Diabetes, 50: 521–533.

CHAPTER 12

CARDIOMYOCYTE DIFFERENTIATION

DINENDER K. SINGLA[1], SHREEYA JAYARAMAN,[2,3]
JIANHUA ZHANG,[2,3] TIMOTHY J. KAMP[2,3]

[1]*Cardiovascular Research Institute, University of Vermont, Colchester, VT 05446, USA*
[2]*WiCell Research Institute, University of Wisconsin, Madison, WI 53715, USA*
[3]*Division of Cardiovascular Medicine, University of Wisconsin, Madison, WI 53792, USA*

1. INTRODUCTION

The differentiation of human embryonic stem cells (hESCs) into cardiomyocytes (CMs) holds great appeal for a wide variety of applications. This is of particular importance because other sources of human CMs are quite limited given the obvious challenges of getting samples from patients and the lack of robust immortalized human cardiac cell lines. Although research employing animal CMs has provided major advances, ready access to human CMs may produce data more directly applicable to human cardiac biology and disease. Therefore, *in vitro* differentiated hESC-derived CMs (hESC-CMs) provide a useful model for research applications focused on understanding cardiac contractility, electrophysiology, pharmacology, toxicology, development, etc. Likewise, hESC-CMs hold significant interest for therapeutic applications aimed at repairing diseased and damaged heart muscle.

Insights obtained from studies of heart development during normal embryogenesis provide the critical background upon which techniques to differentiate *in vitro* hESCs into CMs can be understood. Efforts utilizing hESCs build on extensive research over the prior two decades understanding and optimizing mouse embryonic stem cell (mESC) cardiac differentiation. However, the methods for obtaining CMs from ESCs *in vitro* are relatively inefficient and continue to be refined, in part because the understanding of normal cardiac development is incomplete. The purpose of the present chapter is to describe the existing methodologies to differentiate hESCs into CMs and to characterize the properties of the resulting myocytes.

J.R. Masters et al (eds.), Embryonic Stem Cells, 211–234.

2. CARDIAC DEVELOPMENT

The formation of the heart during normal embryogenesis has been extensively characterized in a variety of model systems including chick, frog, zebrafish, and mouse (Olson and Srivastava 1996; Bruneau 2002; Zaffran and Frasch 2002). Even studies in insects such as *Drosophila* have provided critical insights into cardiac development (Azpiazu and Frasch 1993). Early cardiogenesis in vertebrates and insects share common conserved features including critical inductive tissue interactions across primary germ layers. The vertebrate heart arises from lateral plate mesoderm cells in response to essential inductive signaling events mediated by soluble, small molecules released in a precisely timed and spatially regulated fashion (Zaffran and Frasch 2002). The rostral endoderm adjacent to the cardiac mesoderm provides essential inductive signals for cardiogenesis including bone morphogenetic proteins (BMPs) (Schultheiss et al. 1997). Inhibitory signaling for cardiogenesis comes from the neuroectoderm in the form of specific Wnt signaling molecules (Marvin et al. 2001). Gradients of Wnt signaling are critical in restricting cardiogenesis to specific mesodermal regions. Likewise, roles for fibroblast growth factor (FGF) signaling and Notch signaling have been described in early cardiogenesis (Barron et al. 2000). The understanding of all of the specific signaling molecules and their temporal and spatial expression patterns required for cardiogenesis is incomplete. Nevertheless, several key molecules have been identified as critical in cardiac differentiation, and these provide useful tools for optimizing *in vitro* differentiation of ESCs to CMs.

3. LESSONS LEARNED FROM MOUSE ESC CARDIAC DIFFERENTIATION

mESCs were first isolated in 1981 (Evans and Kaufman 1981; Martin 1981), and these cells have been extensively utilized as an *in vitro* system to generate CMs. The *in vitro* differentiation of mESCs into CMs was originally described using an initial aggregation step to form structures referred to as embryoid bodies (EBs) (Doetschman et al. 1985). The EBs typically include derivatives of all three primary germ layers and can form specialized cell types such as CMs (Boheler et al. 2002). The EB system enables inductive signaling essential for cardiogenesis to occur; however, there is substantial variability from EB to EB and only a fraction exhibit cardiogenesis. Multiple studies have identified critical parameters influencing the ability of mESCs to differentiate into CMs in EBs including: (1) the starting number of ESCs initially in the aggregates; (2) the specific medium utilized including serum and growth factors; (3) the mESC line; and (4) the time of EB plating. By optimizing these factors, multiple laboratories have been able to obtain spontaneously contracting CMs from mESCs (Boheler et al. 2002).

The CMs obtained from mESCs have been identified and characterized using gene expression studies, immunohistochemistry for cardiac-specific proteins, ultrastructure analysis, and functional studies evaluating the contractile and electrophysiological properties of the cell (Boheler et al. 2002). Furthermore, distinct types of CMs have been observed including nodal-like, ventricular-like, atrial-like, and Purkinje-like myocytes. The CMs mature during time in culture from primitive small spherical cells with poorly organized myofilaments to more elongated cells with well-organized bundles of myofilaments. Although the EB system using mESCs has provided a reliable methodology to obtain CMs, it is largely inefficient with the CMs forming a small minority of the cells present and with EBs containing a variety of different CM cell types.

Research focused on improving the reproducibility and efficiency of obtaining CMs from mESCs has explored a number of different approaches. A variety of different signaling molecules linked to cardiogenesis have been tested for their ability to enhance cardiac differentiation of mESCs in EBs. Given the critical role of BMPs in cardiac development (Winnier et al. 1995; Zhang and Bradley 1996), both agonists and antagonists for this signaling pathway have been studied, and depending on the time of application during EB formation both BMP antagonists and agonists have been identified as promoting cardiogenesis (Behfar et al. 2002; Yuasa et al. 2005). The BMP antagonist Noggin has shown the greatest published efficiency at inducing cardiogenesis from mESCs if the cells are exposed at the preEB stage but not later, after EB formation (Yuasa et al. 2005). Studies of other signaling molecules including IGF-1, FGF, oxytocin, erythropoietin, and retinoic acid have demonstrated some increase in efficiency of generation of CMs from EBs, but the effects were relatively meager compared to the recent study using Noggin (Behfar et al. 2002; Yuasa et al. 2005). Using the less-defined approach of coculture, explants of chick precardiac endoderm and mesoderm have also resulted in efficient differentiation of mESCs into CMs with all of the EBs showing spontaneous contractions and 86% of the cells being CMs (Rudy-Reil and Lough 2004). Screens testing small molecules applied to undifferentiated mESCs have also identified hits which induce cardiogenesis including ascorbic acid and cardiogenols (Takahashi et al. 2003; Wu et al. 2004). The results from several different laboratories suggest that promising approaches are emerging to induce cardiac differentiation *in vitro*, but most of these results have not been widely reproduced in multiple laboratories and with multiple mESC lines.

Because cardiogenesis in EBs with most protocols has been relatively inefficient, methods to enrich or isolate CMs from other cell types have been developed. Pioneering work by Field and colleagues described the use of genetically engineered mESCs containing a transgenic cardiac-specific promoter (α-MHC) driving the expression of an antibiotic resistance gene (neomycin resistance) to select CMs differentiating *in vitro* from mESCs (Klug et al. 1996). By exposing the differentiating EBs to neomycin, an enrichment of the cells to >99% CMs was possible (Klug et al. 1996). Furthermore, the approach utilizing the α-MHC-neomycin resistance-targeted mESCs has been extrapolated to protocols generating large numbers of CMs in bioreactors (~10^9 CMs/2L bioreactor) (Schroeder et al. 2005). Concurrent work by Metzger and associates used the cardiac α-actin promoter for driving a reporter β-galactosidase to identify CMs differentiating from mESCs (Metzger et al. 1996). Thus, strategies utilizing several different cardiac-specific promoters including α-MHC, α-actin, and Nkx2.5 have been successfully used to identify and isolate CMs differentiating from mESCs (Klug et al. 1996; Kolossov et al. 1998; Hidaka et al. 2003), but it is critical to appreciate that a range of cellular phenotypes have been determined in the isolated cells including atrial, nodal, and ventricular myocytes. The different cardiac cell types are anticipated based on the fact that the promoters utilized in these studies are active throughout the heart. To obtain ventricular myocytes specifically, two groups have created genetically engineered mESCs lines containing reporter genes driven by the rat myosin light chain 2v (Myl2) promoter to obtain ventricular-specific expression of CFP or eGFP in differentiating mESCs (Meyer et al. 2000; Muller et al. 2000). Evaluation of CMs identified using this strategy have shown they are primarily ventricular CMs. These studies in mESCs have proven the potential utility of using genetically engineered cell lines with cell type specific reporters or antibiotic resistance genes to obtain more homogenous populations of CMs.

4. hESC LINES AND CELL CULTURE MAINTENANCE

hESCs were first successfully isolated from surplus *in vitro* fertilization embryos in 1998 (Thomson et al. 1998), and it was quickly evident that these cells exhibited some differences from mESCs that could impact the *in vitro* differentiation of hESCs to CMs. For example, hESCs cannot be maintained undifferentiated using leukemia inhibitor factor (LIF), in contrast to mESCs. Also, the population doubling time was different with mESCs doubling every 8–15 h and hESCs doubling every 25–30 h (Snir et al. 2003). Another practical difference is that the hESCs do not survive well if enzymatically isolated into single cells. Therefore, the commonly used hanging drop methodology for mESC EB formation and cardiac differentiation is not possible for hESCs as it requires enzymatic digestions of the hESC colonies to single cells. The initial experience with hESC cardiac differentiation highlights these differences as factors promoting cardiogenesis from mESCs, including DMSO, RA, and BMP2, have not been effective in inducing cardiac differentiation of hESCs (Kehat et al. 2001, 2002; Xu et al. 2002a, b; Mummery et al. 2003).

At present, there are many hESC lines that have been established around the world. The National Institutes of Health Registry lists 78 hESC lines that were derived before August 9, 2001, and are approved for US federally funded research. Of those lines, approximately 22 are currently available to investigators. In addition, other lines continue to be derived, but the combination of public and private efforts makes a precise estimate of the current number of hESC lines difficult to ascertain. Of the likely few hundred lines of hESCs isolated to date, only ten have published evidence documenting the ability to form CMs (see Table 1). In addition, no rigorous comparisons between the lines in their efficiency of forming CMs have been described, although it seems likely that differences exist. Recently established embryonic stem cell banks will compare and contrast the available hESC lines, including their propensity for cardiogenesis.

Table 1. hESC lines demonstrated to differentiate into CMs

	H1	H7	H9	H9.1	H9.2	H13	H14	hES2	hES3	hES4
Kehat et al. 2001					+					
Xu et al. 2002	+	+	+	+	+					
He et al. 2003	+	+	+				+			
Mummery et al. 2003										+
Kamp lab unpublished						+				
Passier et al. 2005								+	+	+

Table 2. Medium for hESC maintenance culture on MEFs

Final concentration	Amount for 500 mL stock solution	Source
80% DMEM-F12	400 mL	Invitrogen
20% KO serum replacer	100 mL	Invitrogen
1% nonessential amino acids	5.0 mL	Invitrogen
1 mM L-glutamine[a]	2.5 mL	Invitrogen
0.1 mM β-mercaptoethanol	Part of L-glutamine	Sigma
4 ng/mL bFGF[b]	1.0 mL	Invitrogen

[a]L-glutamine stock solution; 5 ml of 200 mM L-glutamine + 7 μL 14.3 M β-mercaptoethanol
[b]bFGF stock; bFGF = 10 μg, 0.1% fraction V BSA in PBS = 5 mL (store at −20/−70°C)

Maintaining hESCs on feeder layers of mouse embryonic fibroblasts (MEFs) or feeder-free using conditioned medium have both been utilized successfully to provide hESCs for differentiation into CMs (Kehat et al. 2001, 2002; Xu et al. 2002a, b; He et al. 2003). Table 2 provides a standard medium which can be utilized to culture hESCs on MEFs. hESCs are passaged every 5–6 days using Collagenase IV (0.05 g of collagenase IV, Invitrogen, Catalog # 17104-019 in 50 mL DMEM-F12 medium) to dissociate the colonies as described elsewhere in this book. There are no direct comparisons of different maintenance culture conditions and the ability of hESCs to generate CMs *in vitro*, but one study has suggested that as passage number increases for H9.2 hESCs, that the propensity to form CMs increases (Segev et al. 2005).

5. EBs FOR CARDIAC DIFFERENTIATION

The most common methodology for inducing cardiogenesis from hESCs has been the formation of EBs comparable to the technique pioneered with mESCs (see Figure 1). Multiple laboratories have described hESC-CMs arising from EBs and have characterized them based on their gene and protein expression patterns as well as functional properties (Kehat et al. 2001; Xu et al. 2002a, b; He et al. 2003) It has also been possible to generate CMs from hESCs without using EBs by utilizing a feeder layer of a visceral endoderm-like cell line called END-2

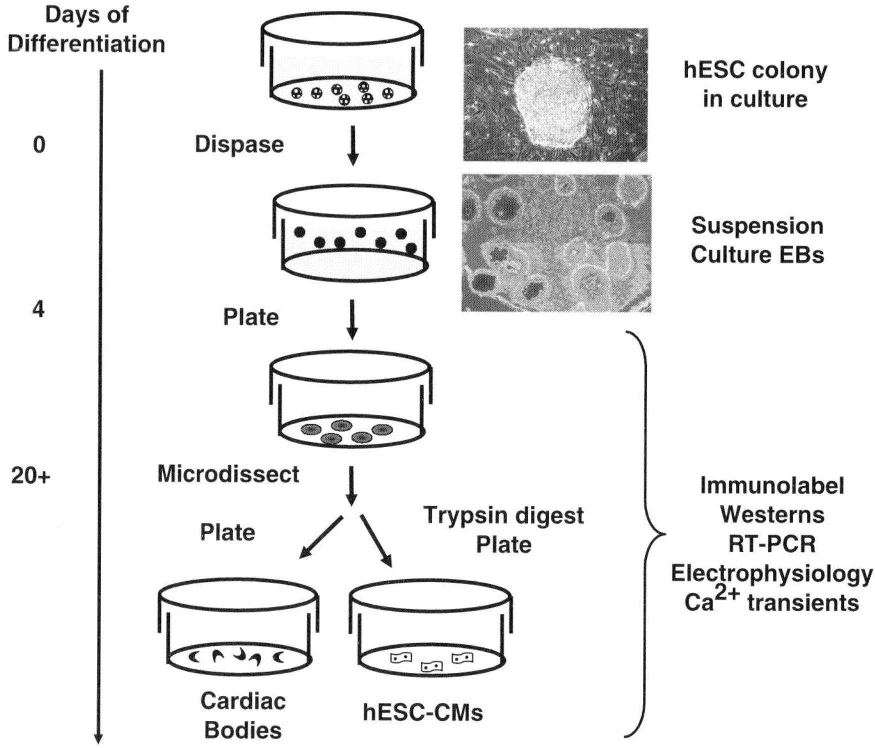

Figure 1. Schematic of hESC cardiac differentiation via EB protocol and analysis of resulting cardiomyocytes (CMs). hESCs maintained in culture are dissociated with dispase on day 0 of the protocol and cell aggregates are put into suspension culture until day 4 to form suspension EBs. The EBs are then plated on gelatin-coated plates and allowed to differentiate with contracting outgrowths appearing in the range of 8–20 days of culture. The contracting EB outgrowths can then be microdissected and further cultured as cardiac bodies or undergo enzymatic isolation to obtain isolated hESC-CMs. These preparations can be characterized with immunolabeling, Western blots, RT-PCR, electrophysiology, or Ca^{2+} transients. Images show an undifferentiated hESC colony and a day 3 suspension EB.

(Mummery et al. 2003). However, the present chapter will focus on the more widely utilized EB approach. In addition, the protocols and techniques are less refined for hESC differentiation to CMs compared to mESC cardiac differentiation due to the shorter period of study and general lack of genetically engineered hESC lines to aid in the isolation and purification of specific cell lineages.

5.1 EB Formation Protocol (see Figure 1)

5.1.1 Materials

1. Standard hESC cultures maintained in the hESC culture medium (Table 2) on MEF feeder layers in 6-well plates (Nunc, Fisher Scientific Catalog # 14-832-11)
2. Six-well plates [Corning (Costar) 3471 low attachment plates]

3. EB differentiation medium
   - DMEM/F12 (Invitrogen Catalog # 11330-032)
   - FBS (20% tested for CM differentiation; Invitrogen or Hyclone)
   - L-Glutamine (2 mmol/L) (Invitrogen Catalog # 25030-081)
   - β-mercaptoethanol (0.1 mM) (Sigma Catalog # M-7522)
   - Nonessential amino acids (1%) (Invitrogen Catalog # 11140-050)
4. Dispase solution
   - Dissolve 1 mg/mL dispase (Invitrogen) in hES cell culture medium
5. Gelatin, Type A (Sigma Catalog # G-1890)

5.1.2 Procedures

Day 0:

- Dissociate mature hESC colonies (generally 5–6 day old cultures) by aspirating medium and adding 1 mL of prewarmed (37°C) dispase solution/well in a 6-well plate. Incubate in the 37°C CO_2 incubator for 20–30 min. Inspect by swirling dish to determine when all colonies are free-floating and then stop the incubation.
- Transfer free-floating colonies (3,000–8,000 hESCs/colony) to a 15 mL conical tube gently. Do not pipet up and down.
- Rinse each well with 1 mL of EB medium and add to 15 mL tube.
- Let the colonies settle by gravity.
- Gently aspirate the dispase-containing medium.
- Rinse the colonies 3–4 more times with 5 mL EB medium and let the colonies settle by gravity.
- Resuspend the cells in 6 mL of EB medium (1 mL/starting number of wells) and plate into ultra low attachment 6-well Corning plate by adding 2 mL of EB medium to each well first and then 1 mL of cells in EB medium to each well. Be gentle as aggregates of cells easily break apart. Then incubate in 37°C CO_2 incubator.

Day 1–3:

- Change the EB medium on day 1 (not day 2 or 3) by pipetting the cells out of the well into a 15 mL conical tube, gravity settle, aspirate medium, and resuspend to 6 mL with EB medium. Add 4 mL/well EB medium to the low attachment 6-well plate, and then transfer 1 mL/well suspended EBs back into low attachment 6-well plate to the final volume of 5 mL/well.
- Prepare gelatin-coated plates
  a. Add 0.5 g gelatin to 500 mL endotoxin-free water (0.1% solution) in autoclavable glass bottles (see notes). Gelatin will not dissolve initially at room temperature. Do not allow water or gelatin solution to sit unsterilized for longer than 2 h.
  b. Autoclave 0.1% gelatin for 30 min. Gelatin will solubilize and remain a liquid. Store at room temperature.
  c. At least 1 day prior to plating suspension EBs, coat wells with gelatin solution by placing at least 1 mL per well in a standard attachment 6-well plate. Tilt plate in several directions so that liquid covers the entire surface area.

d. Place plates in 37°C incubator overnight.
e. Immediately prior to plating suspension EBs, aspirate remaining gelatin solution.

Day 4:

- Transfer suspension EBs into 50 mL conical tube. Let them settle by gravity. Aspirate 21 mL of old medium and leave 9 mL of the old medium in the tube. Add 1.5 mL/well fresh EB differentiation medium to gelatin-coated 6-well plate. Distribute suspension EBs in 1.5 mL/well to the gelatin-coated 6-well plate, to the final volume of 3 mL/well.

Day 5:

- Gently add 1 mL/well EB medium.

Day 6:

- Change the complete EB differentiation medium daily by aspirating the old medium and refeed with 3 mL EB medium to each well. For the first 20 days medium is changed daily. After that, medium can be changed at lower frequency depending on the density of EBs.

5.1.3 Notes

1. Each well of 6-well low attachment plates contains 50–100 suspension EBs for a total of 300–600 EBs per 6-well plate.
2. Contracting areas typically begin to appear ~8 days after EB formation with more appearing until ~20 days after EB formation (Segev et al. 2005).
3. Optimization of serum for cardiac differentiation is essential for success utilizing the EB methods. New lots of serum must be tested side-by-side with an effective lot to identify empirically those lots which promote or permit cardiogenesis. There is tremendous variability between lots and typical lot matching approaches have not been successful in identifying cardiogenesis-promoting lots.
4. Glass bottles used for 0.1% gelatin solution should be cleaned with NaOH when first obtained, and then dedicated to sterile gelatin solution only. These bottles should never be cleaned with detergent.

5.2 Microdissection and Culture of Contracting Cardiac Bodies

After the first 3 weeks in culture, the contracting outgrowths from EBs start to become overgrown by more rapidly dividing non-CM cells in the EB. Therefore, simple microdissection of the contracting outgrowths from EBs and replating enables longer-term culture and enriches the culture in CMs. The electrically coupled, contracting collection of CMs are referred to as cardiac bodies and can be maintained in culture for weeks to months. Alternative approaches using gentle enzymatic digestion of EBs followed by Percoll density gradient centrifugation have been described to obtain cardiac bodies (Xu et al. 2002a, b). However, we will focus only on microdissected methodology.

5.2.1 Material

1. One 6-well of mature contracting EBs from protocol 5.1
2. Scalpel (Feather sterile stainless steel, disposable scalpel, No. 10)
3. Conical tubes (15 mL)
4. Water bath (37°C)
5. EB differentiation medium (see protocol 5.1)
6. 0.1% gelatin (see protocol 5.1)
7. 24-well plates (Nunc, Fisher Scientific Catalog # 12-565-75)
8. Coverslips # 1, 15 mm (Nunc, Fisher Scientific Catalog # 12-565-75), or other glass coverslip of choice

5.2.2 Procedure

1. Prepare gelatin-coated coverslips
   - Spray forceps with 70% ethanol and air-dry in the hood. Autoclave 15 mm coverslips in a covered beaker. Use the forceps to pick up coverslips and place them in the wells of the plate.
   - Add 0.5 mL/well of 0.1% gelatin solution on coverslips in 24-well plate. Place plates in 37°C CO_2 incubator overnight.
2. Using a colony marker with a 2X objective, mark the beating EB areas.
3. Place plate on the microscope inside static enclosure (Picking hood). The interior of the static enclosure should be sterilized with UV light for 20 min prior to use.
4. Focus and adjust magnification so an entire beating area is visible in the field of view.
5. Dissect out beating areas using sterile scalpel under the microscope and leave the dissected cardiac bodies in well.
6. Bring the plate from the static enclosure to the tissue culture hood.
7. Use 5 mL pipet to transfer the dissected cardiac bodies from the wells to a 15 mL tube.
8. Remove 2–3 cardiac bodies using a 5 mL pipet and add to each well of 24-well plate containing gelatin-coated coverslips. Bring volume of EB differentiation medium to 1 mL per well.

5.2.3 Notes

1. Attached beating cardiac bodies remain viable and most are spontaneously active for many weeks in culture (12 weeks or more). Because the microdissected outgrowths eliminate most of the rapidly proliferative cells, there is less problem with overgrowth of other cells during prolonged culture.
2. Immunostaining with anti-cardiac troponin I suggests that in the range of 40% of the cells obtained from microdissected outgrowths are CMs.

5.3 Enzymatic Isolation and Culture of Single CMs from EB Protocol

For some applications, it is preferable to be able to obtain isolated single hESC-CMs. Such single CMs are useful for immunocytochemistry, cellular electrophysiology, flow cytometry, and other studies. Using relatively standard enzymatic isolation techniques on microdissected EBs, viable single hESC-CMs can be obtained. We prefer to plate hESC-CM on matrigel-coated coverslips for longer-term culture and electrophysiology measurements, but standard short-term culture on gelatin-coated coverslips are adequate for applications such as immunocytochemistry.

5.3.1 Materials

1. Microdissected ESC cardiac bodies as described in protocol 5.2
2. Trypsin 0.05%—EDTA (Invitrogen Catalog # 25300-054)
3. Conical tubes (15 mL)
4. Water bath (37°C)
5. EB differentiation medium (see protocol 5.1)
6. Growth factor reduced matrigel (BD 354230) 10 mL stored at −20°C
7. Coverslips (Fisher brand microscope round cover glass #12-545-83 15CIR-1D, #1 × 15 mm)
8. 12-well or 24-well plates (12-well plate, Nunc, Fisher Scientific Catalog # 12-565-321; 24-well plate, Nunc, Fisher Scientific Catalog # 12-565-75)
9. 100–1,000 μL micropipets

5.3.2 Procedures

1. Prepare coverslips 1–3 days before EB processing
   - For gelatin-coated coverslips see protocol 5.2.
   - For matrigel-coated coverslips:
     a. Thaw matrigel (0.5 mL is enough for 6 coverslips) at 4°C for 12–24 h. Try to use thawed Matrigel in less than 48 h or it will start to gel (even at 4°C).
     b. Add 80 μL matrigel to the center of each coverslip. Do this rapidly because the matrigel will gel if kept warm for very long.
     c. Immediately wrap plate with parafilm and store at 4°C at least overnight so that the matrigel proteins coat the coverslip, and use the coated coverslips within 2 or 3 days.
2. Pipet microdissected beating outgrowths obtained above into 15 mL tube.
3. Centrifuge at 1,000 rpm for 1 min so that the dissected cardiac bodies settle to the bottom of the tube.
4. Aspirate down to the pellet.
5. Add 2 mL of prewarmed trypsin (37°C) to 10–12 microdissected cardiac bodies (0.5 mL/2–3 cut out EBs) to the tube.
6. Pipet up and down to resuspend the pellets.
7. Incubate the tube in 37°C water bath for 5 min, and then pipet up and down to resuspend the cells.

8. Repeat last step—heating for 5 min and resuspend the cells.
9. Add 2 mL of EB differentiation medium to the tube; the FBS in the medium inactivates the trypsin.
10. Spin at 1,000 rpm for 5 min.
11. Rinse again with 4 mL of EB differentiation medium and let undigested material settle to the bottom of the tube.
12. Pull off the cell suspension and add to a separate 15 mL tube.
13. Remove 20 μL cell suspension and add it directly to the hemacytometer chamber
14. Use a hemacytometer chamber with a microscope using a 10X objective lens to count cells.
15. After counting, spin down the cells at 1,000 rpm for 5 min.
16. Aspirate down to the pellet and bring it up in a volume desired to add to individual wells containing the coverslips coated with 0.1% gelatin or matrigel.
17. Plate CMs on coverslips
    - For matrigel-coated coverslips:
        a. At a convenient point during the trypsin digestion, remove the coverslips from 4°C.
        b. Using a 1,000 μL pipet, quickly remove the matrigel and pipet into a discard tube.
        c. Immediately add 80 μL of the EB differentiation medium and let the plate sit in the hood.
        d. When the cells are ready to plate, use a 1,000 μL pipet to remove the medium from the coverslips and discard.
        e. Plate 10,000–20,000 cells/80 μL into the center of each individual coverslip on the matrigel-coated area in EB differentiation medium.
        f. Incubate the plate overnight in a CO_2 incubator at 37°C.
        g. The next day add 1 mL of the EB differentiation medium to each well in the plate.
    - For gelatin-coated coverslips:
        a. Immediately prior to plating CMs, aspirate remaining gelatin solution.
        b. Plate 50,000–100,000 cells/15 mm coverslip in 1 mL/well of EB differentiation medium in a 24-well plate.
        c. Incubate the plate in a CO_2 incubator at 37°C.
18. Change EB differentiation medium every other day.

5.3.3 Notes

1. Plated cells resume spontaneous contractions typically 1–2 days after plating.
2. Matrigel will gel if it gets warm and since the volume is small (75–80 μL), you must work quickly.

3. Each matrigel aliquot has 500 μL, enough for 6 coverslips at 75–80 μL per coverslip
4. If you want to immunostain the coverslips, use a 24-well plate in which 1 coverslip fits snugly into one well.

6. CHARACTERIZATION OF hESC-CMs

A variety of approaches have been applied to characterize the hESC-CMs. The presence of hESC-CMs in culture is typically evident by the development of spontaneously contracting outgrowths from EBs. Thus, a highly localized region of the EB undergoes cardiogenesis which can be recognized by spontaneous contractions, or as shown in Figure 2 as a highly localized area of intense immunolabeling for a cardiac-specific protein such as cardiac troponin I. The first evaluation of cardiogenesis from hESCs simply involves microscopically determining the time course of appearance and abundance of spontaneously contracting EBs. The percentage of contracting EBs has ranged from a few percent up to 70% of the EBs, with a more typical number being ~20% (Kehat et al. 2001; Xu et al. 2002a, b; He et al. 2003; Segev et al. 2005). Additional information can be obtained by determining the rate of EB contraction; however, it is critical to maintain the EBs at a constant temperature near 37°C as the rate slows and contractions stop as EBs cool to room temperature. The observed rates of spontaneous contractions near 37°C have ranged from 10 bpm to ~120 bpm, and furthermore, some EBs are not continuously contracting but show more episodic patterns of contractions likely related to the complex geometry and electrical interconnections in the three dimensional aggregate (He et al. 2003). Thus, simple

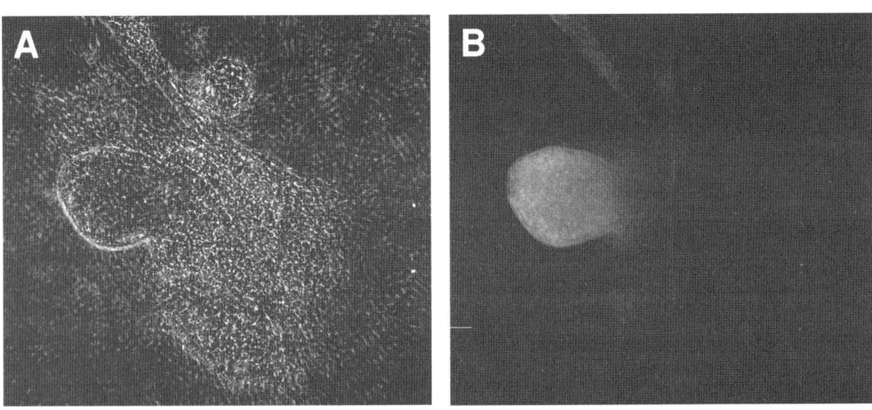

Figure 2. EBs develop outgrowths containing spontaneously contracting cardiomyocytes identified with immunolabeling of the cardiac-specific protein troponin I. Panel A demonstrates a phase contrast image of a fixed EB that was immunolabeled with an antibody to myofilament protein cardiac troponin I. Panel B shows the immunofluorescence image of the same EB with prominent cardiac troponin I immunofluorescence in the large outgrowth, but not elsewhere in the EB. Scale bar 300 μm.

observations of the cultures provide the first opportunity for evaluation of the success of inducing cardiogenesis, but more sophisticated analysis of cardiac differentiation can be performed evaluating the gene and protein expression time courses and determining the functional properties of the resulting hESC-CMs as described in the following protocols.

6.1 RT-PCR for Gene Expression

Standard reverse transcription-polymerase chain reaction (RT-PCR) provides a sensitive method to evaluate for changes in gene expression during differentiation. However, it is essential to realize that as differentiation progresses, multiple cell types are present in the EB, contributing to the observed measurements.

6.1.1 Materials required

1. EBs formed using protocol 5.1 and sample at time points of choice
2. TRIzol reagent (Invitrogen Life Technologies)
3. DNase I, Amplification Grade (Invitrogen Life Technologies)
4. SuperScript III First-Strand Synthesis System for RT-PCR (Invitrogen Life Technologies)
5. *Taq* DNA Polymerase (Promega)
6. Taq Extender PCR Additive (Stratagene)
7. PCR Nucleotide mix (Roche Applied Science)
8. Relevant PCR primers with examples shown in Table 3
9. PCR thermal cycler, e.g., Mastercycler gradient thermal cycler (Eppendorf)
10. Agarose (Sigma Aldrich)
11. SYBR Green I Nucleic Acid Stain (Invitrogen Life Technologies)
12. 100 bp DNA Ladder (Promega)
13. 50X Tris-Acetate-EDTA (TAE) buffer: Tris base (242 g); glacial acetic acid (57.1 mL); 0.5M EDTA pH 8.0 (100 mL); distilled water (to make 1 L)
14. 6X Loading dye: Bromophenol blue (0.25 g); Xylene cyanol FF (0.25 g); Ficoll Type 400 (15 g); distilled water (to make 100 mL)

6.1.2 Procedures

1. Collect 4–5 EBs with beating areas (typically present in one well of 6-well plate).
2. Extract RNA using TRIzol reagent according to the manufacturer's instructions.
3. Treat 1 μg of RNA with DNase I, Amplification Grade.
4. Use 1 μg of DNase-treated RNA to generate first-strand cDNA synthesis using SuperScript III First-Strand Synthesis System for RT-PCR as per the manufacturer's instructions.
5. Each PCR reaction mix contains sdWater (10.25 μL), dNTPs (4.00 μL), 15 μM forward and reverse primers (2.50 μL, each), *Taq* DNA polymerase (0.25 μL), *Taq* extender (0.5 μL), *Taq* extender buffer (2.50 μL), and 5 μL of cDNA.

Table 3. RT-PCR primers

Gene	Function	Primers (5′ – 3′)	Amplicon size
Oct4 (Mummery et al. 2003)	TF marker of pluripotency	GAGAACAATGAGAACCTTCAGGAGA (sense), TTCTGGCGCCGGTTACAGAACCA (antisense)	215 bp
Nkx2.5 (Passier et al. 2005)	Cardiac TF	GGTGGAGCTGGAGAAGACAGA (sense), CGACGCCGAAGTTCACGAAGT (antisense)	536 bp
GATA-4 (Passier et al. 2005)	Cardiac TF	ACCAGCAGCAGCGAGGAGAT (sense), GAGAGATGCAGT-GTGCTCGT (antisense)	512 bp
α-MHC (Bodmer 1993; Passier et al. 2005)	Cardiac myofilament	GGGGACAGTGGTAAAAGCAA (sense), TCCCTGCGTTCCACTATCTT (antisense)	542 bp
α-actinin (Mummery et al. 2003)	Cardiac myofilament	GGCGTGCAGTACAACTACGTG (sense), AGTCAATGAGGTCAGGCCGGT (antisense)	580 bp
ANF (Andrée et al. 1998; Mummery et al. 2003)	Cardiac cytosolic protein	GAACCAGAGGGGAGAGACAGAG (sense), CCCTCAGCTTGCTTTTTAGGAG (antisense)	406 bp
Phospholamban (Mummery et al. 2003)	Cardiac SR protein	ACAGCTGCCAAGGCTACCTA (sense), GCTTTTGACGTGCTTGTTGA (antisense)	191 bp
MLC-2a (Schneider and Mercola 2001; Mummery et al. 2003)	Atrial ventricular myofilament	GAGGAGAATGGCCAGCAGGAA (sense), GCGAACATCTGCTCCACCTCA (antisense)	449 bp
MLC-2v (Mummery et al. 2003)	Ventricular myofilament	First round GCGCCAACTCCAACGTGTTCT (sense), GTGATGATGTGCACCAGGTTC (antisense) Nested PCR AGGAGGCCTTCACTATCATGG (sense), GTGATGATGTGCACCAGGTTC (antisense)	444 bp
β-actin (Mummery et al. 2003)	Constitutive protein	CCTGAACCCTAAGGCCAACCG (sense), GCTCATAGCTCTTCTCCAGGG (antisense)	400 bp
β-tubulin (Mummery et al. 2003)	Constitutive protein	TGGCTTTGCCCCTCTCACCA (sense), CGGCGGAACATGGCAGTGAA (antisense)	369 bp

TF = transcription factor; SR = sarcoplasmic reticulum

6. Use initial cycling conditions of: 94°C, 3 min, followed by 35 cycles at 94°C, 45 s, 62°C, 90 s, 72°C, 60 s, and a final extension cycle of 7 min at 72°C.
7. The PCR products are analyzed by agarose gel electrophoresis. Briefly, agarose is dissolved in 1X TAE buffer (10 mL of 50X TAE buffer and diluted with distilled water to make 500 mL) by heating in a microwave until fully dissolved. SYBR Green (0.1%) is added and the mixture is poured into a gel tank and allowed to set. Approximately 1–1.5% gels are used for visualizing bands of 200–1,000 bps, and a 2% gel is used for visualizing lower band sizes.
8. PCR products are mixed with 6X loading buffer. The DNA marker and PCR products are then loaded into the gel.
9. The gel is then run at an appropriate voltage for the duration needed for markers to be clearly separated. Bands are visualized and photographed.

6.2 Immunolabeling

Immunofluorescence or immunohistochemistry techniques can be used to identify protein expression patterns in single cells isolated from the EBs.

6.2.1 Materials

1. 4% Paraformaldehyde (PFA): Dissolve 4 g PFA in Phosphate Buffer Saline (PBS), adjust to 100 mL with PBS, heat the mixture to 95°C, stir until the solution becomes clear, and bring to room temperature. PFA is toxic. Gloves should be used to handle the PFA and work must be conducted under the fume hood.
2. 0.1% Nonidet P (NP)-40 in PBS or 0.02% Triton-X100 in PBS to permeabilize the cells
3. 0.05% trypsin in cell culture medium
4. 0.3% gelatin: Add 0.3 g of gelatin in 100 mL PBS, heat in microwave for 2–5 min, cool at room temperature and filter (0.22 μm) sterilize
5. 10% normal goat serum or 0.5–1% bovine serum albumin (BSA) in PBS is used to block nonspecific binding of antibodies
6. 0.5–1% BSA in PBS for dilution of antibodies
7. Counterstain to visualize cell nuclei: Hoechst 33258 or DAPI (Molecular Probe)
8. Mounting Medium: Vectashield (Vector Laboratories)
9. Epifluorescence microscope or confocal microscope with appropriate filter sets for chosen fluorophores

6.2.2 Procedures

1. Use isolated cardiac bodies or hESC-CMs on coverslips.
2. Fix cells in 4% PFA for 15 min and permeabilize with 0.1% NP-40 or 0.02% Triton-X 100 for 5–15 min at 4°C.
3. Block using 0.5% BSA in PBS for 30 min at room temperature.
4. Incubate with primary antibodies (Table 4) at starting dilutions suggested overnight at 4°C.

Table 4. Antibodies for immunolabeling

Antibodies	Species	Source	Dilution
Cardiac transcription factors			
Nkx2.5	Rabbit IgG	Santa Cruz	1:200
GATA-4	Rabbit IgG	Santa Cruz	1:100
Cardiac myofilament proteins			
α-actinin	Mouse IgG_1	Sigma	1:400
Cardiac actin	Mouse IgG	Sigma	1:1,000
Cardiac troponin-I	Mouse IgG	Chemicon	1:400
Sarcomeric myosin	Mouse IgG_{2b}	Hybridoma Bank	1:500
Muscle cell-to-cell coupling proteins			
Connexin-43	Mouse IgG_1	Santa Cruz	1:40
N-cadherin	Rabbit IgG	R&D System	1:800

5. Wash the cells with PBS 2–3 times for 5 min each wash and then incubate with secondary antibodies (anti-mouse or anti-goat as appropriate) Alexa Fluor 568 or Texas Red-conjugated with IgM or IgG (Molecular Probe or Amersham) for 1–2 h.
6. Perform nuclear staining using Hoechst 33258 or DAPI (Molecular Probes).
7. Negative controls are performed either incubating with primary or secondary antibody alone.
8. Coverslips are mounted with antifade medium (Vector Laboratories).
9. Image the cells with standard epifluorescence microscopy or confocal microscopy.

6.3 Western blot

6.3.1 Materials

1. 0.25% trypsin/EDTA (Invitrogen)
2. RIPA buffer: 50 mM Tris-HCl, pH 7.4, NP-40 (1%), sodium deoxycholate 0.25%, 150 mM NaCl/1 mM EDTA/2 mM sodium orthovanadate/5 mM sodium fluoride/1 mM PMSF and mammalian protease inhibitor cocktail (Sigma)
3. 10% Sodium Dodecyl Sulphate (SDS): dissolve 10 g of SDS in DDH_2O
4. Polyacrylamide gel either commercially available or using standard techniques
5. Electrophoresis apparatus – gel tank, power supply
6. Washing solution: Tris buffered saline (TBS)—Tween20; Tris-base: 2.42 g, Nacl: 8 g, dissolve in 1 L of DDH_2O and adjust the pH: 7.6 with 1 M HCl and add 1 mL of Tween20
7. BSA: dissolve 5 g of BSA in 100 mL of TBS

8. Polyvinyl difluoride (PVDF) membrane (Bio-Rad)
9. Primary antibody: (see Table 4 as most of listed antibodies work for both immunocytochemistry and immunoblotting)
10. Secondary antibody: Horseradish peroxidase anti-mouse IgG
11. Visualizer: chemiluminescence system (Amersham or Upstate cell signaling solutions)
12. X-ray film (Sigma)
13. Table-top centrifuge

6.3.2 Procedures

1. Isolate EBs, cardiac bodies, or digested cells.
2. Suspend EBs in modified RIPA buffer and allowed to lyse for 30 min on ice.
3. Centrifuge the cell homogenates for 15 min at 14,000 g at 4°C to pellet the insoluble debris. Retain the supernatant as the cellular lysate.
4. Measure protein concentration of the lysates using a standard protein assays such as the Bradford assay (Biorad reagent).
5. Perform SDS-polyacrylamide gel electrophoresis by loading 10–40 μg protein on 10–15% gel (gel concentration dependent on target proteins).
6. Transfer to polyvinyl difluoride membranes (Bio-Rad).
7. For blocking, incubate the blots in 5% BSA at 4°C overnight or 2 h at room temperature.
8. Incubate with the primary antibody diluted in TBS for 2 h at room temperature or at 4°C overnight.
9. Wash three times using TBS Tween20 for 20 min each at room temperature using Orbitron rotator III.
10. Incubate blots with secondary antibody horseradish peroxidase anti-mouse IgG diluted in TBS for 1–2 h at room temperature.
11. Incubate blots with solutions from chemiluminescence kit (Amersham) for 5 min. (Note: avoid air bubbles.)
12. Transfer blots were wrapped in the saran wrap and mounted on the x-ray cassette (avoid any saran wrap wrinkles) or other imaging equipment.

6.4 EB Contraction

Measurement of the contractile performance of cardiac muscle provides important information regarding the functional properties of the muscle. A first approach is to evaluate changes in unloaded shortening, such as that found in spontaneously contracting EBs. Using microdissected cardiac bodies plated on coverslips, videomicroscopy with edge-detection hardware and software can be used to track the magnitude of contractions and changes in the contractions in response to stimuli such as pharmacological agents. Figure 3 demonstrates the effect of the nonselective β-AR agonist isoproterenol (ISO) on the contraction amplitude of cultured cardiac bodies.

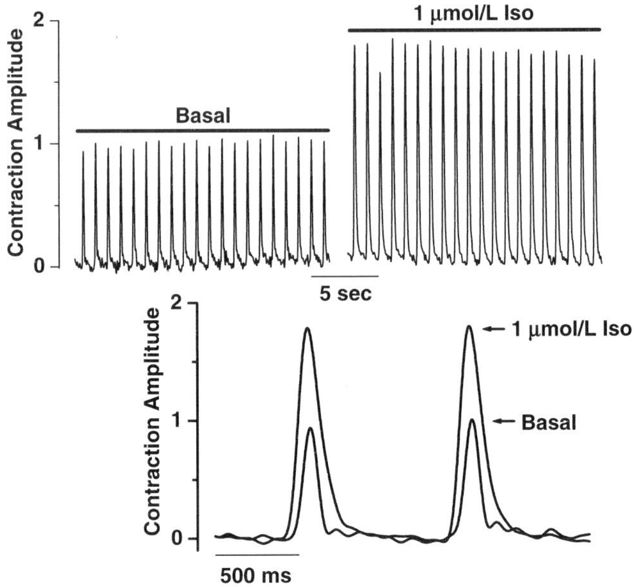

Figure 3. Response of cardiac body contractions measured with videomicroscopy to β-AR stimulation with isoproterenol (ISO). An isolated cardiac body was field stimulated at 1 Hz and contraction amplitude was measured in arbitrary units at baseline and after exposure to 1.0 μM ISO. Larger contractions are observed after perfusion with ISO. (Reprinted from He et al., 2003, Circulation Research, 93: 32–39 with permission.)

6.4.1 Materials

1. Microdissected cardiac bodies or EBs with contracting areas plated on 15 mm gelatin-coated coverslips
2. Tyrodes solution containing (mmol/L) 140 NaCl, 1 $MgCl_2$, 10 HEPES, 10 Glucose, 1.8 $CaCl_2$, pH 7.4 with NaOH
3. Inverted microscope with temperature controlled cellular perfusion chamber that can accommodate 15 mm coverslips
4. CCD camera (e.g., CCD BW Cameral NL-2332, National Electronics) with edge detection hardware (e.g., Video Edge Detector VED 105, Crescent Electronics) and videomonitor (e.g., Sony BW Video Monitor PVM-9)
5. Electrical field stimulation apparatus including platinum bath electrodes and electronic field stimulator (e.g., Grass SD-9 stimulator)
6. Analog to digital converter and computerized data acquisition software

6.4.2 Procedures

1. Place coverslip with cultured cardiac body into perfusion chamber and continuously perfuse at 37°C with Tyrodes solution.
2. Use videomicroscopy and center the field of view on the edge of the contracting cardiac body and measure the amplitude of the contractions. The contractions

can be continuously recorded during interventions such as drug perfusion. The complete procedural details of videomicroscopy and edge-detection can be found elsewhere.

3. To control the rate of contraction of the cardiac bodies, electrical field stimulation can be employed to stimulate the preparation at rates greater than the intrinsic rates (e.g., 10 ms duration pulses at 30–50 V are typically effective to entrain the cardiac body).

6.4.3 Notes

Each experiment serves as its own control given the variability in the absolute magnitude of the contractions observed because of the differences in geometry, orientation, and size of each cardiac body. Efforts at producing oriented cardiac fibers for more precise, standardized contractile measurements are an important future direction.

6.5 Electrophysiology

The electrophysiological properties of native cardiac muscle have been characterized in detail. The electrical impulse responsible for the heartbeat can be recorded on the surface electrocardiogram. Similarly, spontaneously contracting EBs exhibit regular electrical activity, which can be recorded by extracellular field potentials. Such recordings can be performed using specialized culture dishes which have an embedded multielectrode array (MEA) attached to an amplifier. The technical details can be found elsewhere (Kehat et al. 2002; Xue et al. 2005). MEA recordings of hESC-derived EBs in culture have demonstrated that the hESC-CMs form a functional syncytium with stable patterns of focal activation and conduction (Kehat et al. 2002). From these data, one can also easily determine the rate of spontaneous activity. This system also allows one to test the impact of perfusion of test compounds or other interventions on the rate of contraction and conduction patterns. An alternative approach is the use of voltage-sensitive fluorescent dyes such as di4-ANNEPs and optical recordings of membrane potential changes (Xue et al. 2005).

The electrical activity in the heart is generated at the cellular level by the well-orchestrated activity of multiple ion channels, ion exchangers, and electrogenic pumps to produce the prototypical changes in cellular membrane potential referred to as an action potential (AP). The cardiac AP has been studied in native CMs for four decades (Schram et al. 2002). These studies have demonstrated that different types of CMs in the heart exhibit different cellular APs based on differences in the underlying ionic conductances. Therefore, the AP provides a complex functional signature of the cardiac cell type under study.

The AP in cardiac myocytes can be measured using a variety of approaches, which will be discussed but not described in detail here. Using sharp high-resistance KCl microelectrodes, APs can be recorded by impaling multicellular cardiac muscle preparations. Intracellular recordings from cardiac bodies differentiated from hESCs using sharp KCl electrodes have demonstrated that multiple types

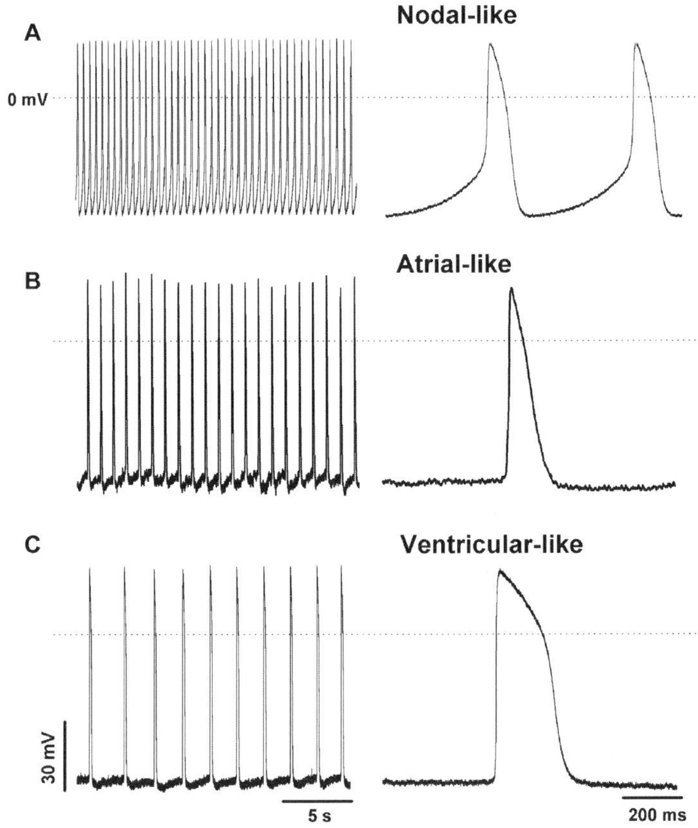

Figure 4. Intracellular recordings of membrane potential from hESC-derived cardiac bodies demonstrate spontaneous action potentials. Three major types of AP waveforms were observed in cultured cardiac bodies: (**A**) nodal-like; (**B**) embryonic atrial-like; and (**C**) embryonic ventricular-like. (Reprinted from He et al., 2003, Circulation Research, 93: 32–39 with permission.)

of cardiac myocytes can be detected including atrial, nodal, and ventricular-like cells as shown in Figure 4 (He et al. 2003). The properties of these APs include a relatively depolarized membrane potential and slow upstrokes which are typical of embryonic rather than adult CMs. Alternatively, intracellular recordings can be made using the ruptured patch clamp technique, and investigators using this technique have also provided evidence for multiple types of CMs arising from differentiating hESCs (Mummery et al. 2003). Thus recordings of the spontaneous or stimulated APs in hESC-CMs provide critical functional information defining the phenotype of the cells present. Additional electrophysiological characterization of the hESC-CMs using enzymatically isolated single cells and whole-cell patch clamp techniques can provide detailed information on the specific ionic currents present in the cells (Satin et al. 2004). Thus, cellular electrophysiology approaches provide a powerful technique to rigorously characterize the functional properties of live hESC-CMs. Furthermore, measuring changes in the electrophysiological properties or ionic currents in response to drugs or other interventions will provide a powerful method to examine the responses of human CMs to these interventions.

6.6 Intracellular Ca^{2+} Transients

Excitation–contraction coupling in CMs involves the regular cycling of intracellular Ca^{2+}. The AP-induced rise in intracellular Ca^{2+} triggers activation of the myofilaments that leads to mechanical contraction. The depolarization of each cardiac AP is associated with the influx of Ca^{2+} resulting mainly from the activation of sarcolemmal L-type Ca^{2+} channels. In adult mammalian ventricular myocytes, the Ca^{2+} influx into the myoplasm via the L-type Ca^{2+} channels serves as a trigger to induce release of intracellular Ca^{2+} stores from the sarcoplasmic reticulum referred to as Ca-induced Ca^{2+} release (Bers 2002). The intracellular Ca^{2+} transients underlying the contraction of native CMs have been extensively studied using fluorescent indicators such as Fura-2, but the methodology is beyond the scope of this chapter. Initial studies have likewise demonstrated Ca^{2+} transients as a characteristic feature of hESC-CMs (Kehat et al. 2001; Dolnikov et al. 2006). Close examination of the properties of the Ca^{2+} transient from hESC-CMs maintained from a few days to 8 weeks have revealed that the Ca transient is due to influx of extracellular Ca^{2+} with little if any release of intracellular stores. This has been attributed to immature sarcoplasmic reticulum in these cells and is comparable to findings in native animal CMs isolated early in development in which myocardial contraction is due more to influx of extracellular Ca^{2+} than intracellular release (Pegg and Michalak 1987; Dolnikov et al. 2006). Therefore, the regular Ca^{2+} transient observed in contracting hESC-CMs provides clear functional evidence identifying the cell as a CM and helps define its level of maturity and excitation–contraction properties.

7. CONCLUSIONS AND FUTURE

The differentiation of hESCs into CMs is readily possible using standard EB techniques. The resulting hESC-CMs have been extensively characterized and exhibit properties typical of embryonic CMs as manifest by relatively depolarized membrane potentials, slow AP upstrokes, and Ca^{2+} cycling dependent solely on influx of extracellular Ca^{2+}. Multiple types of embryonic-type CMs have been observed suggesting that the hESCs can differentiate into nodal, atrial, and ventricular CMs. Future approaches to obtain more homogenous, defined populations of CMs from the hESCs will be of importance. Additionally, efforts at obtaining CMs with a more mature phenotype will be important. At present the process of cardiogenesis in EBs is relatively inefficient with regard to the number of cells produced. Initial efforts at extrapolating some of the approaches utilizing various cytokines and small molecules found to induce mESC cardiogenesis have not yet proven successful with hESCs; however, these studies are early and it is likely that advances will be forthcoming. In addition, techniques exploiting genetically engineered hESC lines such as those that have been successful with mESCs to obtain more pure populations of hESC-CMs have not yet been described. In part, this likely reflects the greater degree of difficulty of transducing or genetically engineering hESCS, but such direct extrapolations of mESC techniques are also anticipated in the near future. Finally, most of the studies with hESC differentiation to CMs have not utilized approaches and techniques necessary to provide cells safe for clinical applications. As the field advances, utilizing hESC lines free of animal contaminants and differentiation procedures with defined medium also free of animal products will be essential to provide cells appropriate for clinical applications.

REFERENCES

Andrée, B., Duprez, D., Vorbusch, B., Arnold, H.H., and Brand, T. (1998) BMP-2 induces ectopic expression of cardiac lineage markers and interferes with somite formation in chicken embryos. Mech. Dev., 70: 119–131.

Azpiazu, N. and Frasch, M. (1993) Tinman and bagpipe: two homeo box genes that determine cell fates in the dorsal mesoderm of Drosophila. Genes Dev., 7: 1325–1340.

Barron, M., Gao, M., and Lough, J. (2000) Requirement for BMP and FGF signaling during cardiogenic induction in non-precardiac mesoderm is specific, transient, and cooperative. Dev. Dyn., 218: 383–393.

Behfar, A., Zingman, L.V., Hodgson, D.M., Rauzier, J.M., Kane, G.C., Terzic, A., and Puceat, M. (2002) Stem cell differentiation requires a paracrine pathway in the heart. FASEB J., 16: 1558–1566.

Bers, D.M. (2002) Cardiac excitation-contraction coupling. Nature, 415: 198–205.

Bodmer, R. (1993) The gene tinman is required for specification of the heart and visceral muscles in Drosophila. Development, 118: 719–729.

Boheler, K.R., Czyz, J., Tweedie, D., Yang, H.T., Anisimov, S.V., and Wobus, A.M. (2002) Differentiation of pluripotent embryonic stem cells into cardiomyocytes. Circ. Res., 91: 189–201.

Bruneau, B.G. (2002) Transcriptional regulation of vertebrate cardiac morphogenesis. Circ. Res., 90: 509–519.

Doetschman, T.C., Eistetter, H., Katz, M., Schmidt, W., and Kemler, R. (1985) The in vitro development of blastocyst-derived embryonic stem cell lines: formation of visceral yolk sac, blood islands and myocardium. J. Embryol. Exp. Morphol., 87: 27–45.

Dolnikov, K., Shilkrut, M., Zeevi-Levin, N., Gerecht-Nir, S., Amit, M., Danon, A., Itskovitz-Eldor, J., and Binah, O. (2006) Functional properties of human embryonic stem cell-derived cardiomyocytes: intracellular Ca2+ handling and the role of sarcoplasmic reticulum in the contraction. Stem Cells, 24: 236–245.

Evans, M.J. and Kaufman, M.H. (1981) Establishment in culture of pluripotential cells from mouse embryos. Nature, 292: 154–156.

He, J.Q., Ma, Y., Lee, Y., Thomson, J.A., and Kamp, T.J. (2003) Human embryonic stem cells develop into multiple types of cardiac myocytes: action potential characterization. Circ. Res., 93: 32–39.

Hidaka, K., Lee, J.K., Kim, H.S., Ihm, C.H., Iio, A., Ogawa, M., Nishikawa, S., Kodama, I., and Morisaki, T. (2003) Chamber-specific differentiation of Nkx2.5-positive cardiac precursor cells from murine embryonic stem cells. FASEB J., 17: 740–742.

Kehat, I., Gepstein, A., Spira, A., Itskovitz-Eldor, J., and Gepstein, L. (2002) High-resolution electrophysiological assessment of human embryonic stem cell-derived cardiomyocytes: a novel in vitro model for the study of conduction. Circ. Res., 91: 659–661.

Kehat, I., Kenyagin-Karsenti, D., Snir, M., Segev, H., Amit, M., Gepstein, A., Livne, E., Binah, O., Itskovitz-Eldor, J., and Gepstein, L. (2001) Human embryonic stem cells can differentiate into myocytes with structural and functional properties of cardiomyocytes. J. Clin. Invest., 108: 407–414.

Klug, M.G., Soonpas, M.H., Koh, G.Y., and Field, L.J. (1996) Genetically selected cardiomyocytes from differentiating embryonic stem cells form stable intracardiac grafts. J. Clin. Invest., 98: 216–224.

Kolossov, E., Fleischmann, B.K., Liu, Q., Bloch, W., Viatchenko-Karpinski, S., Manzke, O., Ji, G.J., Bohlen, H., Addicks, K., and Hescheler, J. (1998) Functional characteristics of ES cell-derived cardiac precursor cells identified by tissue-specific expression of the green fluorescent protein. J. Cell Biol., 143: 2045–2056.

Martin, G.R. (1981) Isolation of a pluripotent cell line from early mouse embryos cultured in medium conditioned by teratocarcinoma stem cells. Proc. Natl. Acad. Sci. USA, 78: 7634–7638.

Marvin, M.J., Di Rocco, G., Gardiner, A., Bush, S.M., and Lassar, A.B. (2001) Inhibition of Wnt activity induces heart formation from posterior mesoderm. Genes Dev., 15: 316–327.

Metzger, J.M., Lin, W.I., and Samuelson, L.C. (1996) Vital staining of cardiac myocytes during embryonic stem cell cardiogenesis in vitro. Circ. Res., 78: 547–552.

Meyer, N., Jaconi, M., Landopoulou, A., Fort, P., and Puceat, M. (2000) A fluorescent reporter gene as a marker for ventricular specification in ES-derived cardiac cells. FEBS Lett., 478: 151–158.

Muller, M., Fleischmann, B.K., Selbert, S., Ji, G.J., Endl, E., Middeler, G., Muller, O.J., Schlenke, P., Frese, S., Wobus, A.M., Hescheler, J., Katus, H.A., and Franz, W.M. (2000) Selection of ventricular-like cardiomyocytes from ES cells in vitro. FASEB J., 14: 2540–2548.

Mummery, C., Ward-van Oostwaard, D., Doevendans, P., Spijker, R., van den, B.S., Hassink, R., van der, H.M., Opthof, T., Pera, M., de la Riviere, A.B., Passier, R., and Tertoolen, L. (2003) Differentiation of human embryonic stem cells to cardiomyocytes: role of coculture with visceral endoderm-like cells. Circulation, 107: 2733–2740.

Olson, E.N. and Srivastava, D. (1996) Molecular pathways controlling heart development. Science, 272: 671–676.

Passier, R., Oostwaard, D.W., Snapper, J., Kloots, J., Hassink, R.J., Kuijk, E., Roelen, B., de la Riviere, A.B., and Mummery, C. (2005) Increased cardiomyocyte differentiation from human embryonic stem cells in serum-free cultures. Stem Cells, 23: 772–780.

Pegg, W. and Michalak, M. (1987) Differentiation of sarcoplasmic reticulum during cardiac myogenesis. Am. J. Physiol., 252: H22–H31.

Rudy-Reil, D. and Lough, J. (2004) Avian precardiac endoderm/mesoderm induces cardiac myocyte differentiation in murine embryonic stem cells. Circ. Res., 94: e107–e116.

Satin, J., Kehat, I., Caspi, O., Huber, I., Arbel, G., Itzhaki, I., Magyar, J., Schroder, E.A., Perlman, I., and Gepstein, L. (2004) Mechanism of spontaneous excitability in human embryonic stem cell derived cardiomyocytes. J. Physiol., 559: 479–496.

Schneider, V.A. and Mercola, M. (2001) Wnt antagonism initiates cardiogenesis in *Xenopus laevis*. Genes Dev., 15: 304–315.

Schram, G., Pourrier, M., Melnyk, P., and Nattel, S. (2002) Differential distribution of cardiac ion channel expression as a basis for regional specialization in electrical function. Circ. Res., 90: 939–950.

Schroeder, M., Niebruegge, S., Werner, A., Willbold, E., Burg, M., Ruediger, M., Field, L.J., Lehmann, J., and Zweigerdt, R. (2005) Differentiation and lineage selection of mouse embryonic stem cells in a stirred bench scale bioreactor with automated process control. Biotechnol. Bioeng., 92: 920–933.

Schultheiss, T.M., Burch, J.B., and Lassar, A.B. (1997) A role for bone morphogenetic proteins in the induction of cardiac myogenesis. Genes Dev., 11: 451–462.

Segev, H., Kenyagin-Karsenti, D., Fishman, B., Gerecht-Nir, S., Ziskind, A., Amit, M., Coleman, R., and Itskovitz-Eldor, J. (2005) Molecular analysis of cardiomyocytes derived from human embryonic stem cells. Dev. Growth Differ., 47: 295–306.

Snir, M., Kehat, I., Gepstein, A., Coleman, R., Itskovitz-Eldor, J., Livne, E., and Gepstein, L. (2003) Assessment of the ultrastructural and proliferative properties of human embryonic stem cell-derived cardiomyocytes. Am. J. Physiol. Heart. Circ. Physiol., 285: H2355–H2363.

Takahashi, T., Lord, B., Schulze, P.C., Fryer, R.M., Sarang, S.S., Gullans, S.R., and Lee, R.T. (2003) Ascorbic acid enhances differentiation of embryonic stem cells into cardiac myocytes. Circulation, 107: 1912–1916.

Thomson, J.A., Itskovitz-Eldor, J., Shapiro, S.S., Waknitz, M.A., Swiergiel, J.J., Marshall, V.S., and Jones, J.M. (1998) Embryonic stem cell lines derived from human blastocysts. Science, 282: 1145–1147.

Winnier, G., Blessing, M., Labosky, P.A., and Hogan, B.L. (1995) Bone morphogenetic protein-4 is required for mesoderm formation and patterning in the mouse. Genes Dev., 9: 2105–2116.

Wu, X., Ding, S., Ding, Q., Gray, N.S., and Schultz, P.G. (2004) Small molecules that induce cardiomyogenesis in embryonic stem cells. J. Am. Chem. Soc., 126: 1590–1591.

Xu, C., Police, S., Rao, N., and Carpenter, M.K. (2002a) Characterization and enrichment of cardiomyocytes derived from human embryonic stem cells. Circ. Res., 91: 501–508.

Xu, R.H., Chen, X., Li, D.S., Li, R., Addicks, G.C., Glennon, C., Zwaka, T.P., and Thomson, J.A. (2002b) BMP4 initiates human embryonic stem cell differentiation to trophoblast. Nat. Biotechnol., 20: 1261–1264.

Xue, T., Cho, H.C., Akar, F.G., Tsang, S.Y., Jones, S.P., Marban, E., Tomaselli, G.F., and Li, R.A. (2005) Functional integration of electrically active cardiac derivatives from genetically engineered human embryonic stem cells with quiescent recipient ventricular cardiomyocytes: insights into the development of cell-based pacemakers. Circulation, 111: 11–20.

Yuasa, S., Itabashi, Y., Koshimizu, U., Tanaka, T., Sugimura, K., Kinoshita, M., Hattori, F., Fukami, S., Shimazaki, T., Ogawa, S., Okano, H., and Fukuda, K. (2005) Transient inhibition of BMP signaling by Noggin induces cardiomyocyte differentiation of mouse embryonic stem cells. Nat. Biotechnol., 23: 607–611.

Zaffran, S. and Frasch, M. (2002) Early signals in cardiac development. Circ. Res., 91: 457–469.

Zhang, H. and Bradley, A. (1996) Mice deficient for BMP2 are nonviable and have defects in amnion/chorion and cardiac development. Development, 122: 2977–2986.

CHAPTER 13

HUMAN EMBRYONAL CARCINOMA (EC) CELLS: COMPLEMENTARY TOOLS FOR EMBRYONIC STEM CELL RESEARCH

PETER D. TONGE AND PETER W. ANDREWS
The Centre for Stem Cell Biology and the Department of Biomedical Science, University of Sheffield, Western Bank, Sheffield S10 2TN, UK

1. INTRODUCTION

The study of embryonic stem (ES) cells has been closely related to the study of teratocarcinomas and embryonal carcinoma (EC) cells (Andrews, 2002). EC cells provided the paradigm for the concept of a cancer stem cell and of a stem cell capable of initiating multiple pathways of differentiation. It was experience with mouse EC cells, coupled with evidence of their close relationship to the inner cell mass (ICM) cells of the blastocyst stage of mouse embryos, which allowed Evans and Kaufman (1981) and Martin (1981) independently to derive lines of mouse ES cell lines. Although human ES cells were derived much later (Thomson et al. 1998; Reubinoff et al. 2000), prior studies of human EC cells had provided many of the markers that were used to characterize these cells. However, since EC cells are tumor cells with grossly abnormal karyotypes and often with reduced pluripotency compared to ES cells, one view might be that the value of EC cells as an experimental tool vanished once ES cells became available. An alternative view is that they do retain distinct experimental advantages and remain complementary to ES cells in the study of pluripotency.

The pluripotency of ES cells provides both advantages and disadvantages as experimental tools. The advantage is obvious; indeed it provides the *sine qua non* for their study. However, because of their pluripotency and uncontrolled spontaneous differentiation, ES cell cultures are typically heterogeneous. Moreover, the culture conditions for ES cells can be demanding, often requiring the presence of feeders or expensive growth factors. By contrast, EC cells with reduced potency, and some being nullipotent, are considerably easier to culture in large amounts. Mostly they can be grown without feeder cells, in relatively simple media, and their cultures may also be much less heterogeneous and so easier to

J.R. Masters et al (eds.), Embryonic Stem Cells, 235–253.

standardize. Consequently, studies with EC cells may be more readily reproducible, robust and interpretable than corresponding work with ES cells. The disadvantages of EC cells, of course, are that they are tumor cells, adapted to tumor growth, genetically abnormal and often with reduced capacity for differentiation, so that some caution is necessary in drawing wider conclusions. Nevertheless, while presenting a caricature of normality (Pierce 1975), EC cells can offer a simplified system in which to develop tools and strategies for investigating the biology of ES cells.

2. THE HISTORY OF TERATOCARCINOMAS AND EMBRYONAL CARCINOMAS

Teratomas are histologically complex tumors that may contain a wide variety of cells types (Damjanov 1993a, b). Their most common manifestation in females is ovarian cysts that appear to arise from parthenogenetically activated oocytes. In this situation, following initiation of embryogenesis, the parthenogenetic and ectopic embryo becomes progressively disorganized but continues to grow to form a large mass that includes an array of haphazardly arranged tissues. These tumors are usually benign, although they can grow to very large sizes. Differentiated testicular tumors also occur, but testicular germ cell tumors are usually malignant. Teratomas and teratocarcinomas have fascinated clinicians for hundreds of years, and pathologists have developed various hypotheses to explain their origins and complex histology (Damjanov and Solter 1974, Wheeler 1983). However, their experimental study was not possible until, in 1954, Stevens discovered that male mice of the 129 strain develop spontaneous teratocarcinomas at an appreciable frequency (Stevens and Little 1954).

The pioneering research of Stevens and also Pierce during the 1950s and 1960s established our basic understanding of these tumors. From the work of Stevens it became clear that the testicular tumors are initiated from primordial germ cells (PGC) that appear to be susceptible to malignant transformation only within a small window of 2–3 days after migrating into the genital ridge at 11 days of fetal development (Stevens 1967). In a separate landmark study, Pierce and his colleagues were able to show that a single EC cell when injected into a new host had the capability of regenerating a whole teratocarcinoma with its wide diversity of tissues, so providing the first demonstration of the stem cell nature of cancer (Kleinsmith and Pierce 1964). The early phase of the experimental study of teratocarcinomas was concluded by the first derivation of EC cell lines from teratocarcinomas *in vitro* (Finch and Ephrussi 1967; Kahan and Ephrussi 1970). This led to further studies that confirmed the stem cell status of EC cells with demonstrations that clonal EC cell lines could remain undifferentiated under certain culture conditions *in vitro*, but would differentiate extensively if their culture conditions were modified, or if they were re-implanted into a mouse, where they would form a teratocarcinoma (Jakob et al. 1973; Martin and Evans 1974; Nicolas et al. 1975).

Teratocarcinomas in humans exhibit more complexity than their murine counterparts. They can contain elements of choriocarcinoma and yolk sac carcinoma, which are highly malignant and correspond to the extraembryonic tissues of the trophoblast and yolk sac respectively (Damjanov 1993a, b). Although yolk sac tumors occur in conjunction with teratocarcinomas in the mouse, trophectoblastic differentiation is not seen. Another marked species difference is the frequent presence of seminoma in the human but not murine tumors. Seminomas and nonseminomas are classed as germ cell tumors (GCT) in recognition of their presumed germ cell origins. Nevertheless, whereas this has been demonstrated experimentally in the laboratory mouse, the consensus view that human GCT arise by a defect in PGC development during fetal life is based largely upon circumstantial arguments (Skakkebaek 1972; Skakkebaek et al. 1987).

3. HUMAN EC CELL LINES

A large number of cell lines have been derived from human testicular GCT and most are composed of human EC cells (Andrews and Damjanov 1994). Strikingly, no *bona fide* seminoma cell line has ever been derived. Initially it was assumed that human EC cells would resemble mouse EC cells and early studies reported coexpression of similar markers (Hogan et al. 1977; Holden et al. 1977). However, it eventually became evident that whereas the morphology of human and mouse EC cells is similar, and they express high levels of some characteristic markers, such as alkaline phosphatase and Oct4, they express quite different patterns of surface antigens (Andrews et al. 1982; Przyborski et al. 2000). Most notable amongst these differences is the expression of stage specific embryonic antigen-1 (SSEA1) by mouse but not human ES cells, and SSEA3 and SSEA4 by human, but not mouse EC cells, even though all these antigens may be expressed by other types of mouse and human cells (Knowles et al. 1978; Solter and Knowles 1978; Andrews et al. 1982, 1996; Shevinsky et al. 1982; Kannagi et al. 1983). Other differences included the expression of Thy-1 and major histocompatibility complex (MHC) antigens by human but not murine EC cells (Andrews et al. 1980, 1996).

A significant concern from these observations was that human and mouse EC cells might correspond to quite different normal cell types within the embryo. It was well established that the antigen expression pattern of mouse EC cells closely resembles that of the ICM cells of the mouse blastocyst (Jacob 1978) and, indeed, the developmental potential of mouse EC cells also closely resembled these embryonic cells, confirmed by the formation of chimeras after EC cells were introduced into mouse blastocysts that were then allowed to implant and to develop to term (Brinster 1974; Mintz and Illmensee 1975; Papaioannou et al. 1975). Human EC cells also exhibit a distinct difference in potency from their murine counterparts since they can differentiate into trophectoderm (Andrews et al. 1980, 1982; Damjanov and Andrews 1983). The question therefore existed as to whether human EC cells are equivalent in phenotype to human ICM cells; one notion was that they might reflect an earlier stage of embryonic development (Andrews et al. 1980). However, more recent access to human embryos has now allowed a demonstration that in terms of antigen expression, human EC cells do resemble cells of the human ICM (Henderson et al. 2002), while the surface antigen phenotype of human ES cells closely resembles that of human EC cells (Draper et al. 2002). Evidently, the differences between human and mouse EC and ES cells reflects differences between the embryology of these species (Figure 1).

Human EC cells possess a very similar gene expression profile to human ES cells (Sperger et al. 2003), and so a gene knockdown or overexpression may be expected to produce a similar phenotype in both types of cell. An example is the transcription factor Oct4, which is required for the maintenance of the undifferentiated state of mouse ES cells; when its expression is lowered, the cells differentiate into trophectoderm (Niwa et al. 2000). Oct4 is also expressed by human EC (Figure 2) and ES cells, so to test whether Oct4 has a similar role in human EC and ES cells we first developed techniques for RNA interference (RNAi) using the 2102Ep and NTERA2 human EC cell lines. In both cases, RNAi knockdown of Oct4 expression resulted in differentiation of the cells (Matin et al. 2004); a similar result was also obtained with human ES cells H7 and H14 (Hay et al. 2004; Matin et al. 2004). In the case of 2102Ep EC cells and human ES cells, as well as two other human EC cell lines, 1777N and TERA1, knockdown of Oct4 expression resulted in the appearance of trophectodermal-like cells (Matin et al. 2004; Andrews et al. 2005), as occurred in mouse ES cells. Thus, the function of Oct4 seems to be similar in both human EC and ES cells, and similar to its function in mouse ES cells. One caveat, however, was provided by the human EC cell line, NTERA2. These EC cells also differentiated in response to Oct4 knockdown, but they did not yield trophectoderm (Matin et al. 2004). This appears to indicate some subtle difference between the NTERA2 cells and other human EC and ES cells, which might reflect their origins from a

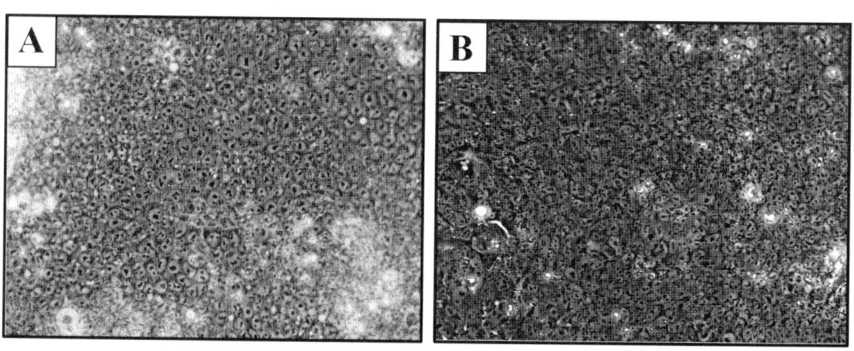

Figure 1. Human EC cells, NTERA2 (**A**), appear morphologically very similar to human cells, Sheff6 (**B**) (Centre for Stem Cell Biology, Sheffield).

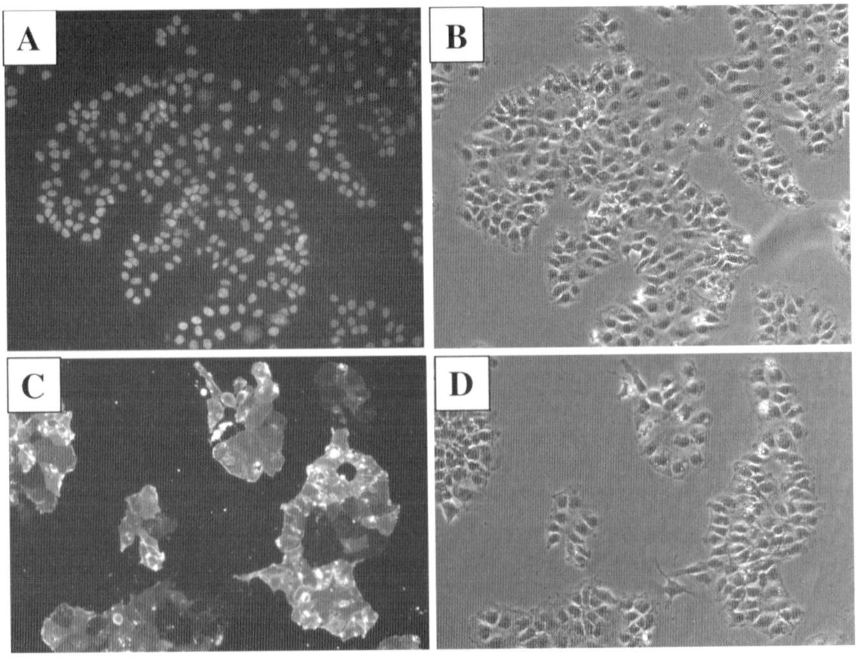

Figure 2. Human EC cells (NTERA2) express markers associated with undifferentiated cells. Oct-4 expression (**A**) is found in the majority of cells, corresponding phase contrast (**B**), while SSEA-3 (**C**) is expressed at variable levels on the majority of cells, corresponding phase contrast (**D**).

tumor, or might reflect some, as yet unknown, aspect of early pluripotent cells in the human embryo. Whatever the cause, the observation does indicate the need for caution in comparing the results of studies between EC and ES cells, notwithstanding their many similarities.

4. HUMAN EC CELLS AND DIFFERENTIATION

Very few human EC cell lines show any significant capacity for differentiation. Several form xenograft tumors in athymic (*nu/nu*) "nude," or SCID mice, and these tumors are typically composed entirely of EC cells, as recognized by histopathologists with experience of human GCT (Andrews et al. 1982). Only a small number of lines have shown significant evidence of differentiation in xenograft tumors with the formation of teratocarcinomas (Andrews et al. 1984; Teshima et al. 1988; Hata et al. 1989; Pera et al. 1989). Of these, perhaps the most widely studied is the TERA2 cell line and particularly its subline NTERA2 (Andrews et al. 1984). Single cell clones of TERA2 and NTERA2 form similar teratocarcinomas, formally confirming the stem cell characteristics of these human EC cells (Andrews et al. 1984; Thompson et al. 1984).

In culture many human EC cell lines show some limited capacity for differentiation when cultured at low-cell densities, while maintaining their EC phenotype if cultured at high cell densities. For example, the human teratocarcinoma cell line 2102Ep is composed of EC cells, and forms xenograft tumors consisting of EC without overt signs of differentiation (Andrews et al. 1982). In culture, the cells retain an EC phenotype expressing marker antigens such as SSEA3 (Figure 2), SSEA4, and TRA-1–60 if they are plated at high cell densities (>65,000 cells per cm^2), whereas, if cultures are plated at much lower densities (~1,500 cells per cm^2), a significant number of the cells adopt a markedly different morphology, being much larger and flatter than typical EC cells, and express the surface antigen SSEA1, which is absent from human EC cells. These SSEA1(+) cells synthesize fibronectin, which is not produced by the undifferentiated EC cells (Andrews 1982), and low-density cultures produce trophoblastic giant cells (Damjanov and Andrews 1983).

Although limited differentiation of this type may be commonly seen in human EC cell lines, few lines show strong evidence of substantial somatic differentiation *in vitro*. One line, GCT27, must be cultured on feeder cells to maintain its undifferentiated state, and will differentiate in the absence of feeders in a way similar to ES cells (Pera et al. 1989). Some other lines have been reported to differentiate in response to specific inducers, e.g., NTERA2 and NCCIT which respond to retinoic acid (Andrews 1984; Damjanov 1993a, b).

NTERA2 was a subline of TERA2 recovered from a xenograft tumor of TERA2 produced in an athymic (*nu*/*nu*) mouse (Andrews et al. 1984). NTERA2 itself was originally derived from a lung metastasis, in a young man with testicular cancer (Fogh and Trempe 1975). Clonal sublines of NTERA2 were then produced by micromanipulation of single cells; a number of such single cell clones were derived, notably NTERA2 cl.D1 (abbreviated NT2/D1) which has been widely used by various investigators. Like TERA2 itself, these single-cell cloned lines produce xenograft tumors with the features of teratocarcinomas and a wide variety of tissue types as well as undifferentiated stem cells. In culture these cells differentiate in response to several inducers, most notably all-trans retinoic acid (Andrews 1984), hexamethylene bis-acetamide (HMBA) (Andrews et al. 1986, 1990), BUdR (Andrews et al. 1986), and bone morphogenetic protein-7 (BMP7) (Andrews et al. 1994). These agents also induce differentiation of human ES cells (Draper et al. 2002; Xu et al. 2002; zur Nieden et al. 2005). The need for controlling BMP signaling in the maintenance of undifferentiated human ES cells remains to be clarified (Hovatta et al. 2003; Xu et al. 2005).

In response to retinoic acid, almost all cells in a culture of NTERA2 differentiate, rapidly losing expression of markers of the undifferentiated state, notably the surface antigens SSEA3, SSEA4, and TRA-1-60, and acquiring expression of other surface antigen markers, particularly ganglioside-associated antigens (Fenderson et al. 1987). Neurons are prominent amongst the differentiated derivatives but represent only a small proportion of the total differentiated cell population, which are mostly uncharacterised. Studies of sublines of retinoic acid-resistant NTERA2 cells have suggested that retinoic acid acts primarily through the retinoic acid receptor gamma (RARγ) (Moasser et al. 1994).

The Notch and Wnt families, two sets of genes that play a role in controlling proliferation and differentiation in a variety of stem cell systems, for example in neural differentiation system (Ciani and Salinas 2005; Yoon and Gaiano 2005), are expressed in undifferentiated EC and ES cells and during their differentiation (Walsh and Andrews 2003). However, one noticeable difference between NTERA2 and various human ES cells is the absence of *Wnt-1* expression in NTERA2 EC cells. In fact, Wnt signaling appears to drive differentiation of EC cells as demonstrated by the differentiation of P19 mouse EC cells when Wnt-1 is overexpressed (Tang et al. 2002). Whether perturbation of Wnt signaling in human EC cells has comparable effects, is as yet unknown. Several members of the Notch receptor family (*Notch-1*, *-2*, *-3*) and their ligands (*Delta1*, *Jagged1*) are expressed by human EC cells (Walsh and Andrews 2003). Our initial data indicate a requirement of Notch signaling for maintenance and proliferation of undifferentiated human EC cells, which might in part account for their requirement for a high cell density and, most likely homotypic cell:cell contact to maintain their undifferentiated state (Andrews et al. 1982, 1984). During the differentiation of NTERA2 cells there are marked changes in the expression of members of the Notch and Wnt signaling pathways, particularly with strong upregulation of one *Wnt* gene, *Wnt2b*, soon after exposure to retinoic acid (Wakeman et al. 1998; Walsh and Andrews 2003). It seems likely that regulation of these genes contributes to lineage selection once differentiation is initiated.

One notable feature of retinoic acid induced differentiation of NTERA2 cells is the induction of *Hox* gene expression (Mavilio et al. 1988). Further studies of NTERA2 cells revealed for the first time that retinoic acid induces *Hox* gene expression in a concentration and time-dependent manner that relates to the position of the individual genes in the *Hox* clusters, high concentrations being required for induction of the more 5′ located genes (Mavilio et al. 1988; Bottero et al. 1991). During development, the *Hox* genes are differentially expressed in overlapping domains along the anterior–posterior axis of the developing embryo, with the more 5′ genes progressively restricted to more posterior locations, producing a precise Hox code, which if perturbed leads to transformations and alterations of segmental identity (Niederreither et al. 2000; Begemann et al. 2001). Neural cells appear to initially possess an anterior character and then become posteriorized in response to posteriorizing signals (Slack and Tannahill 1992). An important aspect of posteriorization is the transcriptional activation of the appropriate *Hox* genes, which subsequently regulate downstream genes that influence a cell's path of development and its ultimate differentiated phenotype. The identification of functional retinoic acid response elements (RAREs) within *Hox* gene regulatory regions suggests that retinoic acid directly mediates *Hox* gene expression (Studer et al. 1994; Dupe et al. 1997). Together these observations suggest that high concentrations of retinoic acid-mediated differentiation of EC cells bias neuronal phenotypes toward posterior fates. Indeed, posteriorization of cell phenotype by retinoic acid has been demonstrated in mouse ES cells (Wichterle et al. 2002; Irioka et al. 2005).

Like retinoic acid, BUdR also induces neural differentiation (Andrews et al. 1990), but this has been little studied. By contrast HMBA and BMP largely induce nonneural lineages, and the patterns of marker antigen induced are quite distinct, especially in response to BMP (Andrews et al. 1990, 1994; Qualtrough 1998). Four members of the BMP family (BMP2, 4, 6, and 7) all induce differentiation of NTERA2 cells, but with different levels of effectiveness, BMP7 being most effective. The observed pattern of differentiation is quite distinct to that observed with retinoic acid, in terms of cell surface antigen expression and cell morphology, and is especially marked by the induction of α–Smooth Muscle actin, which is not normally expressed in retinoic acid treated cells (Qualtrough 1998).

The reasons why most human EC cell lines fail to differentiate in response to agents like retinoic acid or BMP is largely unknown. In one study it was observed that hybrids between NTERA2 (pluripotent) EC and 2102Ep (nullipotent) EC cells, retained the ability to differentiate in response to retinoic acid, although they exhibited little or no ability to produce neurons (Duran et al. 2001; Bahrami et al. 2005). At the same time, the 2102Ep cells expressed RARγ, and responded to retinoic acid by induction of RARβ, though without differentiation. Thus the reasons for 2102Ep nullipotency are complex: evidently the retinoic acid response machinery is present, while the ability of the hybrid cells to differentiate implies that the 2102Ep cells have lost expression of some key component required for differentiation. Nevertheless, the absence of neural differentiation in the hybrids also suggests that the 2102Ep cells have acquired expression of a specific factor capable of inhibiting that particular pathway.

5. MODELS OF NEURONAL DIFFERENTIATION

EC cells satisfy some of the criteria required of a cell line that is to be used for studying neuronal differentiation. EC cells divide rapidly, are susceptible to transfection and are able to terminally differentiate to yield a multitude of cell types.

Unlike human ES cell lines, not all human EC cell lines behave in the same way and consequently particular cell lines have become favorites for specific lines of research. The NTERA2 cell line has been frequently studied with relation to neural differentiation, primarily because upon retinoic acid exposure it reliably yields post-mitotic neurons (Figure 3), which develop elaborate neurite processes similar to those produced by primary neurons in culture (Pleasure et al. 1992). It is primarily for this reason that the NTERA2 clone D1 line is the most widely characterized human EC cell line (Andrews 1984).

A classic inducer of EC cell differentiation (Strickland and Mahdavi 1978), exposure of NTERA2 cells to retinoic acid, causes a rapid loss of stem cell marker expression (Oct4, SSEA3, TRA-1-60 etc) which is replaced by the

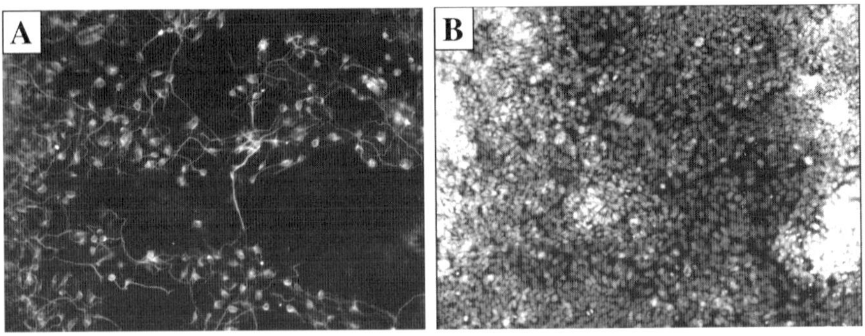

Figure 3. Neuronally differentiated NTERA2 EC cells. TUJ1 positive cells (**A**) possess a polarized morphology. Nuclear stain (**B**) of the same field, Hoechst.

expression of ganglioside surface antigens (Fenderson et al. 1987) and characteristic neural markers (neuroD, B-III tubulin and neurofilaments) (Andrews 1984; Pleasure et al. 1992; Przyborski et al. 2000). As NTERA2 EC cells progress from a pluripotent ground state toward a mature neuron they recapitulate *in vivo* development, expressing a succession of characteristic neural markers (Przyborski et al. 2003). By following a four-week treatment of retinoic acid with successive replating in the presence of mitotic inhibitors it is possible to isolate a pure population of neurons (Leypoldt et al. 2001). These NTERA2-derived neurons have been extensively analyzed and it appears that they are functionally mature, to the extent that they express a variety of neurotransmitter phenotypes (catecholinergic, cholinergic, GABAergic and serotonergic)(Guillemain et al. 2000) and form functional synapses (Hartley et al. 1999).

Serum free conditions have proven to be permissive for neuronal differentiation of murine and human, ES and EC cells (Okabe et al. 1996; Zhang et al. 2001). Using serum free media and cell aggregation, conditions originally utilized to maintain neural stem cells as "neurospheres"(Carpenter et al. 1999), derivatives of NTERA2 exhibiting characteristics of radial glial cells (BLBP, Pax6 and 3CB2 expression) have been obtained (Marchal-Victorion et al. 2003). Use of these conditions significantly boosts the number of NTERA2 neurons yielded from about 5% to over 30%. Efforts to drive neural differentiation efficiently have also produced protocols utilizing the coculture of undifferentiated cells with other cell lines (Kawasaki et al. 2000; Saporta et al. 2004), although the neuralizing factors produced by those cells remain unidentified.

In contrast to human ES and mouse EC cells, NTERA2 cells unexpectedly do not express *Sox1* although they do express *Sox2* (Stevanovic 2003). Sox1 is a transcription factor that is expressed along the entire anteroposterior axis of the mouse neural tube (Pevny et al. 1998), within dividing neuroepithelial cells. Differentiating mouse P19 EC cells express *Sox1*, while the overexpression of *Sox1* in undifferentiated P19 EC cells imparts a neural fate without the requirement of RA (Pevny et al. 1998). Whether the ability of NTERA2 cells to differentiate into neurons in the absence of *Sox1* expression represents some aberration due to its tumor origins, or whether NTERA2 cells represent some specific physiological aspect of human neural stem cells, as yet unrecognized *in vivo*, remains unknown. In NTERA2 cells there may well be functional redundancy of the *Sox* genes, as another *SoxB* family transcription factor, *Sox3* is greatly up regulated upon retinoic acid treatment (Stevanovic 2003).

Astrocytic cells have been reported from retinoic acid differentiated NTERA2 cells and it is thought that they arise after the initial phase of neuronal generation (Bani-Yaghoub et al. 1999), as is observed during *in vivo* development (Jacobson 1991). In addition, cells expressing markers of the oligodendrocytic lineage (GalC and CNPase) can be found in cultures but only in very low numbers (Ferrari et al. 2000; Marchal-Victorion et al. 2003). The few oligodendrocytes that are found can either be due to a lack of appropriate conditions required for oligodendrocyte production, or a reduced potential to give rise to oligodendrocytes. In contrast to NTERA2, human ES cells possess the ability to efficiently yield oligodendrocytes and astrocytes (Reubinoff et al. 2001; Zhang et al. 2001), as expected with their superior differentiation potential.

Cell aggregation is a familiar method for differentiating human EC and ES cells. The use of cell aggregation to induce the differentiation of mouse EC cells was first utilized by Martin and Evans (1975). Since then, cell aggregation has been incorporated in differentiation protocols for many EC (F9, P19 and NTERA2) and ES cell lines. The benefit of using cell aggregation most likely derives from increased cell contacts, promoting intercellular signaling, an important aspect of *in vivo* development. Undifferentiated NTERA2 EC cells, like human ES cells, express the connexin 43 protein and, consequently, possess functional gap junctions (Bani-Yaghoub et al. 1997; Wong et al. 2004). Connexins are expressed by neurons, astrocytes and oligodendrocytes and it has been shown, *in vivo*, that neuroblasts and proliferating cells of the ventricular zone are coupled whereas the differentiated neurons are not (Bittman et al. 1997). In NTERA2 cells, connexin 43 expression becomes markedly reduced upon retinoic acid induced differentiation (Bani-Yaghoub et al. 1997). Blockade of gap junction communication with specific inhibitors during differentiation of NTERA2 (and P19) cell differentiation greatly reduces the yield of neurons (Bani-Yaghoub et al. 1997; Bani-Yaghoub et al. 1999). These observations suggest a crucial role for gap junction communication during the intermediate stages of neural differentiation, perhaps being required to maintain the proliferating neuroblasts, and prevent terminal differentiation.

The reliability and ease of neural differentiation upon retinoic acid exposure, and the expression of neuroepithelial markers (nestin) within undifferentiated NTERA2 EC cells raised the suggestion that the cell line is a committed human neuronal precursor cell line which has retained stem cell characteristics (Pleasure and Lee 1993). However, this is certainly not the case: the surface antigen and transcription factor expression profile of NTERA2 EC cells is comparable to that of other undifferentiated human EC and ES cells. Further, extensive nonneural differentiation is evident in xenograft tumors of NTERA2 cells (Andrews et al. 1984) and it is clear that other cell types can be induced by agents such as HMBA and BMP. Even in retinoic acid-induced cultures, the differentiated cells are quite heterogeneous and we have isolated neuronal and nonneural subsets based upon expression of the surface antigen ME311 (absent from the neural lineage (Fenderson et al. 1987)) and have generated neural and nonneural cDNA libraries (Ackerman et al. 1994). The propensity to yield neurons is shared by both human ES cells and pluripotent human EC cells, which is consistent with the notion that neural differentiation represents the default pathway of early ES cells (Hemmati-Brivanlou and Melton 1997; Tropepe et al. 2001).

6. THERAPEUTIC POTENTIAL

Upon transplantation, NTERA2-derived neurons successfully engraft in to the central nervous system (CNS) of rodent models. Neurons derived from the NTERA2 cell line survive more than a year in host rodent brains and improve motor and cognitive impairments in rodent models of ischemic stroke, with no development of cancer (Lee et al. 2000). NTERA2 neurons have also been shown to survive for more than 2 years in the human brain of a stroke patient. Although no improvements to the patient's motor deficits were reported (Nelson et al. 2002), there were no undesired side effects observed, including no formation of malignant tumors. It seems unlikely that the use of highly aneuploid cells derived from a malignant cancer cell line can provide a satisfactory route for routine treatment of patients, but these studies do at least indicate the feasibility of the approach.

Undoubtedly, effective therapy for neurodegenerative diseases requires methods for obtaining particular neuronal phenotypes. Although human ES cells will be the better source for eventual applications, studies with EC cells may nevertheless contribute to the development of techniques. Much current work has focused on the differentiation of dopaminergic neurons, which could be used in the treatment of Parkinson's disease. In fact, the dopaminergic properties of NTERA2-derived neurons have been well documented, as they have been shown to express dopamine receptors (Sodja et al. 2002), DAT (Zigova et al. 2000), to synthesize and release dopamine (Iacovitti et al. 2001) and express the transcription factor, Nurr1 (Misiuta et al. 2003), all features of midbrain dopaminergic neurons. These NTERA2-derived dopaminergic cells have also been shown to be functional with application of the D1 agonist (SKF-81297) resulting in elevated cellular levels of cyclic AMP content, demonstrating viable dopamine receptors (Sodja et al. 2002). Other researchers have similarly succeeded in deriving dopaminergic neurons from human ES cells (Schulz et al. 2004; Park et al. 2005), and in some studies it has been found that the coculture of human ES cells with stromal cells is an efficient technique for driving them along a neural lineage (Kawasaki et al. 2000). Notably, NTERA2 responds in a very similar fashion to human ES cells to differentiation factors secreted by the

PA6 stromal cell line, as both yield dopaminergic neurons expressing TH and TUJ1 under these conditions (Schwartz et al. 2005). Thus, the similarities in response indicate that the simpler NTERA2 system can indeed complement work with human ES cells to develop useful technologies for eventual applications in regenerative medicine.

7. CONCLUSION

Perhaps due to the relative ease with which human EC cells can be maintained, most studies of these cells to date have ignored the analysis of self-renewal mechanisms and instead focused on identifying markers of the stem cells and directing differentiation of the cells. Thus many of the surface antigens currently used to define human ES cells were first characterized by studies in human EC cells (Draper et al. 2002). NTERA2 EC cells have also become a familiar tool for studying neurogenesis and demonstrating the use of novel techniques for cell culture and differentiation. These have included cell growth in reduced gravity environments (Saporta et al. 2004), construction of precise cellular structures utilizing inkjet printers (Xu et al. 2006) and induction of differentiation by novel factors (milk growth factor) (Kanda et al. 2005). Nevertheless, the evident similarities in the mechanisms that control their self-renewal, do mean that human EC cells can remain useful tools in further work to elucidate mechanisms that function to control self-renewal and commitment to differentiation in human ES cells.

Although EC cells are unlikely to provide routine sources of differentiated cells for regenerative medicine, they remain a source of information pertinent to developing the relevant technology for ES cell-based derivation of cells for transplantation. Importantly, a related use of EC and ES cells is likely to be in high-throughput screening for drug discovery and toxicology. For this purpose, human EC cells may offer the distinct advantages that come from their robust and simple growth requirements (no requirements for feeders or expensive growth factors), compared to those needed to maintain and differentiate ES cells.

Whereas EC cells may be expected to provide complementary tools to ES cells for a wide range of eventual applications, from a different perspective, ES cells may provide, perhaps unexpectedly, new insights into EC cells and cancer biology. Teratocarcinomas epitomize the idea that cancers are diseases in which the mechanisms that control the balance between cell differentiation and cell proliferation are perturbed. In these tumors, the EC cells seem to be the cells that are primarily responsible for the malignant characteristics of the tumor, whereas their differentiated derivatives are largely benign in character. A corollary of this view is the notion that EC cells in tumors will be subject to strong selection for genetic variants that limit their ability to differentiate. Thus it is perhaps not surprising that many EC cell lines have indeed limited

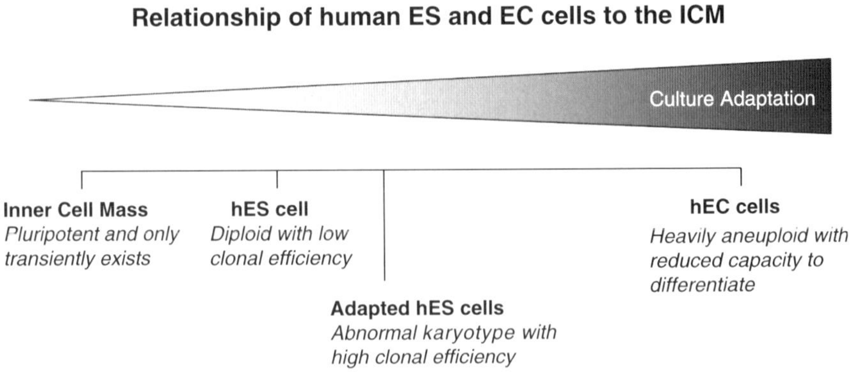

Figure 4. Relationship of human ES and EC cells to the ICM.

capacity for differentiation. Human EC cells are, in fact, highly aneuploid, and include amplifications and deletions of various chromosomal regions (Chaganti et al. 1993; Rosenberg et al. 1999). Of these changes, gain of the chromosomal arm 12p is the most common genetic irregularity in testicular germ cell tumors (Kraggerud et al. 2002), along with copy number increases of 17q (Skotheim et al. 2002) (Figure 4).

Interestingly, human ES cells have also been observed to undergo karyotypic changes, particularly involving the gain of 17q and chromosome 12 (Draper et al. 2004), while mouse ES cells have also been noted to become increasingly aneuploid as time in culture increases, and their aneuploidy is thought to be a major reason why some mES cells fail to contribute to chimeras (Longo et al. 1997). One might imagine then that ES cells in culture are subject to similar selection pressures to EC cells within tumors: like the derivatives of EC cells, the differentiated derivatives of ES cells have a limited life span and their production inevitably limits the ability of undifferentiated ES cells to repopulate a culture after passaging. Consequently, ES cells that acquire genetic changes limiting their differentiation will tend to accumulate over time. That the same karyotypic changes are seen in EC cells from teratocarcinomas and ES cells on prolonged passage supports this view: presumably overexpression of a gene or genes located on these chromosomes can give selective advantages to the undifferentiated stem cell. One consequence of this observation is that while EC cells might be useful complementary tools for the study of ES cell biology, the adaptation of ES cells upon prolonged culture may provide a unique tool for tumor biology, providing insights into the mechanisms that promote tumor progression.

Acknowledgments

We are grateful to many of our colleagues for help and advice. This work was supported in part by grants from the JDRF, the MRC, the BBSRC and Yorkshire Cancer Research.

REFERENCES

Ackerman, S.L., Knowles, B.B., et al. (1994) Gene regulation during neuronal and non-neuronal differentiation of NTERA2 human teratocarcinoma-derived stem cells. Brain Res. Mol. Brain Res., 25(1–2): 157–162.

Andrews, P.W. (1982) Human embryonal carcinoma cells in culture do not synthesize fibronectin until they differentiate. Int. J. Cancer, 30(5): 567–571.

Andrews, P.W. (1984) Retinoic acid induces neuronal differentiation of a cloned human embryonal carcinoma cell line in vitro. Dev. Biol., 103(2): 285–293.

Andrews, P.W. (2002) From teratocarcinomas to embryonic stem cells. Philos. Trans. R. Soc. Lond. B, Biol. Sci., 357: 405–417.

Andrews, P.W., Bronson, D.L., et al. (1980) A comparative study of eight cell lines derived from human testicular teratocarcinoma. Int. J. Cancer, 26(3): 269–280.

Andrews, P.W., Casper, J., et al. (1996) Comparative analysis of cell surface antigens expressed by cell lines derived from human germ cell tumours. Int. J. Cancer, 66(6): 806–816.

Andrews, P.W. and Damjanov, I. (1994) Cells from human germ-cell tumours. In: Atlas of Human Tumor Cell Lines (Eds.: Hay, R.J., Park, J.G., and Gazdar, A.), Academic Press, London, pp. 443–476.

Andrews, P.W., Damjanov, I., et al. (1994) Inhibition of proliferation and induction of differentiation of pluripotent human embryonal carcinoma cells by osteogenic protein-1 (or bone morphogenetic protein-7). Lab Invest., 71(2): 243–251.

Andrews, P.W., Damjanov, I., et al. (1984) Pluripotent embryonal carcinoma clones derived from the human teratocarcinoma cell line Tera-2. Differentiation in vivo and in vitro. Lab Invest., 50(2): 147–162.

Andrews, P.W., Gonczol, E., et al. (1986) Differentiation of TERA-2 human embryonal carcinoma cells into neurons and HCMV permissive cells. Induction by agents other than retinoic acid. Differentiation, 31(2): 119–126.

Andrews, P.W., Goodfellow, P.N., et al. (1982) Cell-surface antigens of a clonal human embryonal carcinoma cell line: morphological and antigenic differentiation in culture. Int. J. Cancer, 29(5): 523–531.

Andrews, P.W., Matin, M.M., et al. (2005) Embryonic stem (ES) cells and embryonal carcinoma (EC) cells: opposite sides of the same coin. Biochem. Soc. Trans., 33(Pt 6): 1526–1530.

Andrews, P.W., Nudelman, E., et al. (1990) Different patterns of glycolipid antigens are expressed following differentiation of TERA-2 human embryonal carcinoma cells induced by retinoic acid, hexamethylene bisacetamide (HMBA) or bromodeoxyuridine (BUdR). Differentiation, 43(2): 131–138.

Bahrami, A.R., Matin, M.M., et al. (2005) The CDK inhibitor p27 enhances neural differentiation in pluripotent NTERA2 human EC cells, but does not permit differentiation of 2102Ep nullipotent human EC cells. Mech. Dev., 122(9): 1034–1042.

Bani-Yaghoub, M., Bechberger, J.F., et al. (1997) Reduction of connexin43 expression and dye-coupling during neuronal differentiation of human NTera2/clone D1 cells. J. Neurosci. Res., 49(1): 19–31.

Bani-Yaghoub, M., Bechberger, J.F., et al. (1999) The effects of gap junction blockage on neuronal differentiation of human NTera2/clone D1 cells. Exp. Neurol., 156(1): 16–32.

Bani-Yaghoub, M., Felker, J.M., et al. (1999) Human NT2/D1 cells differentiate into functional astrocytes. Neuroreport, 10(18): 3843–3846.

Begemann, G., Schilling, T.F., et al. (2001) The zebrafish neckless mutation reveals a requirement for raldh2 in mesodermal signals that pattern the hindbrain. Development, 128(16): 3081–3094.

Bittman, K., Owens, D.F., et al. (1997) Cell coupling and uncoupling in the ventricular zone of developing neocortex. J. Neurosci., 17(18): 7037–7044.

Bottero, L., Simeone, A., et al. (1991) Differential activation of homeobox genes by retinoic acid in human embryonal carcinoma cells. Recent Results Cancer Res., 123: 133–143.

Brinster, R.L. (1974) The effect of cells transferred into the mouse blastocyst on subsequent development. J. Exp. Med., 140(4): 1049–1056.

Carpenter, M.K., Cui, X., et al. (1999) In vitro expansion of a multipotent population of human neural progenitor cells. Exp. Neurol., 158(2): 265–278.

Chaganti, R.S., Rodriguez, E., et al. (1993) Cytogenetics of male germ-cell tumors. Urol. Clin. North Am., 20(1): 55–66.

Ciani, L. and Salinas, P.C. (2005) WNTs in the vertebrate nervous system: from patterning to neuronal connectivity. Nat. Rev. Neurosci., 6(5): 351–362.

Damjanov, I. (1993a) Pathogenesis of testicular germ cell tumours. Eur. Urol., 23(1): 2–5; discussion 6–7.

Damjanov, I. (1993b) Teratocarcinoma: neoplastic lessons about normal embryogenesis. Int. J. Dev. Biol., 37(1): 39–46.

Damjanov, I. and Andrews, P.W. (1983) Ultrastructural differentiation of a clonal human embryonal carcinoma cell line in vitro. Cancer Res., 43(5): 2190–2198.

Damjanov, I. and Solter, D. (1974) Experimental teratoma. Curr. Top. Pathol., 59: 69–130.

Draper, J.S., Pigott, C., et al. (2002) Surface antigens of human embryonic stem cells: changes upon differentiation in culture. J. Anat., 200(Pt 3): 249–258.

Draper, J.S., Smith, K., et al. (2004) Recurrent gain of chromosomes 17q and 12 in cultured human embryonic stem cells. Nat. Biotechnol., 22(1): 53–54.

Dupe, V., Davenne, M., et al. (1997) In vivo functional analysis of the Hoxa-1 3′ retinoic acid response element (3′RARE). Development, 124(2): 399–410.

Duran, C., Talley, P.J., et al. (2001) Hybrids of pluripotent and nullipotent human embryonal carcinoma cells: partial retention of a pluripotent phenotype. Int. J. Cancer, 93(3): 324–332.

Evans, M.J. and Kaufman, M.H. (1981) Establishment in culture of pluripotential cells from mouse embryos. Nature, 292: 154–156.

Fenderson, B.A., Andrews, P.W., et al. (1987) Glycolipid core structure switching from globo- to lacto- and ganglio-series during retinoic acid-induced differentiation of TERA-2-derived human embryonal carcinoma cells. Dev. Biol., 122(1): 21–34.

Ferrari, A., Ehler, E., et al. (2000) Immature human NT2 cells grafted into mouse brain differentiate into neuronal and glial cell types. FEBS Lett., 486(2): 121–125.

Finch, B.W. and Ephrussi, B. (1967) Retention of multiple developmental potentialities by cells of a mouse testicular teratocarcinoma during prolonged culture in vitro and their extinction upon hybridization with cells of permanent lines. Proc. Natl. Acad. Sci. USA, 57(3): 615–621.

Fogh, J. and Trempe, G. (1975) New human tumor cell lines. In: Human Tumor Cells In Vitro (Eds. Fogh, J.). Plenum Press, NY, pp. 115–159.

Guillemain, I., Alonso, G., et al. (2000) Human NT2 neurons express a large variety of neurotransmission phenotypes in vitro. J. Comp. Neurol., 422(3): 380–395.

Hartley, R.S., Margulis, M., et al. (1999) Functional synapses are formed between human NTera2 (NT2N, hNT) neurons grown on astrocytes. J. Comp. Neurol., 407(1): 1–10.

Hata, J., Fujita, H., et al. (1989) [Differentiation of human germ cell tumor cells]. Hum. Cell, 2(4): 382–387.

Hay, D.C., Sutherland, L., et al. (2004) Oct-4 knockdown induces similar patterns of endoderm and trophoblast differentiation markers in human and mouse embryonic stem cells. Stem Cells, 22(2): 225–235.

Hemmati-Brivanlou, A. and Melton, D. (1997) Vertebrate embryonic cells will become nerve cells unless told otherwise. Cell, 88(1): 13–17.

Henderson, J.K., Draper, J.S., et al. (2002) Preimplantation human embryos and embryonic stem cells show comparable expression of stage-specific embryonic antigens. Stem Cells, 20(4): 329–337.

Hogan, B., Fellous, M., et al. (1977) Isolation of a human teratoma cell line which expresses F9 antigen. Nature, 270(5637): 515–518.

Holden, S., Bernard, O., et al. (1977) Human and mouse embryonal carcinoma cells in culture share an embryonic antigen (F9). Nature, 270(5637): 518–520.

Hovatta, O., Mikkola, M., et al. (2003) A culture system using human foreskin fibroblasts as feeder cells allows production of human embryonic stem cells. Hum. Reprod., 18(7): 1404–1409.

Iacovitti, L., Stull, N.D., et al. (2001) Differentiation of human dopamine neurons from an embryonic carcinomal stem cell line. Brain Res., 912(1): 99–104.

Irioka, T., Watanabe, K., et al. (2005) Distinct effects of caudalizing factors on regional specification of embryonic stem cell-derived neural precursors. Brain Res. Dev. Brain Res., 154(1): 63–70.

Jacob, F. (1978) The Leeuwenhoek lecture, 1977. Mouse teratocarcinoma and mouse embryo. Proc. R. Soc. Lond. B. Biol. Sci., 201(1144): 249–270.

Jakob, H., Boon, T., et al. (1973) [Teratocarcinoma of the mouse: isolation, culture and properties of pluripotential cells]. Ann. Microbiol. (Paris), 124(3): 269–282.

Jacobson, M. (1991) Developmantal Neurobiology. Plenum press, New York.

Kahan, B.W. and Ephrussi, B. (1970) Developmental potentialities of clonal in vitro cultures of mouse testicular teratoma. J. Natl. Cancer Inst., 44(5): 1015–1036.

Kanda, Y., Katsura, K., et al. (2005) Milk growth factor (MGF)-induced differentiation of NT2/D1 cells. Neurosci. Lett., 384(3): 260–264.

Kannagi, R., Cochran, N.A., et al. (1983) Stage-specific embryonic antigens (SSEA-3 and -4) are epitopes of a unique globo-series ganglioside isolated from human teratocarcinoma cells. EMBO J., 2(12): 2355–2361.

Kawasaki, H., Mizuseki, K., et al. (2000) Induction of midbrain dopaminergic neurons from ES cells by stromal cell-derived inducing activity. Neuron, 28(1): 31–40.

Kleinsmith, L.J. and Pierce, G.B., Jr. (1964) Multipotentiality of single embryonal carcinoma cells. Cancer Res., 24: 1544–1551.

Knowles, B.B., Aden, D.P., et al. (1978) Monoclonal antibody detecting a stage-specific embryonic antigen (SSEA-1) on preimplantation mouse embryos and teratocarcinoma cells. Curr. Top. Microbiol. Immunol., 81: 51–53.

Kraggerud, S.M., Skotheim, R.I., et al. (2002) Genome profiles of familial/bilateral and sporadic testicular germ cell tumors. Genes Chromosomes Cancer, 34(2): 168–174.

Lee, V.M., Hartley, R.S., et al. (2000) Neurobiology of human neurons (NT2N) grafted into mouse spinal cord: implications for improving therapy of spinal cord injury. Prog. Brain Res., 128: 299–307.

Leypoldt, F., Lewerenz, J., et al. (2001) Identification of genes up-regulated by retinoic-acid-induced differentiation of the human neuronal precursor cell line NTERA-2 cl.D1. J. Neurochem., 76(3): 806–814.

Longo, L., Bygrave, A., et al. (1997) The chromosome make-up of mouse embryonic stem cells is predictive of somatic and germ cell chimaerism. Transgenic Res., 6(5): 321–328.

Marchal-Victorion, S., Deleyrolle, L., et al. (2003) The human NTERA2 neural cell line generates neurons on growth under neural stem cell conditions and exhibits characteristics of radial glial cells. Mol. Cell Neurosci., 24(1): 198–213.

Martin, G.R. (1981) Isolation of a pluripotent cell line from early mouse embryos cultured in medium conditioned by teratocarcinoma stem cells. Proc. Natl. Acad. Sci. USA, 78: 7634–7636.

Martin, G.R. and Evans, M.J. (1974) The morphology and growth of a pluripotent teratocarcinoma cell line and its derivatives in tissue culture. Cell, 2(3): 163–172.

Martin, G.R. and Evans, M.J. (1975) Differentiation of clonal lines of teratocarcinomas cells: formation of embryoid bodies in vitro. Proc. Natl. Acad. Sci. USA, 72: 1441–1445.

Matin, M.M., Walsh, J.R., et al. (2004) Specific knockdown of Oct4 and beta2-microglobulin expression by RNA interference in human embryonic stem cells and embryonic carcinoma cells. Stem Cells, 22(5): 659–668.

Mavilio, F., Simeone, A., et al. (1988) Activation of four homeobox gene clusters in human embryonal carcinoma cells induced to differentiate by retinoic acid. Differentiation, 37(1): 73–79.
Mintz, B. and Illmensee, K. (1975) Normal genetically mosaic mice produced from malignant teratocarcinoma cells. Proc. Natl. Acad. Sci. USA, 72(9): 3585–3589.
Misiuta, I.E., Anderson, L., et al. (2003) The transcription factor Nurr1 in human NT2 cells and hNT neurons. Brain Res. Dev. Brain Res., 145(1): 107–115.
Moasser, M.M., DeBlasio, A., et al. (1994) Response and resistance to retinoic acid are mediated through the retinoic acid nuclear receptor gamma in human teratocarcinomas. Oncogene, 9(3): 833–840.
Nelson, P.T., Kondziolka, D., et al. (2002) Clonal human (hNT) neuron grafts for stroke therapy: neuropathology in a patient 27 months after implantation. Am. J. Pathol., 160(4): 1201–1206.
Nicolas, J.F., Dubois, P., et al. (1975) [Mouse teratocarcinoma: differentiation in cultures of a multipotential primitive cell line]. Ann. Microbiol. (Paris), 126(1): 3–22.
Niederreither, K., Vermot, J., et al. (2000) Retinoic acid synthesis and hindbrain patterning in the mouse embryo. Development, 127(1): 75–85.
Niwa, H., Miyazaki, J., et al. (2000) Quantitative expression of Oct-3/4 defines differentiation, dedifferentiation or self-renewal of ES cells. Nat. Genet., 24(4): 372–376.
Okabe, S., Forsberg-Nilsson, K., et al. (1996) Development of neuronal precursor cells and functional postmitotic neurons from embryonic stem cells in vitro. Mech. Dev. 59(1): 89–102.
Papaioannou, V.E., McBurney, M.W., et al. (1975) Fate of teratocarcinoma cells injected into early mouse embryos. Nature, 258(5530): 70–73.
Park, C.H., Minn, Y.K., et al. (2005) In vitro and in vivo analyses of human embryonic stem cell-derived dopamine neurons. J. Neurochem., 92(5): 1265–1276.
Pera, M.F., Cooper, S., et al. (1989) Isolation and characterization of a multipotent clone of human embryonal carcinoma cells. Differentiation, 42(1): 10–23.
Pevny, L.H., Sockanathan, S., et al. (1998) A role for SOX1 in neural determination. Development, 125(10): 1967–1978.
Pierce, G.B. (1975) Teratocarcinomas: introduction and perspectives. In: Teratomas and Differentiation (Ed.: Sherman, M.I. and Solter, D.) Academic Press, New York, pp. 3–12.
Pleasure, S.J. and Lee, V. M. (1993) NTera 2 cells: a human cell line which displays characteristics expected of a human committed neuronal progenitor cell. J. Neurosci. Res., 35(6): 585–602.
Pleasure, S.J., Page, C., et al. (1992) Pure, postmitotic, polarized human neurons derived from NTera 2 cells provide a system for expressing exogenous proteins in terminally differentiated neurons. J. Neurosci., 12(5): 1802–1815.
Przyborski, S.A., Morton, I.E., et al. (2000) Developmental regulation of neurogenesis in the pluripotent human embryonal carcinoma cell line NTERA-2. Eur. J. Neurosci., 12(10): 3521–3528.
Przyborski, S.A., Smith, S., et al. (2003) Transcriptional profiling of neuronal differentiation by human embryonal carcinoma stem cells in vitro. Stem Cells, 21(4): 459–471.
Qualtrough, J.D. (1998) Bone Morphogenetic Proteins in Human Embryonal Carcinoma Cells. Thesis. Sheffield University Library.
Reubinoff, B.E., Itsykson, P., et al. (2001) Neural progenitors from human embryonic stem cells. Nat. Biotechnol., 19(12): 1134–1140.
Reubinoff, B.E., Pera, M.F., et al. (2000) Embryonic stem cell lines from human blastocysts: somatic differentiation in vitro. Nat. Biotechnol., 18(4): 399–404.
Rosenberg, C., Schut, T.B., et al. (1999) Chromosomal gains and losses in testicular germ cell tumors of adolescents and adults investigated by a modified comparative genomic hybridization approach. Lab. Invest., 79(12): 1447–1451.
Saporta, S., Willing, A.E., et al. (2004) Rapid differentiation of NT2 cells in Sertoli-NT2 cell tissue constructs grown in the rotating wall bioreactor. Brain Res. Bull., 64(4): 347–356.
Schulz, T.C., Noggle, S.A., et al. (2004) Differentiation of human embryonic stem cells to dopaminergic neurons in serum-free suspension culture. Stem Cells, 22(7): 1218–1238.

Schwartz, C.M., Spivak, C.E., et al. (2005) NTera2: a model system to study dopaminergic differentiation of human embryonic stem cells. Stem Cells Dev., 14(5): 517–534.

Shevinsky, L.H., Knowles, B.B., et al. (1982) Monoclonal antibody to murine embryos defines a stage-specific embryonic antigen expressed on mouse embryos and human teratocarcinoma cells. Cell, 30(3): 697–705.

Skakkebaek, N.E. (1972) Possible carcinoma-in-situ of the testis. Lancet, 2(7776): 516–517.

Skakkebaek, N.E., Berthelsen, J.G., et al. (1987) Carcinoma-in-situ of the testis: possible origin from gonocytes and precursor of all types of germ cell tumours except spermatocytoma. Int. J. Androl., 10(1): 19–28.

Skotheim, R.I., Monni, O., et al. (2002) New insights into testicular germ cell tumorigenesis from gene expression profiling. Cancer Res., 62(8): 2359–2364.

Slack, J.M. and Tannahill, D. (1992) Mechanism of anteroposterior axis specification in vertebrates. Lessons from the amphibians. Development, 114(2): 285–302.

Sodja, C., Fang, H., et al. (2002) Identification of functional dopamine receptors in human teratocarcinoma NT2 cells. Brain Res. Mol. Brain Res., 99(2): 83–91.

Solter, D. and Knowles, B.B. (1978) Monoclonal antibody defining a stage-specific mouse embryonic antigen (SSEA-1). Proc. Natl. Acad. Sci. USA, 75(11): 5565–5569.

Sperger, J.M., Chen, X., et al. (2003) Gene expression patterns in human embryonic stem cells and human pluripotent germ cell tumors. Proc. Natl. Acad. Sci. USA, 100(23): 13350–13355.

Stevanovic, M. (2003) Modulation of SOX2 and SOX3 gene expression during differentiation of human neuronal precursor cell line NTERA2. Mol. Biol. Rep., 30(2): 127–132.

Stevens, L.C. (1967) Origin of testicular teratomas from primordial germ cells in mice. J. Natl. Cancer Inst., 38(4): 549–552.

Stevens, L.C. and Little, C.C. (1954) Spontaneous testicular teratomas in an inbred strain of mice. Proc. Natl. Acad. Sci. USA, 40(11): 1080–1087.

Strickland, S. and Mahdavi, V. (1978) The induction of differentiation in teratocarcinoma stem cells by retinoic acid. Cell, 15(2): 393–403.

Studer, M., Popperl, H., et al. (1994) Role of a conserved retinoic acid response element in rhombomere restriction of Hoxb-1. Science, 265(5179): 1728–1732.

Tang, K., Yang, J., et al. (2002) Wnt-1 promotes neuronal differentiation and inhibits gliogenesis in P19 cells. Biochem. Biophys. Res. Commun., 293(1): 167–173.

Teshima, S., Shimosato, Y., et al. (1988) Four new human germ cell tumor cell lines. Lab. Invest., 59(3): 328–336.

Thompson, S., Stern, P.L., et al. (1984) Cloned human teratoma cells differentiate into neuron-like cells and other cell types in retinoic acid. J. Cell Sci., 72: 37–64.

Thomson, J.A., Itskovitz-Eldor, J., et al. (1998) Embryonic stem cell lines derived from human blastocysts. Science, 282(5391): 1145–1147.

Tropepe, V., Hitoshi, S., et al. (2001) Direct neural fate specification from embryonic stem cells: a primitive mammalian neural stem cell stage acquired through a default mechanism. Neuron, 30(1): 65–78.

Wakeman, J.A., Walsh, J., et al. (1998) Human Wnt-13 is developmentally regulated during the differentiation of NTERA-2 pluripotent human embryonal carcinoma cells. Oncogene, 17(2): 179–186.

Walsh, J. and Andrews, P.W. (2003) Expression of Wnt and Notch pathway genes in a pluripotent human embryonal carcinoma cell line and embryonic stem cell. APMIS, 111(1): 197–210; discussion 210–211.

Wheeler, J.E. (1983) History of teratomas. In: The Human Teratomas: Experimental and Clinical Biology (Ed.: Damjanov, I., Knowles, B.B., and Solter, D.), Humana Press, Clifton, NJ, pp. 1–22.

Wichterle, H., Lieberam, I., et al. (2002) Directed differentiation of embryonic stem cells into motor neurons. Cell, 110(3): 385–397.

Wong, R.C., Pebay, A., et al. (2004) Presence of functional gap junctions in human embryonic stem cells. Stem Cells, 22(6): 883–889.

Xu, R.H., Chen, X., et al. (2002) BMP4 initiates human embryonic stem cell differentiation to trophoblast. Nat. Biotechnol., 20(12): 1261–1264.

Xu, R.H., Peck, R.M., et al. (2005) Basic FGF and suppression of BMP signaling sustain undifferentiated proliferation of human ES cells. Nat. Methods, 2(3): 185–190.

Xu, T., Gregory, C.A., et al. (2006) Viability and electrophysiology of neural cell structures generated by the inkjet printing method. Biomaterials, 27(19): 4181–4186.

Yoon, K. and Gaiano, N. (2005) Notch signaling in the mammalian central nervous system: insights from mouse mutants. Nat. Neurosci., 8(6): 709–715.

Zhang, S.C., Wernig, M., et al. (2001) In vitro differentiation of transplantable neural precursors from human embryonic stem cells. Nat. Biotechnol., 19(12): 1129–1133.

Zigova, T., Barroso, L.F., et al. (2000) Dopaminergic phenotype of hNT cells in vitro. Brain Res. Dev. Brain Res., 122(1): 87–90.

zur Nieden, N.I., Kempka, G., et al. (2005) Induction of chondro-, osteo- and adipogenesis in embryonic stem cells by bone morphogenetic protein-2: effect of cofactors on differentiating lineages. BMC Dev. Biol., 5(1): 1.

CHAPTER 14

QUALITY CONTROL OF HUMAN STEM CELL LINES

GLYN N. STACEY

The UK Stem Cell Bank, Division of Cell Biology and Imaging National Institute for Biological Standards and Control, South Mimms, Herts, UK

1. CHALLENGES IN CELL CULTURE

Cell culture-based methodologies clearly have a significant and expanding role in research and also in the manufacture and testing of new biological medicines. However, it is vitally important to remember that cell cultures are prone to a number of effects and variables not found in well-defined laboratory reagents (Stacey 2002). In cell culture there are inherent risks of genetic and phenotypic instability, cross-contamination, and microbial contamination that could invalidate experimental data. Furthermore, cell cultures need constant and careful attention to ensure that the cells used in experimental work perform consistently and provide reliable results. These challenges are especially critical in the case of stem cell lines which means that quality control of stem cell lines is essential for high-quality stem cell research. Quality control strategies to ensure best practice and reliable data from human stem cell lines will be the subject of the following sections.

2. PERCEPTIONS OF QUALITY

The term "quality" is sometimes interpreted to mean the highest grade achievable, however, a more pragmatic and practical approach is to relate quality in cell culture to the standard required for a particular intended use, i.e., it must be "fit for purpose" (Stacey and Phillips 1999). For stem cell lines the principle of fitness for purpose is a useful notion as it draws attention to the needs and expectations of the final users and the different applications they have for the cells. Clearly there will be significant differences between the users carrying out basic research and those developing therapies at the level of clinical trials where the culture history, precise conditions of derivation, and records of the banking process, environment and safety testing will all be critical (Cobo et al. 2005; Healy et al. 2005).

J.R. Masters et al (eds.), Embryonic Stem Cells, 255–276.

Quality control refers to a series of checks and tests performed at different points in any process to ensure that an acceptable product arises from the process. However, quality control is only part of overall quality assurance for cell lines which includes:

- Evaluation and quality control measures for cells and critical reagents coming into the laboratory
- Control of the laboratory environment, equipment and procedures
- Control of data arising from cell culture
- Control of the delivery of research materials, including cells, to other laboratories (Stacey 2004)

For human stem cell lines there are certain core quality criteria to address for general biomedical research purposes and these will be the focus for this review of quality control issues and methods.

3. FUNDAMENTAL ELEMENTS OF QUALITY CONTROL FOR STEM CELL LINES

There are some central key issues for quality control which are consistent for all cell cultures including cultures of bacteria, fungi, algae, and animal cell lines (e.g., WFCC 1999). These can be assimilated into three critical characteristics of cell cultures that are fundamental to assure the quality of any cell culture work:

- Identity, i.e., the cells are what they are purported to be
- Purity, i.e., freedom from microbiological contamination
- Stability on growth or passage *in vitro*

The following sections will explore how quality control procedures for stem cell lines help to deliver these fundamental criteria and also maintain the key characteristics of stem cell lines.

4. CELL CHARACTERISATION

4.1 Phenotypic Characterisation Using Antibody Markers

Since the original publication on the isolation of human embryonic stem (hES) cell lines (Thomson et al. 1998), variations of the methodology have arisen in different laboratories, including the method of a cell line's derivation, its maintenance, and subculture. This variation has raised questions about whether the hES lines so far derived all have the same characteristics and what might be the critical common features of hES cells. Some central issues for standardisation and characterisation of hES cells have been developed (Loring and Rao 2006), drawing on published data and experience with a cross section of the available hES lines. The conclusion is that an hES cell line should express certain phenoptypic markers including OCT-4, Nanog, SSEA-3, SSEA-4, TRA-1-81, TRA 160 and alkaline phosphatase and, unlike mouse embryonic stem (ES) cells, should be negative for SSEA-1. The expression of these markers is consistent with that seen in embryonal carcinoma cell lines which appear to be the malignant equivalent of hES cells and which were used to develop a range of antibodies now used to characterise hES cells (Pera et al. 2000; Andrews et al. 2001; Draper et al. 2002). In general the markers identify an undifferentiated state in the culture and when differentiation occurs the presence of certain antigens is altered and notably OCT-4 (which is associated with the ability of an hES cell to self-renew) is lost and changes in the glycosylated state of the SSEA-associated glycoprotein give rise to altered levels of reaction with the anti-SSEA antibodies.

In reality hES cultures often contain a proportion of differentiated cells which will vary to some degree from one time point in culture to another. Whilst much work has been done to try to elucidate the key molecules and pathways involved in maintaining the undifferentiated hES cell state, the full range of effects that subtle differences in culture conditions and cell passaging procedures might have on stem cell cultures has yet to be determined. Careful monitoring of the phenotype of stem cell lines is therefore an important control for experimental work and is most commonly achieved by flow cytometry, although immunohistology of cells provides additional useful information on location of positive cells within hES cell colonies and subcellular location of antibody reactivity.

Flow cytometric methods may vary significantly between different centres and comparisons of such data should take into consideration the instrument set-up and method of quantifying fluorescence. It is important to establish appropriate positive and negative controls in both flow cytometry and immunocytochemistry experiments to exclude non-specific cross-reactions (e.g., known positive controls, anti-mouse antibody negative control). It is also wise to check new sources or new batches of antibody to check isotype, titre, and specificity. The embryonal carcinoma cell line 2102Ep, selected for its stability in culture, can be cultured and tested in parallel with hES cells and has been adopted in this way as a reference cell line in an international collaborative project on hES cell characterisation (Andrews et al. 2005). Centrally prepared stocks of this cell line distributed to participants in the project have been used to provide data in parallel with local hES cell lines as a generic control for phenotypic marker flow cytometry studies. Bone marrow stem cell fixed cell preparations, which have good stability at room temperature, have been trialled for standardisation of haematopoietic stem cell quantitation (Edwards et al. 2005) and could prove valuable in the future for standardisation of stem cell lines.

In addition to the standard cell markers used for hES cells described above there are many new markers being investigated for their relevance in stem cell biology and numerous methods for reverse transcriptase-polymerase chain reaction (RT-PCR) detection of target RNAs have been published. The role that these methods will play in quality control regimes for stem cell lines is yet to be determined but it is important to constantly review the development of such tests to ensure that current best practice is sustained for sources of stem cell lines.

4.2 Pluripotency

The capacity of human stem cell lines to generate almost all the cell types of the human body is obviously the primary characteristic of interest. Whilst this capability is achievable for mouse ES cells through germline reconstitution experiments the same experiments for human cells are not possible for obvious ethical reasons. There are limited options to determine pluripotency with hES cells which include the preparation of embryoid bodies (EBs) showing evidence of the three known germ layers (endoderm, ectoderm, and mesoderm), production of teratinocarcinomas in mice revealing representative tissues from all three germ layers and finally *in vitro* differentiation into cell populations also representative of the three germ layers. It is important to remember that these experimental procedures provide evidence for pluripotency but do not confirm the ability of stem cells to regenerate all the cells and tissue of the human body. As known in well-established tumorigenicity assays with continuous cell lines such as HeLa and Vero, the formation of tumours in animals is influenced by the age and strain of the test animal and the volume and route of the inoculation. In addition reliable and robust *in vitro* differentiation protocols for hES cells have only recently begun to emerge. Until greater experience and standardisation is achieved in these methods it will be difficult to recommend which approach to take for quality control purposes for hES cells. However, progress with the standardisation and improved efficiency in the preparation of EBs, established for mouse ES cells, may provide some solutions for quality control purposes for hES cells until other methods become optimised (Dang et al. 2002; Kurosawa et al. 2003; Fok and Zandstra 2005; Wang et al. 2005).

4.3 Genetic Characterisation

4.3.1 Karyology

The published approaches to characterisation of hES cells have identified the importance of a diploid karyotype (i.e., 46, X, Y for male and 46, X, X for female) since the appearance of aneuploidy (additional copies of chromosomes) or other chromosomal aberrations are considered to represent cells that have transformed and may no longer retain the characteristics of *de novo* hES cell cultures. It is tempting to talk about such hES cells having a "normal" karyotype but this terminology should be avoided as even in natural human populations the Giemsa-banded karyotype (see below) will show some variations in a proportion of individuals. The most commonly used karyological method involves fixation of condensed metaphase chromosomes (Hsu 1952; Tjio and Leven 1956) followed by treatment with trypsin and staining with Giemsa stain to reveal a characteristic banding pattern on different chromosomes developed by Wang and Federoff (1972). However, other variations on such karyological techniques have been developed as Q banding and R banding, that provide advantages in certain circumstances.

Using basic karyological analysis of metaphase chromosomes, it is possible to determine the species of particular cells by the number, size, and morphology of the chromosomes. When such preparations are "aged" (e.g., by gentle heating) and stained with Giemsa (i.e., G-banding) this identification is made more reliable and also enables identification of subtle genetic changes such as larger deletions and inversions.

Such karyological data does not necessarily give consistent results for each cell. The number of chromosomes detected in each cell often varies and whilst this occurs to a limited extent in tissues and primary cultures it is much more marked in cell lines. Finite cell lines such as human diploid fibroblasts show stability of their karyotype with *in vitro* passage, and whilst the range of chromosome numbers per cell will vary, the modal number (i.e., the most frequent number of chromosomes per cell), which is characteristic of each species, is constant. However, for transformed tumour cells such as the HeLa cell line, the modal number can change with passage in culture (Stacey and Hartung, 2007) and other chromosomal changes may occur (Harris 1964; Rutzky et al. 1980). hES cells were originally reported to consistently reveal diploid karyology. However, more recent detailed studies have shown that karyological abnormalities, such as duplication of chromosomes (aneuploidy) do occur on repeated passage (Draper et al. 2004), and it is important to periodically check the karyotype of cultures and avoid the use of high-passage cultures for key experiments (see section 7).

4.3.2 Authenticity of cell lines

The authentication of a cell line has two primary components (1) provenance, i.e., a traceable and documented origin starting from the laboratory in which they were derived (see section 6) and (2) direct characterisation of the cells which confirms the cells identity. Few cell lines show a unique morphology, and it would be extremely difficult if not impossible to identify a culture simply by microscopic examination. A range of specialised tests are employed to study cell identity (see section 4.3.3).

All too often cells are transferred from one laboratory to another in research collaborations with very little documentation, other than the labelling on the flask or tube of cells. It may be years later that differences in cell performance between laboratories may be observed and resolution of such phenomena is time-consuming. Cells passed repeatedly from one laboratory to another are particularly exposed to the risk of cross-contamination. In the history of cell culture there are many examples of cell line cross-contamination, but only a minority have been published. Isolation of the first human continuous cell line, HeLa, in the early 1950s (Gey et al. 1952), was soon followed by concerns about potential cross-contamination between this line and other newly established human cell lines (Gartler 1967). In a publication by Nelson-Rees et al. in 1981 a large number of examples of cross-contaminated cell lines were identified and, controversially, the originating laboratories were identified. Publications on this topic continue to indicate that new generations of scientists appear to have failed to learn the lessons from their forebears. Much of this problem may be assumed to result from cross-contaminated cells that are freely passed between laboratories and from cell banks. However, even when cells are obtained from the originator, experience has shown that this is not always a guarantee of authenticity. In one study of 252 accessions of lymphoma and leukaemia cell lines at the German culture collection DSMZ, 30% were found to be cross-contaminated and a significant proportion of these had been obtained from the originators (MacLeod et al. 1999). More recent studies have shown that the issue of cross-contamination of cell lines is an all too often unheeded and ongoing threat to the quality of research work involving cell lines (Drexler et al. 2003; Melcher et al. 2005).

4.3.3 Cell line identity testing

Identity testing to try to overcome these problems of cross-contamination has been carried out for some decades using karyology (discussed above) and isoenzyme analysis (O'Brien et al. 1977; Peterson et al. 1984). These techniques provide confirmation of the species of origin of the cells and may also in some circumstances provide specific cell line identification through the detection of unique chromosomal markers and strain specific enzyme profiles (Stacey and Doyle 2000). In addition, other techniques have been successfully employed including human leucocyte antigen molecular typing (Christensen et al. 1993). The original multilocus DNA-fingerprinting technique was discovered in the 1980s (Jeffreys et al. 1985). This and similar multilocus techniques (also based on DNA probes that hybridise with variable number tandem repeats (VNTRs) see Stacey et al. in press) were quickly taken up for cell line identity testing. These methods could provide individual-specific identification for human cell lines and useful identity profiles for a very broad range of species in a single test (Vassart et al. 1987; Gilbert et al. 1990; Hampe et al. 1992; Stacey et al. 1992). Following the discovery of PCR methods for the amplification of short tandem repeat (STR) sequences (Litt and Luty 1992; Tautz 1989), another form of VNTR; reliable multiplexed PCR profiling methods were developed for paternity and forensic testing which have since been applied to cell culture (e.g., Masters et al. 2001; Parson et al. 2005) and such methods have been used for a recent international collaborative study to study identity amongst a large number of hES cell lines (Andrews et al. 2005). Numerous companies now provide relatively cheap DNA profiling services for human cells (see Stacey et al. in press) which makes this technology available to all laboratories using cell lines to enhance the quality of their work.

The culture of hES cells on mouse feeders cells does not seem to present a problem as the primers and targeted loci used in the multiplex PCR methods used for forensic work are selected to avoid cross-reactions with other species. However, use of human feeder cells is becoming increasingly common and may present challenges for human specific DNA profiling of the stem cell line grown on them. Mouse ES cell lines and mouse feeder cells will also require identity testing methods and primer sequences and typing services are available for mouse cell materials (e.g., Charles River www.criver.com). It is also important to remember that whilst a DNA profile provides a DNA "bar code" to confirm identity it is only really valuable when original material from the donor is available for comparison. Furthermore, correct identity does not necessarily mean correct phenotype compared with a sample of the original patient tissue, and cannot assure that key phenotypic characteristics have remained. In this respect proteomic analysis may prove useful to screen for phenotypic consistency and has been used to analyse hES cell cultures (Prowse et al. 2005; Baharvand et al. 2006) and has also been proposed for the quality control of cell lines (Wagg and Lee 2005).

5. MICROBIOLOGICAL CONTAMINATION

Absence of microbiological contamination of cell lines for research use is important since contaminated cultures may pass the contamination to other cell lines in the laboratory and could even represent a risk to laboratory workers. Furthermore they could produce aberrant data due to the biochemical and genetic influence of micro-organisms or may have more subtle effects on the characteristics and performance of the cells. The most common cell culture contaminants are bacteria, fungi, and mycoplasma; but this section will also consider the risk of viral and other potential contamination which could cause effects on stem cell lines that could lead to misleading data.

5.1 Sterility Testing for Bacteria and Fungi

Bacterial contamination from the laboratory environment can be screened for using standard procedures which usually involve the inoculation of culture medium into tryptose soya broth (for aerobic and facultative aerobes) and thioglycollate medium (for facultative aerobes, microaerophilic, and anaerobic organisms) (US Food and Drugs Administration 2005a; European Pharmacopoeia 2006a) and some methods have been published that have been used specifically for testing banks of cell lines (Stacey and Stacey 2000). It should be born in mind that some fastidious organisms that are known to arise in cell culture may not be detected in standard sterility testing protocols (e.g., Mowles et al. 1989; Buehring et al. 1995) and sterility tests may need to be extended to include microbiological growth media that will support the growth of organisms that may be dependent on carbon dioxide or have more complex nutritional requirements. Additional media may therefore be included in sterility screening regimes to selectively culture for fungi (Sabourard's medium) and promote the isolation of more fastidious organisms through enhanced nutrient content (e.g., "chocolate" agar, blood agar, serum-supplemented "broth" media). Such enhancements for cell culture quality control have been reviewed by Cobo et al. 2005.

5.2 Mycoplasma

One of the most common contaminants known in cell culture are mycoplasma. These are micro-organisms, smaller than bacteria, whose natural habitats in mammals are often the mucous epithelia where they typically grow in intimate contact with the host epithelial cells. Improvements in the preparation and quality control of commercial cell culture reagents of animal origin have largely eliminated the original sources of mycoplasma contamination except where primary animal or human tissue is used. However, earlier contamination from tissues and serum gave rise to persistent infections in cell lines and mycoplasma has become established as a relatively common and persistent cell line contaminant (Rottem and Naot 1998). The mycoplasma species most commonly identified in cell cultures are *Mycoplasma orale*, *M. hyorhinis*, *M. argininii*, and *M. fermentans*, but it is also important to note that the closely related *Acholeplasma* spp. are also a potential cell culture contaminant (McGarrity et al. 1993).

The spread of contamination between cell cultures has been promoted by a number of features of these organisms which include:

- Infection does not necessarily affect growth of the cells or cause turbidity in the culture medium and may go unobserved
- A degree of resistance to the antibiotics commonly used in cell culture
- Ability to survive for periods in aerosols and splashes
- Ability to pass through some bacterial filters

Persistent contamination with mycoplasma has been shown to cause a diverse range of damaging and permanent deleterious effects on cell lines and cell culture methods have been identified and examples are given in Table 1 (for reviews see Del Guidice and Gardella 1984; Rottem and Naot 1998).

Table 1. Some examples of publications identifying deleterious effects of mycoplasma contamination in cell culture

Effect of mycoplasma contamination	Example reference
Falsification of tetrazolium dye (MTT) based cytotoxicity assay results	Denecke et al. (1999)
Interference in apoptotic DNA fragmentation assays	Paddenberg et al. (1996)
Enhanced secretion of immune-modulating cytokines by human lung fibroblasts	Fabisiak et al. (1993)
Induction of cytokines in human peripheral blood mononuclear cells	Kita et al. (1992)
Changes in cell line karyology	Polianskaia and Efremova (1993); McGarrity et al. (1984)
Interference in hybrid cell clone selection processes	Boyle et al. (1981)
Interference with identification and isolation procedures for retroviruses	Lipp et al. (1979)
Increased cell death in HIV-1 infected cells	Lemaitre et al. (1992)

A thorough bibliography of the effects of mycoplasma on cell culture has been compiled by Mycoplasma Experience (UK) (http://www.mycoplasma-exp.com).

Clearly the presence of mycoplasma contamination in cell culture is undesirable and it is important for all cell culture laboratories to detect and exclude contamination from their work. This can be achieved by a combination of three approaches. An important first step is to quarantine and test all new cultures coming into the laboratory for mycoplasma. Secondly, any seed stocks of cell lines established for ongoing use should be tested. Finally, a routine testing programme should be put in place to screen all cell lines in culture at regular time points (e.g., monthly) in case the earlier testing fails (e.g., due to low-level contamination) or other contaminated reagents such as culture supernatants, or feeder cells have been used. When positive cultures are discovered the immediate action should be to discard them along with any media and reagents used for the affected cultures. It is possible to eliminate Mycoplasma from cell lines using certain antibiotics (e.g., Ciprofloxacin, Myocoplasma Removal Agent, BM-Cyclin) (Uphoff et al. 1992a). However, success rates for complete eradication are low and some effective antibiotics are known to be genotoxic to mammalian cells (Curry et al. 1996; Shimada and Itoh 1996).

There are numerous published methods and commercial kits available for the detection of Mycoplasma. Table 2 summarises some of the common methods and their relative advantages. The most well-established methods are culture in mycoplasma selective broth and agar and DNA stain of an inoculated indicator cell line such as Vero cells. Both of these methods have been published as pharmacopoeial methods for use in product and cell bank testing (US Food and Drugs Administration 2005b; European Pharmacopoeia 2006b) and figured as the most commonly used methods in research laboratories according to a questionnaire study performed by the European Tissue Culture Society (Stacey et al. 1995). The typical appearance of positive cultures is shown in Figure 1. Recently, PCR methods have probably become the most widespread in routine use but it is important not to assume that such new methods will automatically give improvement on sensitivity or reliability of detection. The use of nested PCR methods may not be helpful as false positives may arise which can cause considerable confusion, waste of laboratory staff time, and lack of confidence in testing data. There are many kits on the market for mycoplasma detection but some methodologies may not detect certain species known to arise in cell culture or may have poor or irreproducible sensitivity (Uphoff et al. 1992b). It is therefore important to select a testing method based on direct comparisons in the laboratory or peer reviewed publications on sensitivity and specificity. It is widely accepted that a standardised broth and agar culture method as given in pharmacopoeial methods is probably the most sensitive detection method validated for work with cell cultures. This involves inoculation of test samples into a mycolasma culture broth medium with thallous acetate added to inhibit bacterial growth. The broths, incubated at 37°C, are observed for a colour change indicating change of pH due to growth of organisms

Table 2. A comparison of some key features of different mycoplasma detection methods

Technique	Advantages	Disadvantages
Inoculation of selective broth and agar subculture	Potentially highly sensitive Confirmation of identity of isolates can be made readily from cultures by colony morphology and biochemical tests or PCR Phamacopoeial method available	Will not detect non-culturable strains Final negative results only available after about 49 days total incubation time
DNA stain of inoculated Vero cells	Results obtained in 3 days Phamacopoeial method available	Requires set up of test cells Requires higher power UV-fluorescence microscopy Small bacteria and cellular DNA fragments may mimic low numbers of mycoplasma
PCR	Results can be obtained within 1 day	Direct PCR may not be more sensitive than DNA stain methods (above) Nested PCR may give rise to false positives
6-methylpurine deoxy deoxyriboside (6-MPDR) added with test sample to 3T3 or Vero culture. Mycoplasma contamination can be detected due to mycoplasma adenosine phosphorylase converting 6-MPDR to toxic metabolytes	Simple end point (cell death)	Requires set up of test cells and 5 days incubation False negatives have been observed when compared with other methods (e.g., Uphoff et al., 1992a, b)
Mycoplasma RNA hybridisation	Sensitivity reported to be high but may vary	Radioactive methods require scintillation counting equipment May be difficult to discriminate between a negative and low-level positive results

and each broth is subcultured (usually at 3–5, 14, and 21 days) onto a selective Mycoplasma agar medium which is incubated and observed for up to 28 days in a microaerophilic atmosphere. Mycoplasma species differ in their growth rates and species such as *M. hominis* (and *Acholeplasma* spp.) may cause a change in broth indicator colour within 2 days whereas species such as *M. fermentans* may not be detected for up to 6 days. However, the *M. hyorhinis* species of

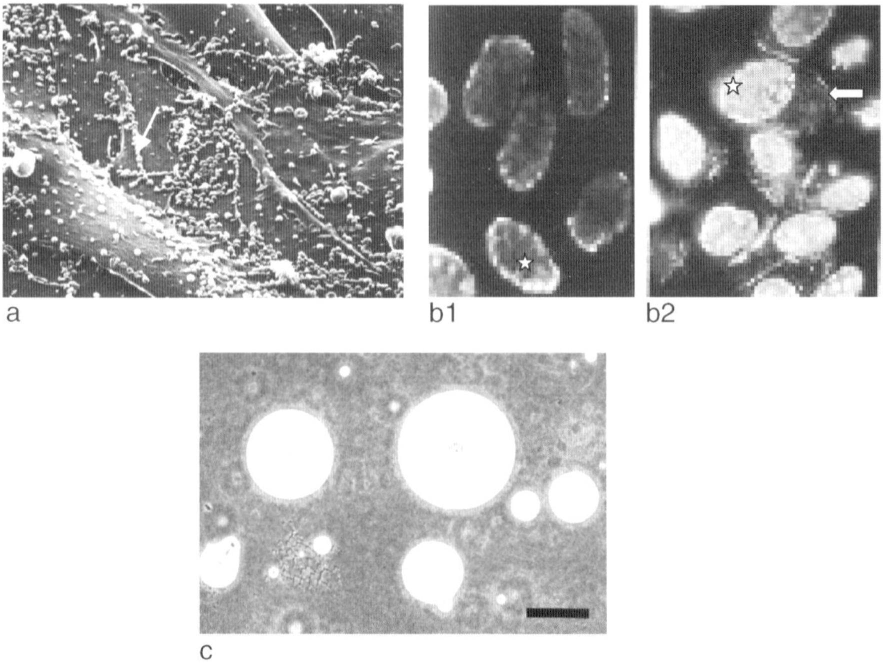

Figure 1. **a)** SEM appearance of mycoplasma organisms on the surface of a contaminated human fibroblast culture (arrow indicates mycoplasma cells) (photomicrograph kindly provided by Dr David Hockley, NIBSC); **b)** DNA stain of Vero cells (star indicates nucleus) **b1)** inoculated with mycoplasma and **b2)** uninoculated control (arrow indicates patch of fluorescing mycoplasma cells and star indicates a Vero cell nucleus); **c)** Photomicrograph of *Acholeplasma lailawii* colonies growing on selective mycoplasma agar medium (bar indicates 1 mm).

Mycoplasma, which is a frequent cell culture contaminant, has historically been the most difficult type to isolate by such culture methods and even with modern improvements in isolation media, strains are still known which cannot grow in the recommended media. Accordingly it is important to have a Mycoplasma testing system that will provide sensitive detection of general mycoplasma contamination but which will also detect "non-culturable" strains. DNA stain of inoculated indicator cells and PCR methods can be used to provide this important supplementary testing. The author has utilised primers for the mycoplasma ribosomal RNA gene (Van Kuppeveld et al. 1994) to establish a method which has proven robust without false positives over a number of years use for routine screening of large numbers of different cell cultures (Stacey 2000). Cell banks are tested by this method but also in parallel by inoculation of selective mycoplasma broth media and subculture onto Mycoplasma agar, as already described, to ensure highest possible sensitivity for detection of culturable strains.

5.3 Virus Contamination

Viruses may be considered obligate parasites of cells and accordingly are absolutely dependent on cells (often a specific type and species of cell) for their growth and replication. They are an ever-present risk when working with any animal-derived materials. Originally contamination of cell cultures arose as a consequence of infected tissues used to prepare primary cell cultures, reagents of animal origin such as serum (Erickson et al. 1991), trypsin (Hallauer et al. 1971) and also possibly via mouth pipetting by laboratory workers.

The nature of the viral contamination risk depends on the type of virus but could include:

- A hazard to health of laboratory workers
- Altered cell biology (e.g., failure to differentiate) or other characteristics of infected cells
- Cross-infection of other cells in the laboratory

Clearly the use of human cells represents a risk from potential infection of the donors and the virological screening of human donors of cells or tissue used to derive human stem cell lines is becoming increasingly comprehensive (European Union 2004; US Food and Drug Administration 2004a). However, it should be born in mind that the donors of embryos frozen some years prior to cell line derivation may not have been tested. Provided good cell culture practices are employed (Coecke et al., 2005; Doblhoff-Dier and Stacey 2006) with appropriate aseptic technique and containment procedures; laboratory workers should not be directly exposed in the unlikely event that a cell line harboured persistent infection with a pathogen. Ideally the human stem cell lines themselves would be tested for potential human pathogens. Approaches to microbiological testing have been reviewed by Cobo et al. (2005). Testing for human pathogens should not be undertaken lightly as this may give recipients of tested cells the perception that the cells are "safe." Generally speaking it may only be practicable to test for relatively few potential contaminants and these tests will have limits on their sensitivity. Thus, testing should be performed by a well-qualified and accredited laboratory using tests qualified for use with cell lines. Probably the key control point for microbiological testing is the master cell bank of each stem cell line (see section 7). If cells are transferred to other workers the exact details of any testing should be provided along with the warning that the cells should continue to be treated as if potentially infectious (i.e., use Good Cell Culture Practice (Coecke et al. 2005)).

Mouse cells can harbour viruses of pathogenic potential in humans (Nicklas et al. 1993; European Medicines Evaluation Agency 1997; Stacey et al. 1998). Thus, mouse ES cell lines and particularly primary cell preparations such as embryonic fibroblast feeder cells could be a source of infectious virus. Animal husbandry controls and colony testing should therefore be in place to ensure that such risks are minimised. Current developments in the use of human feeder cell lines for hES cell culture carry similar risks to the stem cell lines and accordingly similar precautions and safety measures apply (Stacey et al. 2006).

5.4 Other Contaminants

Contamination of bovine serum with bovine spongiform encephalopathy (BSE) associated prion protein has been a cause for concern particularly for British bovine serum and also for other human-derived products (e.g., human serum albumin) due to the apparent transmission of BSE to humans as variant Creutzfeldt–Jacob Disease (vCJD). Fortunately it appears that expansion of the infectious agent in cell culture is generally limited to certain neural tissue-derived cell lines (Chesebro et al. 1993; Bosque and Prusiner 2000; Beranger et al. 2001) and further evidence to support this is that cell culture derived vaccines are not considered to present a risk of infection (Minor et al. 1991). Thus, adventitious expansion of infectious prion protein *in vitro* does not appear to be a significant risk in general cell culture. However, some stem cell culture systems may provide suitable environments for studying their pathology (Milhavet et al. 2006). Reliable tests for prions are not available and where it is desired to try to exclude these agents, as in the case of cell culture-derived products for use in humans, this is achieved primarily through selection of raw materials including measures for donor selection for human-derived materials and certification of sources of raw materials from animals (European Pharmacopoeia 2005).

A variety of other organisms including protists and trypanosomes could theoretically contaminate and survive in cell cultures. It is not feasible to carry out tests that would cover all forms of infection, but where there is a very low risk of such contamination based on a risk assessment of source material (Stacey et al. 1998) standard good laboratory practices, including containment of cell cultures (sealed culture vessels, use of biological safety cabinets, etc.), should prevent rare cases of contaminated cell cultures causing exposure of laboratory staff (Coecke et al. 2005). In any situation where cultures are suspected of harbouring microbial contamination they should be discarded to avoid risk to the quality of the research and to laboratory workers unless the culture is absolutely non-replaceable.

6. CELL LINE PROVENANCE AND TRACEABILITY

The source of any cell preparation or cell line used should be well characterised. For cells and tissues taken directly from animal or humans this may be achieved through careful documentation and tracking of the material and a recommended outline for such data for both primary cultures and cell lines has been given by Coecke et al. (2005). Sourcing cells from unqualified sources can potentially lead to invalid data and wasted time and resources if the cells have been inadvertently switched or cross-contaminated (Stacey et al. 2000). The laboratory that originally isolated the cell line would seem the most desirable source to ensure that the correct cell line is obtained. However, some research laboratories perform little basic quality control and have even been reported to inadvertently provide the wrong cells (MacLeod et al. 1999; Drexler et al. 2003). It is generally a good principle to obtain cell lines from public service culture collections or other *bona fide* biological resource centres that endeavour to ensure that the cells have received at least basic quality control as described in this chapter. However, it is extremely difficult to demonstrate that a particular cell line is authentic unless samples are available for comparison from the original donor patient or animal. Where new cell lines are to be established it is therefore wise to arrange for a sample of original cells or tissue to be retained for genotyping. This can be achieved by setting aside appropriate spare frozen material from early cell line isolation experiments or spotting such early material onto DNA preservation cards (e.g., FTA cards, Whatman, UK).

Numerous initiatives are in progress around the world to isolate new stem cell lines derived under conditions that would permit their use in humans for therapy. In such cases the need for accurate traceability of cultures to their original derivation process will be critical in order to be able to demonstrate compliance with ethical and technical regulation of the use of human tissue and cells and to meet relevant regulation of products derived from human tissues (e.g., European Union 2004; US Food and Drugs Administration 2004a). The fundamental generic requirements for cell culture workers have been reviewed by Coecke et al. (2005).

7. PRINCIPLES OF CELL BANKING

The term "cell bank" has been used widely for a range of activities from supply of cells for local research work, to intensive banking, quality control activities for international distribution of cells, and ultimately the supply of qualified cell lines banked under Good Manufacturing Practices for therapeutic use in humans (e.g., EU Commission of the European Communities 1998; US Food & Drug Administration 2004b, c; Medicines Control Agency 2002). The focus and requirements change considerably between each of these levels with significant differences in resource implications. It is therefore very important to be clear at the outset what the remit for a particular banking operation will be and what formal standards the "bank" will be expected to meet as a consequence of this decision.

Over the many years that micro-organisms and cell cultures have been used in research and industry a fundamental principle has emerged for the establishment of a well characterised cryopreserved master seed stock from which to develop all future cultures. The ability to cryopreserve a batch of vials each containing identical preparations of cells (a cell bank) is key to standardisation in research work using cell lines. Such stocks can also be progressively characterised, safety tested, and made available for use over many decades for the development of safe and standardised cell-derived products and cell therapies. Individual vials of this master cell bank are then used to generate large "working" cell banks that are tested for critical characteristics prior to use. This tiered master-working bank system is central to assuring long-term provision of good quality cells and should be considered best practice for any cell culture laboratory

Table 3. Example of a quality control testing regime for a human stem cell line

Quality control test	Purpose	Master cell bank	Working cell bank
Viability (trypan blue dye exclusion and other appropriate tests)	Ensure cultures readily recoverable	+	+
Morphology	Confirm "typical" cell and colony morphology	+	+
Sterility (bacteria and fungi)	Exclude contamination during banking procedure	+	+
Mycoplasma (e.g., PCR and culture)	Exclude mycoplasma contamination	+	+
Karyology by Giemsa banding	Confirm karyotype and monitor its stability	+	+
DNA profiling	Confirm identity and exclude cross-contamination during banking process	+	+
Immunophenotype (FACS)	Confirm stem cell phenotype	+	+
Isoenzyme analysis	Confirm species of origin	+	–
PCR for viral contamination (key serious human blood born pathogens)	Accredited testing to exclude most common human serious human pathogens	+	–

(Stacey and Doyle 2000; Stacey 2002) and is applicable to feeder cell lines as well as stem cell lines.

The quality control applied to each cell bank should include, as a minimum, some means of determining viability, mycoplasma testing, and a sterility test and these are discussed above. Characterisation of each bank will be dependent on the cell type and key phenotypic and genotypic markers for hES cell line have been discussed already (above). Traditionally the master cell bank has received most detailed characterisation with essential quality control performed on working banks as a minimum. A typical testing regime that might be employed for quality control of stem cell lines is shown in Table 3. Additional characterisation of the working cell bank may be required if instability is suspected in certain characteristics and this should be documented as part of the cell banking process. Release of each cell bank for use should be dependent on the results of the testing regime applied meeting a scientific description (specification) for the each individual cell line.

In the case of hES cell lines some consensus is being drawn on the core characteristics of these cells (e.g., Loring and Rao 2006) which will need to be underpinned through technical standardisation programmes (e.g., Andrews et al. 2005). Coecke and colleagues have recommended that each laboratory should identify a qualified individual to be responsible for checking that all cell stocks used in a laboratory are of a minimum standard to meet Good Cell Culture Practice (Coecke et al. 2005) and promote efficient, effective, and well-standardised research work.

It may not be desirable to establish master and working banks of primary mouse embryonic feeders cells due to the influence that passaging may have on the performance of the cells. However, the preparation of large pooled and homogenised stocks of these cells can improve reliability in the culture of stem cell lines. As a minimum these stocks should be subject to the basic quality control tests and this can be an important precaution to avoid contamination of stem cell lines with bacteria, fungi, and mycoplasma that may occur during processing of animal tissues. Depending on the local animal husbandry standards it may also be advisable to test such stocks for certain mouse viruses that are to be pathogenic for humans (see section 5.4 and for overviews see Stacey et al. 1998; Fleming 2006).

An important supplementary process to the cell banking work already described is to passage cells beyond the expected limit of use to check the stability of their characteristics including the undifferentiated phenotype (i.e., consistency of the undifferentiated phenotype with master cells and lack of differentiation) and also the capacity of the stem cells for pluripotency. Ideally this will involve establishing "extended cell banks" (Stacey 2002) at intervals of around ten passages and then comparing the characteristics of these banks in parallel to determine any drift that may occur in the culture over time.

8. QUALITY CONTROL OF THE CELL CULTURE ENVIRONMENT AND PROCEDURES

As cell-based systems become increasingly complex it will be important to document and control cell culture reagents and materials that influence the growth and response of cells. Critical reagents (those key to cell growth and particularly those most liable to batch variation) should be carefully specified and monitored. Different manufacturing methods for reagents and their purification may affect cells in different ways and the activity of some key biological molecules, such as growth factors, can vary subtly in different preparations or batches (e.g., post-translational modification, aggregation, dissociation, degradation, and contamination) which may affect the cell. It is also important to consider those additional factors, such as gaseous environment and temperature, which will have a direct impact on the growth and response of the cells. Thus, it is wise to apply appropriate calibration and monitoring of carbon dioxide and temperature for cell culture. For a general reference see Coecke et al. (2005).

A further source of variability amongst cell cultures is the method of subculture. Separate workers passaging the same cell line even in the same laboratory may produce different results and cultures can undergo permanent loss of key functions if subjected to suboptimal passaging. Thus it is important to document the key methods of culture maintenance such as preservation, recovery, passage, for the maintenance of stock cultures used for experimental work.

9. CONCLUSIONS

Quality control of stem cell lines is necessary to ensure that cells used in research work give consistent and reliable data. It is important to remember that quality control is only part of a larger quality assurance activity which will differ between research cell lines and those intended for clinical use. However, fundamental principles of Good Cell Culture Practice include the establishment of master and working cell banks. Testing of these banks should be include tests for viability, contamination (STERILITY, MYCOPLASMA), identity and morphology, as a minimum. Other characteristics such as karyology, surface markers, and molecular markers are also key to quality control of human stem cell lines. Ensuring that the cells supplied by biological resource centres are well characterised, reliable, and ethically sourced requires considerable effort and those organisations which are committed to the quality assurance of the cells they release will be vital to promoting high-quality stem cell research in the long term.

REFERENCES

Andrews, P.A., Benvenisty, N., McKay, R., Pera, M.F., Rossant, J., Semb, H., and G.N., Stacey (2005) Commentary: The International Stem Cell Initiative: towards benchmarks for human embryonic stem cell research. Nat. Biotechnol., 23: 795–797.

Andrews, P.W., Przyborski, S.A., and Thomson, J.A. (2001) Embryonal carcinoma cells as embryonic stem cells. In: Stem Cell Biology (Eds.: Marshak, D.R., Gardner, R.L., and Gottlieb, D.), Cold Spring Harbor Monograph Series, Cold Spring Harbor, New York, pp. 231–265.

Baharvand, H., Hajheidari, M., Ashtiani, S.K., and Salekdeh, G.H. (2006) Proteomic signature of human embryonic stem cells. Proteomics, 6: 3544–9354.

Beranger, F., Mange, A., Solassol, J., and Lehmann, S. (2001) Cell culture models of transmissible spongiform encephalopathies. Biochem. Biophys. Res. Commun., 289: 311–316.

Bosque, P.J. and Prusiner, S.B. (2000) Cultured cell sublines highly susceptible to prion infection. J. Virol., 74: 4377–4386.

Boyle, J.M., Hopkins, J., Fox, M., Allen, T.D., and Leach, R.H. (1981) Interference in hybrid clone selection caused by *Mycoplasma hyorhinis* infection. Exp. Cell Res., 132: 67–72.

Buehring, G.C., Valesco, M., and Pan, C.Y. (1995) Cell culture contamination by mycobacteria. In Vitro Cell Dev. Biol. Anim., 31: 735–737.

Chesebro, B., Wehrly, K., Caughey, B., et al. (1993) Foreign PrP expression and scrapie infection in tissue culture cell lines. Dev. Biol. Stand., 80: 131–140.

Christensen, B., Hansen, C., Debiek-Rychter, M., Kieler, J., Ottensen, S., and Schmidt, J. (1993) Identity of tumourigenic uroepithelial cell lines and 'spontaneously' transformed sublines. Br. J. Can., 68: 879–884.

Coecke, S., Balls, M., Bowe, G., Davis, J., Gstraunthaler, G., Hartung, T., Hay, R., Merten, O.-W., Price, A., Shechtman, L., Stacey, G., and Stokes, W. (2005) Guidance on Good Cell Culture Practice: a report of the second ECVAM task force on good cell culture practice. ATLA, 33: 261–287.

Cobo, F., Stacey, G.N., Hunt, C., Cabrera, C., Nieto, A., Montes, R., Cortes, J.L., Catalina, P., Barnie, A., and Concha, A. (2005) Microbiological control in stem cell banks: approaches to standardisation. Appl. Microbiol. Biotechnol., 68: 456–466.

Curry, P.T., Kropko, M.L., Garvin, J.R., Fiedler, R.D., and Thiess, J.C. (1996) In vitro induction of micronulclei and chromosome aberrations by quinolones: possible mechanisms. Mut. Res., 352: 143–150.

Dang, S.M., Kyba, M., Perlingeiro, R., Daley, G.Q., and Zandstra, P.W. (2002) Efficiency of embryoid body formation and hematopoietic development from embryonic stem cells in different culture systems. Biotechnol. Bioeng., 78: 442–453.

Del Guidice, R.A. and Gardella, R.S. (1984) Mycoplasma infection of cell culture: effects, incidence and detection, In: In vitro Monograph 5, Uses and Standardisation of Vertebrate Cell Cultures, Tissue Culture Association, Gaithersberg, MD, USA, 1984, pp. 104–115.

Denecke, J., Becker, K., Jurgens, H., Gross, R., and Wolff, J.E. (1999) Falsification of tetrazolium dye (MTT) based cytotoxicity assay results due to mycoplasma contamination of cell cultures. Anticancer Res., 19: 1245–1248.

Draper, J.S., Smith, K., Gokhale, P., Moore, H.D., Maltby, E., Johnson, J., Meisner, L., Zwaka, T.P., Thomson, J.A., and Andrews, P.W. (2004) Recurrent gain of chromosomes 17q and 12 in cultured human embryonic stem cells. Nat. Biotechnol., 22: 53–54.

Draper, J.S., Pigott, C., Thomson, J.A., and Andrews, P.A. (2002) Surface antigens of human embryonic stem cells: changes upon differentiation in culture. J. Anat., 200: 249–258.

Doblhoff-Dier, O. and Stacey, G.N. (2006) Cell lines: applications and biosafety. In: Biological Safety: Principles and Practice, 4th Edn (Eds.: Flemmings, D.O. and Hunt, D.L.), ASM Press, Washington, DC, pp. 221–240.

Drexler, H.G., Dirks, W.G., Matsuo, Y., MacLeod, R.A. (2003) False leukemia-lymphoma cell lines: an update on over 500 cell lines. Leukemia. 17: 416–426.

Edwards, C., Belgrave, D., Janossy, G., Bradley, N.J., Stebbings, R., Gaines-Das, R., Thorpe, R., Sawle, A., Arroz, M.J., Brando, B., Gratama, J.W., Orfao de Matos, A., Papa, S., Papamichail, M., Lenkei, R., Rothe, G., and Barnett, D. (2005) Multicentre evaluation of stable reference whole blood for enumeration of lymphocyte subsets by flow cytometry. Cytometry B. Clin. Cytom., Jun 22; [Epub ahead of print].

Erickson, G.A., Bolin, S.R., and Landgraf, J.D. (1991) Viral contamination of foetal bovin serum used for tissue culture: risks and concerns. Dev. Biol. Stand., 75: 173–175.

European Medicines Evaluation Agency (1997) Note for guidance on quality of biotechnological products: viral safety evaluation of biotechnology products derived from cell lines of human or animal origin (CPMP/ICH/295/95) European Medicines Evaluation Agency, 7 Westferry Circus, Canary Wharf, London, E14 4HB UK, (http://www.eudra.org/emea.html).

European Pharmacopeia (2006a). European Pharmacopeia section 2.6.1 (Sterility), 5th Edition, Maisonneuve SA, Sainte Ruffine (www.pheur.org).

European Pharmacopeia (2006b). European Pharmacopeia section 2.6.7 (Mycoplasma), 5th Edition, Maisonneuve SA, Sainte Ruffine.

European Pharmacopoeia (2005) Minimising the risk of transmitting animal spongiform encephalopathy agents via human and veterinary medicinal products (5.2.8). European Pharmacopoeia 5.0, 01/2005:50208, pp. 463–471.

European Union (2004) Directive 2004/23/EC of the European Parliament and the Council of 31 March 2004 on setting standards of quality and safety for the donation, processing, preservation, storage and distribution of human tissues and cells. Official Journal of the European Union, L102: 48–58.

EU Commission of the European Communities (1998) The Rules Governing Medical Products in the European Community, Good Manufacturing Practice for Medicinal Products, Volume IV, April 1998, ISBN 9289-20297, with additional Annexes and update of legal references July 2004.

Fabisiak, J.P., Weiss, R.D., Powell, G.A., and Dauber, J.H. (1993) Enhanced secretion of immune-modulating cytokines by human lung fibroblasts during in vitro infection with *Mycoplasma fermentans*. Am. J. Respir. Cell Mol. Biol., 8: 358–364.

Fleming, D.O. (2006) Indigenous and pathogenic agents of research animals. In: Biological Safety: Principles and Practices (Eds.: Fleming, D.O. and Hunt, D.L.), ASM Press, Washington, DC, pp. 19–34.

Fok, E.Y. and Zandstra, P.W. (2005) Shear-controlled single-step mouse embryonic stem cell expansion and embryoid body-based differentiation. Stem Cells, 23: 1333–1342.

Gartler, S.M. (1967) Genetic markers as tracers in cell culture. Natl. Cancer Inst. Monogr., 26: 167–195.

Gey, G.O., Coffman, W.O., and Kubiek, M.T. (1952) Tissue culture studies of proliferative capacity of cervicdl carcinoma and normal epithelium. Cancer Res., 12: 264.

Gilbert, D.A., Reid, Y.A., Gail, M.H., Pee, D., White, C., Hay, R.J., and O'Brien, S.J. (1990) Application of DNA fingerprints for cell line individualisation. Am. J. Hum. Gen. 47: 499–517.

Hallauer, C., Kronauer, G., and Siegl, G. (1971) Parvovirus contaminants of permanent human cell lines I virus isolation from 1960–1970. Arch. Gesamte Virusforsch., 35: 80–90.

Hampe, J., Nurnberg, P., Epplen, C., Jahn, S., Grunow, R., and Epplen, J.T. (1992) Oligonucleotide fingerprinting as a means to identify and survey long term culture B cell hybridomas and T cell lines. Hum. Antibodies Hybridomas, 1992; 3: 186–190.

Harris, M. (1964) Cell Culture and Somatic Variation. Holt, Rinehart and Winston, USA.

Healy, L., Hunt, C., Young, L., and Stacey, G. (2005) The UK Stem Cell Bank: its role as a public research resource centre providing access to well-characterised seed stocks of human stem cell lines. Adv. Drug Deliv. Rev., 57: 1981–1988.

Hsu, T.C. (1952) Mammalian chromosomes in vitro the karyotype of man. J. Hered. 43: 167–172.

Jeffreys, A.J., Wilson, V., and Thein, S.-L. (1985) Individual specific fingerprints of human DNA. Nature, 316: 76–79.

Kita, M., Ohmoto, Y., Hirai, Y., Yamaguchi, N., and Imanishi, J. (1992) Induction of cytokines in human peripheral blood mononuclear cells by mycoplasmas. Microbiol. Immunol., 36: 507–516.

Kurosawa, H., Imamura, T., Koike, M., Sasaki, K., and Amano, Y. A simple method for forming embryoid body from mouse embryonic stem cells. J. Biosci. Bioeng., 96: 409–411.

Lemaitre, M., Henin, Y., Destouesse, F., Ferrieux, C., Montagnier, L., Blanchard, A. (1992) Role of mycoplasma infection in the cytopathic effect induced by human immunodeficiency virus type 1 in infected cell lines. Infect. Immun., 60: 742–748.

Lipp, M., Koch, E., Brandner, G., Bredt, W. (1979) Simulation and prevention of retrovirus-specific reactions by mycoplasmas. Med. Microbiol. Immunol., 167(2): 127–136.

Litt, M. and Luty, J.A. (1989) A hypervariable microsatellite revealed by in-vitro amplification of a dinucleotide repeat within the cardiac muscle actin gene. Am. J. Genet., 44: 397–401.

Loring, J.F. and Rao, M.S. (2006) Establishing standards for the characterization of human embryonic stem cell lines. Stem Cells, 24: 145–150.

MacLeod, R.A.F., Dirks, W.G., Matsuo, Y., Kaufman, M., Milch, H., and Drexler, H.G. (1999) Widespread intra-species cross-contamination of human tumour cell lines arising at source. Int. J. Cancer, 83: 555–563.

Masters, J.R.W., Thompson, J., Daly-Burns, B., Reid, Y.A., Dirks, W.G., Packer, P.I., Toji, L.H., Ohno, T., Tanabe, T.H., Arlett, C.F., Kelland, L.R., Harrison, M., Virmani, A., Ward, T.H., Ayres, K.L., and Debenham, P.G. (2001) Short tandem repeat profiling provides international reference standards for human cell lines. PNAS (USA), 98: 8012–8017.

McGarrity, G.I., Kotani, H., and Butler, G.H. (1993) Mycoplasma and tissue culture cells. In: Mycoplasmas: Molecular Biology and Pathogenesis (Ed.: Maniloff, J.), ASM Press, pp. 445–454.

McGarrity, G.I., Vanaman, V., and Sarama, J. (1984) Cytogenetic effects of infection of cell culture mycoplasmas: a review. In Vitro, 20: 1–18.

Medicines Control Agency (2002) Rules and Guidance for Pharmaceutical Manufacturers and Distributors 2002. Her Majesty's Stationary Office, London.

Melcher, R., Maisch, S., Koehler, S., Bauer, M., Steinlein, C., Schmid, M., Kudlich, T., Schauber, J., Luehrs, H., Menzel, T., and Scheppach, W. (2005) SKY and genetic fingerprinting reveal a cross-contamination of the putative normal colon epithelial cell line NCOL-1. Cancer Genet. Cytogenet., 158: 84–87.

Milhavet, O., Casanova, D., Chevallier, N., McKay, R.D., and Lehmann, S. (2006) Neural stem cell model for prion propagation. Stem Cells, 24: 2284–2291.

Minor, P.D., Will, R.G., and Salisbury, D. (2001) Vaccines and variant CJD. Vaccine 19: 3607.

Mowles, J.M., Doyle, A., Kearns, M.J., and Cerisier, Y. (1989) Isolation of an unusual fastidious contaminant bacterium from an adherent cell line using a novel technique. Advances in animal

cell biology and technology for bioprocesses (Eds.: Spier, R.E., Griffiths, J.B., Stephenne, J., and Crooy, P.J.), Butterworths, Tiptree, pp. 111–114.
Nelson-Rees, W.A., Daniels, D.W., and Flandermeyer, R.R. (1981) Cross-contamination of cells in culture. Science, 212: 446–452.
Nicklas, W., Kraft, V., and Meyer, B. (1993) Contamination of transplantable tumour cell lines and monoclonal antibodies with rodent viruses. Lab. Anim. Sci., 43: 296–300.
O'Brien, S.J., Cliener, G., Olson, R. and Shannon, J.E. (1977) Enzyme polymorphisms as genetic signatures in human cell cultures. Science, 195: 1345–1348.
Parson, W., Kirchebner, R., Muhlmann, R., Renner, K., Kofler, A., Schmidt, S., and Kofler, R. (2005) Cancer cell line identification by short tandem repeat profiling: power and limitations. FASEB J., 19: 434–436.
Pera, M., Reubinoff, B., and Thomson, J.A. (2000) Human embryonic stem cells. J. Cell Sci., 113: 5–10.
Peterson, W.D., Ottenbrit, M.J., and Hukku, B. (1984) Isoenzyme Analysis in Cell Culture Uses Standardisation of Vert. Cultures in vitro, Gaithesberg, USA.
Paddenberg, R., Wulf, S., Heiman, P., Beck, L.A., and Mennherz, H.G. (1996) Internucleosomal DNA fragmentation in cultured cells under conditions reported to induce apoptosis may be caused by mycoplasma endonucleases. Eur. J. Cell Biol., 71: 105–119.
Polianskaia, G.G. and Efremova, T.N. (1993) The effect of mycoplasma contamination and decontamination with ciprofloxacin on the karyotypic structure of the Chinese hamster V-79 lung cell line. Tsitologiia, 35: 71–78.
Prowse, A.B., McQuade, L.R., Bryant, K.J., Van Dyk, D.D., Tuch, B.E., and Gray, P.P. (2005) A proteome analysis of conditioned media from human neonatal fibroblasts used in the maintenance of human embryonic stem cells. Proteomics, 5: 978–989.
Rottem, S. and Naot, Y. (1998) Subversion and exploitation of host cells by mycoplasma. Trends in Microbiol., 6: 436–440.
Rutzky, C.P., Kaye, C.J., Siciliano, M.J., Chao, M., and Kahan, B.D. (1980) Longitudinal karyotype and genetic signature analysis of cultures human colon adenocarcinoma cell lines LS180 and LS174T. Cancer Res., 40: 1443–1448.
Shimada, H. and Itoh, S. (1996) Effects of new quinolone antibacterial agents on mammalian chromosomes. J. Toxicol. Envir. Health, 47: 115–123.
Stacey, G.N. (2000) Detection of mycoplasma by DNA amplification. In: Cell and Tissue Culture for Medical Research (Eds.: Doyle, A. and Griffiths, J.B.), Wiley, Chichester, UK, pp. 58–61.
Stacey, G.N. (2002) Standardisation of cell lines. Dev. Biologicals, 111: 259–272.
Stacey, G. (2004) Validation of cell culture media components. Hum. Fertil., 7: 113–118.
Stacey, G.N., Parodi, B., and Doyle, A. (1995) The European Tissue Culture Society (ETCS) initiative on quality control of cell lines. J. Exp. Clin. Can. Res., 14: 210–211.
Stacey, G.N., Bolton, B.J., Doyle, A., and Griffiths, J.B. (1992) DNA fingerprinting: a valuable new technique for the characterisation of animal cell lines. Cytotechnology, 9: 211–216.
Stacey, G., Byrne, E., and Hawkins, R.J. (in press) DNA fingerprinting and characterisation of animal cell lines. In: Animal Cell Biotechnology: Methods and Protocols, 2nd Edition (Ed.: Joertner, R.), Hmana Press, Totowa, NJ, USA.
Stacey, G.N., Cobo, F., Nieto, A., Talavera, P., Healy, L., and Concha, A. (2006) The development of 'feeder' cells for the preparation of clinical grade hES cell lines: challenges and solutions. J. Biotechnol., 125: 583–588.
Stacey, G. and Doyle, A. (2000) Cell banks: a service to animal cell technology. In: Encyclopedia of Animal Cell Technology, Vol. 1 (Ed.: Spier, R.), Wiley-Interscience, pp. 293–320.
Stacey, G.N. and Hartung, T. (2007) Availability, standardisation and safety of human cells and tissues for drug screening and testing. In: Drug Testing In Vitro: Breakthroughs and Trends in Cell Culture Technology (Eds.: Marx, U. and Sandig, V.), Wiley-VCH, New York, pp. 231–250.
Stacey, G., Masters, J.R.W., Hay, R.J., Drexler, H.G., MacLeod, R.A.F., and Freshney, I.R. (2000) Cell contamination leads to inaccurate data: we must take action now. Nature, 403: 356.

Stacey, G.N. and Phillips, P. (1999) Quality assurance for cell substrates. Dev. Standardisation, 98: 141–151.

Stacey, A. and Stacey, G.N. (2000) Routine quality control testing for cell cultures. In: Methods in Molecular Medicine, Vol. 24: Antiviral Methods and Protocols (Eds.: Kinchington, D. and Schinazi, R.F.), Humana Press, Totowa, pp. 27–40.

Stacey, G.N., Tyrrel, D.A., and Doyle, A. (1998) Source materials. In: Safety in Cell and Tissues Culture (Eds.: Stacey, G.N., Hambleton, P.J., and Doyle, A.), Kluwer Academic, Dordrecht, The Netherlands, pp. 1–25.

Tautz, D. (1989) Hypervariability of simple sequences as a general source of polymorphic DNA markers. Nucleic Acids Res., 17: 6463–6471.

Thomson, J., Itskovitz-Eldor, J., Shapiro, S., et al. (1998) Embryonic stem cell lines derived from human blastocysts. Science, 282: 1145–1147.

Tjio, J.H. and Leven, A. (1956) The chromosome number of men. Hereditas, 42: 1–6.

Uphoff, C.C., Gignac, S.M., and Drexler, H.G. (1992a) Mycoplasma contamination in human cell lines, II Elimination with various antibiotics. J. Immunol. Meth., 149: 55–62.

Uphoff, C.C., Gignac, S.M., and Drexler, H.G. (1992b) Mycoplasma contamination in human cell lines, I Comparison of various detection methods. J. Immunol. Meth., 149: 43–53.

US Food and Drugs Administration (2004a). 21 CFR Parts 16, 1270 and 1271. Current Good Tissue Practice for Human Cell, Tissue, and Cellular and Tissue-Based Products Establishments; Inspection and Enforcement; Final Rule. Department of Health and Human Services, November 24.

US Food and Drug Administration (2004b) Title 21, Code of Federal Regulations, Part 210, Current Good Manufacturing Practice in Manufacturing, Processing, Packing, or Holding of Drugs; General, US FDA.

US Food and Drug Administration (2004c) Title 21, Code of Federal Regulations, Part 211, Current Good Manufacturing Practice for Finished Pharmaceuticals, US FDA.

US Food and Drugs Administration (2005a) Title 21, Code of Federal Regulations, Volume 7, revised April 2005, CFR610.12 (Sterility), FDA, Department of Health and Human Services.

US Food and Drugs Administration (2005b) Title 21, Code of Federal Regulations, Volume 7, revised April 2005, CFR610.30 (Test for Mycoplama), FDA, Department of Health and Human Services.

Van Kuppeveld, F.J.M., Johansson, K.-E., Galama, J.M.D., Kissing, J., Boelske, G., van der Logt, J.T.M., and Melchers, W.J.G. (1994) Detection of mycoplasma contamination in cell cultures by a mycoplasma group-specific PCR. Appl. Env. Micro., 60: 149–152.

Vassart, G., Georges, M., Monsieur, R., Brocas, H., Lequarre, A.S., and Christophe, D. (1987) A sequence in M13 phage detects hypervariable minisatellites in human and animal DNA. Science, 235: 683–684.

Wagg, S.K. and Lee, L.E. (2005) A proteomics approach to identifying fish cell lines. Proteomics, 5: 4236–4244.

Wang, H.C. and Federoff, S. (1972) Banding in human chromosomes treated with trypsin. Nat. New Biol., 235: 52–53.

Wang, X.L., Wang, C.Y., Yu, X.J., Zhao, Y.S., Li, J., Duan, C.M., and Guo, X.M. (2005) Scalable production of embryoid bodies with the rotary cell culture system. Sheng Li Xue Bao. 57: 486–492.

WFCC (1999) Guidelines for the Establishment and Operation of Collections of Cultures of Microorganisms, 2nd Edition, June 1999, http://wdcm.nig.ac.jp/wfcc/publication.html.

INDEX

Human Cell Culture

1. J.R.W. Masters and B. Palsson (eds.): *Human Cell Culture. Vol. I.* 1988
ISBN 0-7923-5143-6

2. J.R.W. Masters and B. Palsson (eds.): *Human Cell Culture, Part 2. Vol. II.* Cancer Cell Lines. 1999 ISBN 0-7923-5878-3

3. J.R.W. Masters and B.O. Palsson (eds.): *Human Cell Culture, Part 3.* Cancer Continuous Cell Lines: Leukemias and Lymphomas. 2000 ISBN 0-7923-6225-X

4. M.R. Koller, B.O. Palsson and J.R.W. Masters (eds.): *Human Cell Culture, Volume IV.* Primary Hematopoietic Cells. 1999 ISBN 0-7923-5821-X

5. M.R. Koller, B.O. Palsson and J.R.W. Masters (eds.): *Human Cell Culture, Volume V.* Primary Mesenchymal Cells. 2001. ISBN 0-7923-6761-8

6. J.R. Masters, B.O. Palsson and J.A. Thomson (eds.): *Human Cell Culture, Volume VI.* Embryonic Stem Cells. 2007. ISBN 0-4020-5982-5

springer.com